Psychiatric Nursing

Psychiatric Nursing

Edited by

Peggy Martin

RGN, RMN, RNT, DipN(Lond)

Formerly Senior Lecturer, Sussex and Kent Institute

Scutari Press
London

© Scutari Press 1995

A division of Scutari Projects Ltd, the publishing company of the
Royal College of Nursing.

First published 1995

British Library Cataloguing in Publication Data

Martin, Peggy
  Psychiatric Nursing
  I. Title
  610.7368

ISBN 1-873853-23-8

Typeset by Parker Typesetting Service, Leicester
Printed and bound in Great Britain by
Bell and Bain Ltd., Glasgow

Contents

Contributors

Liam Clarke RMNH RMN DipEd DipN BA MSc PhD
Lecturer in Mental Health, Institute of Nursing and Midwifery,
University of Brighton

Philip Clegg RMN RGN BA(Hons) MSc PGCEA
Senior Lecturer in Nursing, Leeds Metropolitan University

Gwynneth Down RGN RMN MSc
Senior Nurse Therapist, Greenwich Healthcare, London

Lynn Hamilton RMN
Staff Nurse, Ashen Hill Forensic Unit, East Sussex

Peggy Martin RGN RMN RNT DipN(Lond)
Formerly Senior Lecturer, Sussex and Kent Institute

Bill McGowan MA RMN RGN CertEd Dip. Therapeutic
Community Practice
Lecturer (Mental Health), University of Brighton

Marilyn Paynter SRN RMN RCNT RNT BEd(Hons)
Senior Lecturer in Mental Health, University of Hertfordshire

Lynne Phair RGN RMN DPNS BSc(Hons)
Clinical Leader, Homefield Place Nursing Development Unit

Graham Stew MA RMN RGN DipN CertEd RNT
Senior Lecturer in Nursing Studies, University of Brighton

Sue Torkington BSc DipN RGN RHV FWT PGCEA RNT
Head of Social Sciences applied to Professional Practice, Nightingale
Institute, King's College, London

Stewart Whitehead MA RMN DipCounselling
Centre Manager, Newham Health Care, London

Foreword

The vitality of the nursing profession depends upon the quality of nursing practised by all of its members. The profession endures and advances when nurses are innovative and knowledgeable in their work. Nursing education programmes provide nursing students with opportunities to develop basic skills, clinical competencies and knowledge essential for beginning the practice of nursing. Health care services, however, are growing ever more complex and will continue to change at a quite rapid pace into the twenty-first century. It is incumbent upon all nurses to maintain, refine and expand their capabilities. This is done through continuing education, reflection on work experiences and through reading professional literature.

The aim of this textbook is to provide an informative resource on contemporary mental health nursing for basic students in nursing programmes and for the continuing education of those nurses who opt for a career in this branch of nursing. It provides a broad range of theoretical and practical knowledge and information pertinent to the changing field of psychiatric–mental health nursing.

In the present century psychiatric nursing has moved from simple companionship–custodial care of clients towards a very broad scope of complex, therapeutic modalities of treatment. The results of research in such fields as biology, neurochemistry, genetics, epidemiology, social sciences and in nursing, and the clarification and resolution of legal and ethical issues emerging in relation to psychiatric care, will have an impact upon psychiatric nursing services. It is a responsibility of the nursing profession, and of practising nurses, to comprehend the nature of such trends and developments. Such understanding is necessary to determine the changing directions they may require of nursing in its relations to other professions that provide psychiatric–mental health services. This textbook explores these areas of concern to nurses.

The rising cost of health care is a growing social concern. Custodial psychiatric care was less costly than present-day therapeutic treatment. Consequently, the question now being asked is , 'What are the outcomes attributable to the services provided?' Contemporary research is likely to yield more definitive, cost-effective practices than heretofore. The nursing profession is directing its efforts towards this aim. This nursing text addresses clinical problems and interventions which would lend themselves to outcome studies by nurses.

Psychiatric/mental health nursing demands much of those nurses who choose a career in this specialised area. It requires caring deeply about the well-being and recovery of troubled people; but caring is not enough. It mandates a non-judgmental attitude and presupposes commitment to the personal work that patients must do with nurses to guide them; however, attitude and commitment are not sufficient. Knowledge about problems of clients and of relations between social context and problems and application of knowledge-based practices and outcomes are the keys to beneficial nursing care. This book is a significant resource to that end.

Hildegard E Peplau
Professor Emeritus, Rutgers University

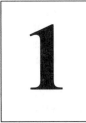

Perspectives in Mental Health

Sue Torkington

Many of the concepts, ideas or notions which inform, support and develop critical debate within psychiatric nursing today lack precision or sharpness of definition. This chapter seeks to examine and clarify some of the issues and bring various perspectives in mental health into sharper focus.

WHAT IS MENTAL HEALTH?

There appears to be no generally accepted definition of mental health. Doona (1979) observes that the problem in defining mental health, and health in general, derives from the fact that 'health' is not a scientific term. Therefore, there are no precise formula, criteria or objectives that can be measured. Leighton (1959) suggests that there are numerous patterns of psychiatric wellness or many mental healths. This view appears to be a positive beginning, because it recognises the dynamic and multifarious nature of mental health and encourages examination of the concept at the individual, interpersonal, environmental and societal level. It is also important to acknowledge that recognition, interpretations and descriptions of mental health will reflect the particular orientation, philosophy and belief system of the investigator. These value positions will be influenced and determined by the individual's age, gender, race and social role, as will the acceptance or rejection of the interpretations and definitions by the observer or recipient.

This argument has been articulated by various groups, each using their own frame of reference. Barker and Peck (1987) express the view of certain women's groups, where accusations are made that mental health is defined by white middle class males. This suggests that the interpretations or diagnoses which emerge do not reflect or support the view of women *per se*, regardless of their racial or social backgrounds.

Ethnic minorities are known to hold beliefs that differ from those of western health professionals about the aetiology and treatment of illness, about the role of religion and the supernatural in illness and its treatment (Faskerud, 1984). Gallagher (1980) also perceives that culture influences the way that mental health is defined and reflects that this influences the symptoms rate.

This is also a recognised phenomenon between different social class groups. Expressing this view more succinctly, Szasz (1972) argues that disturbances described by doctors as mental illness were problems of living which could not be divorced from their social context.

Fernando (1986) reports that the sociological definition perceives mental illness as a form of deviance. If this argument is taken to its logical conclusion, it leads to a view of mental health as an expression of social conformity or normality. Definitions of normality, like definitions of mental health, vary widely; what is viewed as normal in one cultural context may be quite unacceptable in another.

Social definitions of normality and abnormality are based on shared beliefs, behaviours and practices within a cultural group. These provide a model of what is expected of the individual and the family within the social structure and provide guidelines on how to be culturally normal, and also define what is culturally abnormal. Helman (1986) considers that normality is a multidimensional concept: not only is the individual's behaviour important, but also his clothes, hairstyle, smell, gestures, facial expression, tone of voice and use of language. Most cultures have a wide range of social norms which are considered appropriate for different age groups, genders and occupations. Barker *et al* (1989) propose that the medical model of normality implies a belief in a concept of emotional equilibrium drawn explicitly from the biological concept of homeostasis. This is in keeping with the psychoanalytical view which perceives normality as a state of intrapsychic equilibrium: the healthy personality is one free from conflicts among its constituent parts, the id, the ego and the super-ego.

Mosak (1976) suggests that individuals evaluate their own normality by using a number of criteria:

1. Frequency criterion – if most people act or feel the same way then the behaviour or feeling is considered normal.
2. The other as referent – the way other people are perceived as behaving is considered normal.
3. Therapist as referent – the therapist is seen as an example of normality.
4. Self as referent – the self is seen as normal; others are seen as abnormal if they have different views or behaviours.
5. Pre-morbid criterion – a comparison to how one used to feel and how one feels now.

6. Conformity – normality is conforming to the prevailing view of what is appropriate behaviour.
7. Symptomology – being free of symptoms and a medical diagnosis.

Haber *et al* (1978) also consider that most people have a fairly good idea of their own and others' normality using criteria gained from experience and socialisation.

Everest and Harrison (1981) evoke the World Health Organisation definition of mental health which, within the context of the preceding discussion, appears to offer a generalised, flexible and creative view:

> mental health is a condition subject to fluctuation due to biological and social factors, which enable the individual to achieve a satisfactory synthesis of his own potentially conflicting, instinctive drives; to form and maintain harmonious relations with others and to participate in constructive changes in his social and physical environment (Everest and Harrison, 1981).

Peplau (1952) also perceives mental health in a way that is adaptable to differing contexts and interpretations, suggesting that mental health is a word symbol that implies forward movement of personality and other ongoing processes in the direction of creative, constructive, productive, personal and community living.

Various theorists have proposed indicators or characteristics which typify an individual who is mentally well. Roberts (1990) identifies positive mental health indicators such as morale, life satisfaction, self concept and social interaction, while Gallagher (1980) suggests personal happiness, interpersonal adjustment and ability to adjust to change. Similarly Jahoda (1958) describes six characteristics in infancy and childhood that reflect positive mental health:

1. Positive attitude towards oneself.
2. Appropriate growth and development.
3. Ability to integrate and synthesise life events in such a way as to maintain equilibrium and to reduce anxiety or make it tolerable.
4. Autonomy, the ability to make appropriate decisions and to be self directed with specific goals and objectives in mind.
5. The ability to perceive reality without distortion.
6. The ability to love others and to be loved.

Jahoda's ideas can be considered to reflect and support Erikson's (1963) notions on psychosocial development. Erikson (1963) believed it was successful negotiation through each of eight stages that determined how adequate a person would be and how well he would be able to cope with new problems (Hilgard *et al*, 1975).

Various theorists have developed models or theoretical frameworks in which the ideas and issues discussed above can be linked in a logical and sequential way. Ramshorn and Pearlmutter (1982) present a review of four models of mental health: the *normality* model, the *holistic* model, the *wellness* model and the *adaptive* model. The *normality* model proposes several definitions of what is normal. Normality as health is seen as the absence of illness; however, normality may also be conceived as a Utopian state, an idealised, unreachable state of well-being and harmony. Normality as an average is based on a standard or norm of health, while normality as a transactional system stresses process and an individual's growth over time.

The *holistic* model confirms a belief in the unity of mind and body and focuses on the individual's culture, environment and physical, spiritual and mental health. The *wellness* model views mental health in terms of wellness – a dynamic process of maximising one's potential and moving towards a state of complete physical, mental and social well-being. Coping is seen as the mechanism by which one maximises health or wellness. An inability to cope would be viewed as illness. The *adaptive* model also views health as a dynamic process involving change (adaptation) throughout the life span.

Conclusion

What, then, is mental health? The preceding debate has confirmed the view that currently there is no universally accepted definition of mental health. It appears to be agreed that there are multiple factors which influence judgments and interpretations of mental health, such as sex, age, race, social class and occupation. Mental health is defined by some theorists as the absence of mental illness or mental disorder, while at the other end of the semantic scale others define mental health in terms of attributes, such as individuality, creativity and the fulfilment of one's potential. There does appear to be developing realisation that one's state of mental health depends on one's stage in the life cycle, available resources and coping mechanisms. This insight enables an exploration of various influences which may be perceived as at-risk factors across the life span.

FACTORS WHICH MAY COMPROMISE MENTAL HEALTH

It is known that there is an increased incidence of mental health problems following significant life events. Life events, as precipitants of physical and mental illness, have been extensively researched (Brown *et al*, 1973; Goldberg *et al*, 1977; Paykel, 1974). Life events are changes in relationships, interactions, living conditions, employment, health, economic circumstances or life-style that are independent of the individual's control and contribute to their level of stress. Individuals who have experienced one or more stressful life changes within the previous year are at increased risk for onset or relapse of mental illness. Higher than average risks have been identified for widowed, divorced and single individuals (Jablensky, 1986). Macrosocial forces also contribute to mental health problems, for example unemployment (Fleming and Cheshire, 1989), bad housing (Brown and Harris, 1978) and position in the social class structure (Hollingshead and Redlich, 1958).

Butler and Lewis (1982) identify extrinsic and intrinsic factors which affect mental health adversely. Extrinsic factors represent the environmental context and include such things as social status and prestige, role and financial status. Intrinsic factors are those within and unique to the individual such as the nature of the personality, experience of life events, physical changes associated with illness or ageing. This perception is often referred to as the nature–nurture debate, many theorists now concurring that the interaction between biological dispositions and experience in the environment are inseparable. However, genetic factors are known to play a role in some conditions, for example Huntington's chorea, and there has been considerable debate about biochemical explanations for conditions such as schizophrenia.

There appear to be certain periods in the age span when mental health may be compromised. Meredith Davies (1991) considers these to be at puberty, during pregnancy, the menopause, late middle age and retirement. This supports Erikson's (1963) suggestion that a human life is a series of observable stages, each marked by a crisis or a turning point, at which time the individual is simultaneously highly vulnerable to failure and highly open to achievement and heightened potential. Much of the discussion in relevant literature considers the life experiences of infancy (Bowlby, 1969), childhood (Adler, 1964), adolescence (Hill, 1991), adulthood (Sheehey, 1976; Levinson, 1978) and old age (Bowling *et al*, 1991). These periods in the life span, together with the special needs and characteristics of women, offer a logical framework for further debate.

Infancy

Bowlby (1969) was influential in developing the concept of attachment, described as an affectionate tie which develops over time and bonds one person to another. Bowlby (1969) proposed that infants needed to develop a strong attachment or bond with its natural mother and that this quality relationship was necessary for normal healthy social development. It was Bowlby's (1969) view that separation from the mother, particularly in infancy and early childhood, could result in later maladjustment and delinquency. These ideas were, for a short period, undisputed and caused considerable anguish and guilt for working mothers and for those families where children had been separated from mothers because of illness, divorce or death.

Subsequently, other child psychologists entered the debate, for example Tizard, 1979; Rutter, 1981; Sluckin *et al*, 1983, and offered a modified, more moderate view of attachment. Rutter (1981) concluded that secure attachments can be formed with a range of carers and that essential components of these relationships are sensitivity, responsiveness, acceptance and accessibility.

Childhood

Horney (1937) considered that a disturbance in the parent–child relationship can scar the developing personality and cause life-long mental anguish. This notion is supported by the work of others; for instance, Richman *et al* (1982) described a high correlation between maternal psychiatric problems and toddler behaviour problems. Adler (1964) stressed that mental disorders originate from inferiority feelings, caused by an overprotective or neglectful childhood. This conclusion is (in part) supported by Schaffer (1964) who observed that a mother–child relationship which is too cohesive can also jeopardise mental health by creating a personality which is pathologically dependent on others and not able to function adequately alone.

Critical incidents in childhood, such as the birth of a sibling, starting school, bullying, loss of a parent or child abuse, may lead to a variety of behavioural problems, sadness and depression. Some of the most common problems are enuresis (bed-wetting), stealing, disruptive behaviour in school, school non-attendance, aggression and overactivity. Childhood depression may present in a variety of ways; signs of unhappiness may be a solemn face, lack of energy and vitality or a tense manner. Again, the underlying causes may be related to a critical incident (the loss of a parent, family problems, child abuse) or may follow a viral illness such as measles. Graham (1985) suggests that children who have suffered from depression need to be supported by a social network that makes them feel valued, so that the chances of a recurrence can be reduced.

Adolescence

Although adolescent turmoil is a fact, Rutter *et al* (1976) considered that its psychiatric importance has probably been overestimated in the past. The adolescent can show intense emotional extremes, with deep attachments and passionate beliefs, alternating with periods of despairing disinterest, sullenness, withdrawal and loneliness. Lucey and Reder (1991) suggest that these behaviours are not abnormal unless they are extremely prolonged, occur at the expense of other age-appropriate activities or are accompanied by other evidence of arrested emotional development. Depression in adolescence may present in the form of various degrees of misery, pessimism and inertia. Hill (1991) distinguishes three classifications of depression in adolescence: downward mood swings, mild in severity; downcast mood which follows a loss or disappointment; and depression with inappropriate guilt, self-deprecation, serious loss of concentration and morbid preoccupations. Keidal (1983) suggests that suicide and attempted suicide by the depressed adolescent are more common where there is a history of poor communication with parents, alcoholism, child abuse and neglect.

Other problems such as prolonged withdrawal, running away, deliberate self-harm, anti-social acts and eating disorders may be exacerbated if the adolescent does not receive family reassurance and support during these periods of emotional turmoil. Rutter *et al* (1976) warn that it would be unwise to assume that adolescents always 'grow' out of their problems and suggest that careful monitoring of problems is required.

Adulthood

There are predictable times in an adult's life cycle when the individual faces a crisis of decision that determines the future course of events in their lives.

Krauss and Slavinsky (1982) identified four primary tasks of adult development:

1. separating from the family of origin;
2. establishing a family of orientation;
3. establishing an occupational role; and
4. facing the realities of ageing.

At these times there is an increase in the internal stress involved in making such important life decisions and this can make people vulnerable to mental illness.

In early adulthood Erikson (1963) recognises that the key developmental task of the individual is to establish intimacy and solidarity with a partner. Failure to find affiliation and love can result in isolation and a feeling of identity loss. Erikson (1963) suggests that the central task in middle adulthood is one of 'generativity versus stagnation'. Paton and Brown (1991) propose that generativity reflects a concern about providing for others and can take a variety of forms; for example, guiding the next generation or contributing to the development of a profession. The generative person feels at ease with his or her life-style and has a sense of self-acceptance. Stagnation is characterised by self-absorption, and the individual becomes withdrawn and introspective.

Women have life-cycle events in addition to those experienced by men. It has been noted that women are especially vulnerable to mental illness during the premenstrual period (Dalton, 1969). Many studies have concluded that there is an increase in psychiatric morbidity in many women at this time, especially those who are predisposed to neurotic symptoms (Beumont *et al*, 1975; Coppen and Kessel, 1963). Kashiwagi *et al* (1974) also noted a significant association with clinical depression during the premenstrual phase. According to Miles (1981) a similar vulnerability exists during the months following childbirth. Kendall *et al* (1987) have shown a markedly higher rate of psychiatric hospital admission in women for the first 3 months post partum. The most common risk factors are recent stressful life events, poor marital relationship or marital conflict and inadequate social support. Recognition of the disorder by family and professionals is the most important first step, followed by explanation, understanding and support (Platz and Kumar, 1991).

Miles (1981) concludes that hysterectomy is also associated with psychiatric illness. A study of women following hysterectomy demonstrated that psychiatric referral was three times greater among the post-hysterectomy women than in a control group who had had a cholecystectomy. These conclusions are supported by Ballinger (1977) and Richards (1973), who have noted that a markedly inflated risk of depression also occurs after hysterectomy.

There is also considerable debate about the vulnerability of women to mental illness around the time of the menopause. Greene and Cooke (1980), Ballinger (1976) and Weissman and Klerman (1977) have failed to uncover any evidence of a specific menopausal syndrome or involutional melancholia. However, there are life events occurring around this time which may cause depression, self-doubt, regrets and fears of growing old. As Gibbs (1986) reflects, mothers whose children have left home may feel unwell, failure to achieve work ambitions may cause regrets, and those looking after elderly parents may find this a very stressful and sad period of their lives. For some women, these negative attitudes may result in anxiety states or depression.

Retirement and Old Age

Planned and well-resourced retirement heralds a new stage in one's life and can be accompanied by a state of euphoria at the new-found freedom (Atchley, 1976). Sudden or forced retirement has been shown to lead to dissatisfaction and boredom and may result in psychiatric symptoms such as anxiety or depression (Mangen, 1982). Erikson (1963) considers the developmental task for this stage in life is ego integrity versus despair. The individual who has an intact ego is better equipped to deal with ageing and feels completeness and satisfaction. However, failure to attain a sense of ego integrity will result in an individual feeling a sense of despair and a loss of self-esteem.

Various researchers have demonstrated the importance of social networks and support to mental well-being in the elderly (Seeman and Berkman, 1983; Snow and Crapo, 1982; Liang, 1982). Blau (1973) also emphasised the role of a confidant in promoting life satisfaction and reducing psychiatric morbidity; for example, depression. Lowenthal and Haven (1968) have shown that the consequences of a relatively weak set of social networks include mental health problems, while other research has indicated that perceived poor social support can lead to the development of neurotic symptoms (Henderson *et al*, 1981).

Conclusion

The previous discussion has identified, explored and described factors which may compromise mental health. It is evident that significant life events, for example changes in relationships, health, employment and economic circumstances may create the potential for mental health problems to develop. The nature–nurture debate has also been considered, examining the relationship between extrinsic or environmental factors and intrinsic or biopsychological dimensions. Periods in the life span have been explored, raising awareness of those experiences or situations where mental well-being during infancy, childhood, adolescence, adulthood or old age may be compromised. The enhanced insights and understandings, afforded by exploring issues such as these, enable health care practitioners to be more effective in the promotion of mental health.

PROMOTING MENTAL HEALTH

Preventive psychiatry is a term proposed by Caplan (1964) to describe a body of theoretical and practical knowledge that can be used to plan and implement programmes whose goals are the improvement of mental health in the community. A World Health Organisation working party (1973) concluded that the principles of mental health promotion are the same as for health promotion generally; however, there are particular problems in mental health promotion. These are caused by the multifactorial and frequently unknown aetiology of mental disorders and the prejudice and stigma, which hinder early detection of mental illness.

Caplan (1964) initiated a useful taxonomy for considering levels of preventive activity and education, namely *primary*, *secondary* and *tertiary* prevention. This model provides a systematic framework for raising the issues in promoting mental health. However, it has to be acknowledged that the levels are not totally independent nor discrete from each other, and some overlap within the categories does occur.

Primary Prevention

Primary prevention is aimed at healthy people and attempts to reduce the onset of mental health problems by counteracting harmful influences or behaviours before they precipitate or cause illness. Statutory and non-statutory organisations play an important role at all stages in the life span by developing and engaging in strategies which promote mental health. In the antenatal period pregnant women and their partners are encouraged to attend antenatal classes, to help prepare them for the birth of their child and the early years of parenting. This type of preparation informs, affords insight into personal values and needs, helps to reduce anxiety and stress, and creates the potential for realistic expectations and understandings. Health visitors and midwives are involved in these activities but an important role is also played by voluntary groups such as the National Childbirth Trust, which provides antenatal education, preparation and support. Various styles of delivery are now available, and pregnant women and their partners are encouraged to find out and decide which method of delivery they would prefer. This allows for an individualised approach, supports self-choice and independence and enables individuals to retain some control of their experience of childbirth.

In early infancy considerable research and insight has prompted midwives to allow time and support for mothers after delivery to cuddle and touch their babies and to establish eye contact. This is felt to facilitate bonding and a positive start to the mother–child relationship (Field, 1977; Trevarthen, 1977). Mothers whose infants are in special care baby units are now encouraged to stay in the unit, and to care for their baby as much as possible, with support and guidance from staff who are positive and affirming. Parents who are able to touch, cuddle and talk to their baby will establish rapport and are less likely to reject their baby or find it difficult to establish a bond, thus reducing the potential for difficulties in the parent–child relationship in later childhood (Klaus and Kennell, 1982).

During the postnatal period, midwives and health visitors are alert to the possibility of coping difficulties, problems with adjusting to the new role of parent, feelings of loneliness or isolation, and postnatal depression. Supportive and therapeutic inputs through frequent home visits, postnatal support group and provision of services such as home helps may strengthen the individual's coping strategies and help to establish their self-esteem and confidence as a parent. The National Childbirth Trust also offers support through breast feeding counsellors, educational literature and resources such as equipment loans and support groups.

When a baby is stillborn or dies shortly after birth the loss and grief experienced by parents is profoundly distressing. The grieving process has not always been facilitated and supported by skilled help, which has led to many families suffering difficulties in accepting and adjusting to their loss, over a prolonged period. The threat to mental health in this situation has been extensively explored and work by groups such as the Stillbirth and Neonatal Death Society has helped to mitigate some of the pain and unresolved grief by demanding that maternity units provide effective and sensitive help to grieving parents, such as enabling them to hold their baby if they wish, taking photographs of their child, offering advice in respect of funeral arrangements and genetic counselling and giving information about support groups and helpful organisations.

The unexpected death of an apparently healthy infant (sudden infant death syndrome) is another devastating event for parents and families. Overwhelming grief, numb disbelief and feelings of guilt and despair require empathetic, supportive and therapeutic counselling to help ease the emotional pain and trauma. De Salvo Rankin (1983) acknowledges that parents experience severe crisis after a sudden infant death. It can take months to regain family organisation and interpersonal relationships. Parents are frequently offered support by the Foundation for the Study of Infant Deaths, an organisation which has proved invaluable to many parents in enabling adjustment to and acceptance of the loss of their baby.

Parents of low birth weight babies or children with learning or physical disabilities may also experience feelings of disbelief, guilt and loss. In addition to being offered support and counselling, parents need to be encouraged to avoid becoming overprotective and communicating their anxieties to their children (Graham, 1977), as this will stifle development and independence causing frustration, lack of achievement and loss of self-esteem. Parents and siblings of children with special needs require support, information and resources to help them cope positively with their situation. Special educational provision, transport, respite care, counselling and advice are required and may be provided by a variety of professionals and voluntary workers and organisations such as Mencap, the Spastics Society and the Down's Syndrome Association.

Admission to hospital during childhood has been shown to be distressing, with younger children going through a process of protest, despair and denial (Robertson, 1970). Douglas (1975) and Douglas and Gear (1976) found that children who had been admitted to hospital for more than 1 week were more likely to have disturbed behaviour and poorer reading abilities in adolescence. Wolfer and Visintainer (1979) demonstrated that preparing young children and their mothers for admission helped to reduce the child's fears, anxieties and uncooperative behaviour before operations, and problem behaviours after discharge. The National

Association for the Welfare of Children in Hospital (NAWCH) has been exemplary and energetic in its pursuit of better conditions for children in hospital, such as open visiting, parents' rooms, play facilities and appropriate decoration and resources. These facilities all help to make a period in hospital less frightening and more child-centred, thus reducing the potential for separation anxiety.

Research by Brown *et al* (1986) and Harris *et al* (1986) showed that prolonged lack of care in childhood was a causal factor in adult depression. Lack of care could be as a result of parental neglect, indifference or the loss of a parent through death or divorce. A considerable amount of primary mental health education and promotion is carried out by health visitors who identify and assess families where an at-risk situation may be apparent. Using an educational approach health visitors may encourage skills development, for example in play and learning opportunities, home and financial management. Additionally it may be necessary to provide a home help, mothers' group or nursery, where the mother may gain support and new insights. Family units have been developed in many areas to enable an improvement in family relationships and parental skills.

Primary mental health promotion in adolescence necessarily focuses on health education and emotional support, particularly in relation to eating well, drug abuse, preventing teenage pregnancies and emotional conflicts in relationships. The media, including journals, singers, pop groups, radio and television, play a direct (explicit) or indirect (implicit) part in promoting mental health in adolescence, as demonstrated by the recent AIDS awareness concerts and 'soaps' which deal with teenage pregnancy, drug abuse and family problems. Adolescents are vulnerable in many ways because of the need to establish a sense of identity. Erikson (1963) suggests that forging an identity may not always be easy, especially if there is inconsistency in the expression of values, attitudes and behaviours of significant others, particularly parents. This may lead to an identity crisis with some individuals never developing a strong sense of personal identity (Marcia, 1982). Self-image problems may arise from obesity or anorexia, which is commonly associated with psychological disturbances. Similar research by Harford (1976) suggests that drug abuse has its roots in emotional problems stemming from poor family relationships. Counselling, parental education, support groups, health education in schools, colleges and youth organisations all have an important role to play in helping to resolve conflicts and misunderstandings, increase confidence and self-image and develop positive health behaviours and attitudes.

In adulthood primary mental health promotion addresses the need for promoting personal control (for example, through assertiveness training), developing and maintaining healthy and satisfying relationships with significant others, and through managing stress and distressing events. Counselling support through stressful transitions such as marriage break-up, redundancy or serious illness is seen as an important primary preventive measure. This is demonstrated in work by Maguire *et al* (1983), who found that counselling significantly reduced depression and anxiety in women undergoing mastectomy. Maguire's (1983) study showed that counselling enabled enhanced social adjustment adaptation to breast loss and greater satisfaction with breast prosthesis.

Anticipatory guidance and counselling can also be given prior to a transition such as retirement, or after the point of transition such as bereavement. This has been shown to be followed by a significantly lower incidence of psychological disturbances (Egbert *et al*, 1964; Carpenter *et al*, 1968; Parkes, 1977). In addition social support in primary mental health promotion has been extensively examined (Cobb, 1976; Brown and Harris, 1978; Bolton and Oatley, 1987) and in many situations has been found to have a protective impact against depression and loss of self-esteem.

Secondary Prevention

Early identification and intervention are priorities in secondary mental health promotion. Screening and detection of potential or actual problems, before these become established or irreversible, reduce the threat to mental health and prevent more severe disturbances developing. Some factors which may be taken into consideration in early identification are requests for help, decreasing ability to cope with life on a day to day basis and any increasingly stressful situation or crisis.

Requests for help may be explicit; for example, a woman requesting a visit from her GP because she is experiencing panic attacks or becoming increasingly agorophobic. Alternatively requests for help may be implicit. An attempted suicide or shoplifting may, when explored, be symptomatic of an underlying mental health problem. A decreasing ability to cope with life on a day to day basis may be indicative of an anxiety depression or personality disorder. Increasingly stressful situations may lead to an acute breakdown in mental health and a crisis such as rape, child abuse or a personal/family/major disaster requires immediate interventions to enable supportive threapy to begin.

Much of the work in secondary health promotion is facilitated by Community Psychiatric Nurses (CPNs) who have links with primary health care teams and are able to pick up referrals quickly at the first indication of an individual experiencing difficulties. CPNs provide a therapeutic input in a number of ways, by crisis intervention, psychotherapy with individuals, families and groups, and by supervising and evaluating the effects of medication and counselling. A number of voluntary organisations also offer support, such as the Samaritans, Rape Crisis Centres,

Childline, Parentline and MAMA (Meet a Mum Association), a group for mothers with postnatal depression.

Various community projects also play an important role in secondary mental health promotion; for example, the Newpin project in South London aims to befriend mothers in order to reduce the high incidence of maternal depression, child abuse and neglect. Volunteers visit mothers in the scheme several times a week, offering support and encouragement to attend the drop-in centre for training sessions and social contact. Informal evaluation of the scheme has concluded that mothers involved in the Newpin project are engaging in more positive behaviours and relationships with their children (Pound and Mills, 1983).

Tertiary Prevention

Tertiary health promotion focuses on the rehabilitative process. Jarvis (1981) and Schoolcraft (1984) consider that the goals of working with people who have experienced mental health problems are the prevention of long-lasting and debilitating effects; preventing any side-effects of medication; reducing the level of family stress; restoration of the individual to their optimal level of health and facilitating their return to the community after periods of hospitalisation. These goals may be achieved by promoting vocational training and rehabilitation, organising after-care programmes, the provision of good supportive accommodation and a job with a sympathetic employer. Community Psychiatric Nurses follow clients after their discharge from hospital and offer supervision of treatment and individual client/family support. Another important role is in the prevention of stereotyping and alienation of clients with mental health problems, by facilitating communication between clients and their families and other social network systems.

Voluntary organisations also provide a tertiary mental health promotion input; for example, the Mental After Care Association provides residential care and rehabilitation for adults recovering from all forms of mental illness, meeting the needs of individuals by allowing them to exercise choice and encouraging their self-respect.

Conclusion

The promotion of mental health facilitates a substantial reduction of suffering, promotes human potential and reduces the social, emotional, interpersonal and economic damage which results from mental health problems. Prevention in psychiatry has sometimes been viewed with negative scepticism and it has to be acknowledged that certain problems are difficult to prevent. However, even the most intractable conditions such as schizophrenia can have undesirable consequences reduced through secondary and tertiary prevention.

Nurses have an important part to play in this process, By developing their awareness and understanding or perspectives in mental health nurses are better equipped to contribute effectively to primary, secondary and tertiary mental health promotion and to pursue a more pro-active approach to nursing care.

REFERENCES

Adler A (1964) *Problems of Neurosis.* New York: Harper and Row.

Atchley R (1976) *The Sociology of Retirement.* New York: John Wiley.

Ballinger C (1976) Psychiatric morbidity and the menopause: clinical features. *British Medical Journal,* 1: 1183–1185.

Ballinger C (1977) Psychiatric morbidity and the menopause: survey of a gynae-cological outpatient clinic. *British Journal of Psychiatry,* **131**: 83–89.

Barker I and Peck E (eds) (1987) *Power in Strange Places, User Empowerment in Mental Health Services.* Canterbury, Kent: Parker and Company.

Barker P, Baldwin S and Ulas M (1989) Medical expansionism: some implications for psychiatric nursing practice. *Nurse Education Today,* **9**: 192–202.

Beumont P, Richards D and Gelder M (1975) A study of minor psychiatric and physical symptoms during the menstrual cycle. *British Journal of Psychiatry,* **126**: 431–434.

Blau Z (1973) *Old Age in a Changing Society.* New York: Franklin Watts.

Bolton W and Oatley K (1987) A longitudinal study of social support and depression in unemployed men. *Psychological Medicine,* **17**: 453–460.

Bowlby J (1969) *Attachment and Loss, Vol 1. Attachment.* London: Hogarth Press.

Bowling A, Farquhart M and Browne P (1991) Life satisfaction and associations with social network and support variables in three samples of elderly people. *International Journal of Geriatric Psychiatry,* **6**: 549–566.

Brown G and Harris T (1978) *Social Origins of Depression: A Study of Psychiatric Disorder in Women.* London: Tavistock Publications.

Brown G, Harris T and Bifulco A (1986) Long term effect of early loss of parent. In: *Depression in Childhood: Developmental Perspectives,* eds Rutter M *et al.* New York: Guilford Press.

Brown G, Harris T and Peto J (1973) Life events and psychiatric disorders: nature and causal link. *Psychological Medicine,* **3**: 159–176.

Butler R and Lewis M (1982) *Ageing and Mental Health.* St Louis: C V Mosby.

Caplan G (1964) *Principles of Preventive Psychiatry.* New York: Basic Books Inc.

Carpenter J, Aldrich C and Dowerman H (1968) A controlled study of emotional support during pregnancy. *Archives of General Psychiatry,* **19**: 110.

Cobb S (1976) Social support as a moderator of life stress. *Psychosomatic Medicine,* **38**: 300–314.

Coppen A and Kessel N (1963) Menstruation and personality. *British Journal of Psychiatry,* **109**: 711–721.

Dalton K (1969) *The Menstrual Cycle*. Harmondsworth: Penguin.

De Salvo Rankin (1983) Individuals and families caring for the dying. In: *Principles and Practice of Psychiatric Nursing* (2nd edn), eds Stuart G and Sundeen S. St Louis: C V Mosby Co.

Doona M (1979) *Travelbee's Intervention in Psychiatric Nursing*. Philadelphia: F A Davies Co.

Douglas J (1975) Early hospital admissions and later disturbances of behaviour and learning. *Developmental Medicine and Child Neurology*, **17**: 456–480.

Douglas J and Gear T (1976) Children of low birthweight in the 1946 National Cohort. *Archives of Disease in Childhood*, **51**: 820–827.

Egbert L, Battit C, Welch C and Bartloff M (1964) Reduction of post operative pain by encouragement and instruction of patients. *New England Journal of Medicine*, **270**: 825.

Erikson E (1963) *Childhood and Society* (2nd edn). New York: Norton.

Everest R and Harrison T (1981) Introduction. *Nursing*, 1st Series, October, (30): 1300.

Faskerud J (1984) A comparison of perceptions of problematic behaviour by six minority groups and mental health professionals. *Nursing Research*, **33**: 190–197.

Fernando L (1986) What is normal? *Nursing Times*, **82** (3): 58–59.

Field T (1977) Effect of early separation, interactive deficits and experimental manipulations of infant–mother face to face interaction. *Child Development*, **48**: 763–771.

Fleming M and Cheshire N (1989) Unwanted and unwell. *Nursing Times*, **85** (11): 48–49.

Gallagher B (1980) *The Sociology of Mental Illness*. New Jersey: Prentice Hall.

Gibbs A (1986) *Understanding Mental Health*. London: Consumers Association and Hodder and Stoughton.

Goldberg S, Schooler N, Hogarty G and Roper M (1977) Prediction of relapse in schizophrenic outpatients treated by drug and sociotherapy. *American Journal of Psychiatry*, **134**: 171–184.

Graham P (1977) Possibilities for prevention. In: *Epidemiological Approaches in Child Psychiatry*, ed. Graham P. London: Academic Press.

Graham P (1985) Childhood depression in general practice. *Maternal and Child Health*, August 1985, 252–254.

Greene J and Cooke D (1980) Life stress at the climacterium. *British Journal of Psychiatry*, **136**: 486–491.

Haber J, Leach A, Schudy A and Sideleau B (1978) *Comprehensive Psychiatric Nursing*. New York: McGraw Hill.

Harford T (1976) A national study of adolescent drinking behaviour, attitudes and correlates. *Journal for Studies of Alcoholism*, **37**: 1747.

Harris T, Brown G and Bifulco A (1986) Loss of parent in childhood and adult psychiatric disorder: the role of lack of adequate parental care. *Psychological Medicine*, **16**: 641–659.

Helman C (1986) *Culture, Health and Illness.* Bristol: Wright.

Henserson S, Byrne D and Duncan Jones P (1981) *Neurosis and the Social Environment.* London: Academic Press.

Hilgard E, Atkinson R and Atkinson R (1975) *Introduction to Psychology* (6th edn). New York: Harcourt Brace Jovanovich.

Hill P (1991) Emotional disorders in adolescence. *Maternal and Child Health,* May 1991: 157–162.

Hollingshead A and Redlich F (1958) *Social Class and Mental Illness: A Community Study.* New York: Wiley.

Horney K (1937) *The Neurotic Personality of Our Time.* New York: W W Norton.

Jablensky A (1986) Epidemiologic surveys of mental health of geographically defined populations in Europe. In: *Community Surveys of Psychiatric Disorder,* eds Weismann M *et al.* New Brunswick: Rutgers University Press.

Jahoda M (1958) *Current Concepts of Positive Mental Health.* New York: Basic Books Inc.

Jarvis L (1981) *Community Health Nursing: Keeping the Public Healthy.* Philadelphia: F A Davies Co.

Kashwagi T, McClure J and Wetzel R (1974) Premenstrual affective syndrome and psychiatric disorder. *Diseases of the Nervous System,* **37**: 116–119.

Keidal G (1983) Adolescent suicide. *Nursing Clinics of North America,* **18**: 323–332.

Kendall R, Chalmers J and Platz C (1987) Epidemiology of puerperal psychoses. *British Journal of Psychiatry,* **114**: 1325–1335.

Klaus M and Kennell J (1982) *Parent–Infant Bonding.* St Louis: C V Mosby.

Krauss J and Slavinsky A (1982) *The Chronically Ill Psychiatric Patient and the Community.* Boston: Blackwell.

Leighton A (1959) *My Name is Legion.* New York: Basic Books Inc.

Levinson D (1978) *The Season's of a Man's Life.* New York: Knopf.

Liang J (1982) Sex differences in life satisfaction among the elderly. *Journal of Gerontology.* **37**: 100–108.

Lowenthal M and Haven C (1968) Interaction and adaptation: intimacy as a critical variable. *American Sociological Review,* **33**: 20–30.

Lucey C and Reder P (1991) Emotional dilemmas of younger adolescents: the doctor's dilemma too? *Maternal and Child Health,* March 1991: 90–95.

Maguire P, Brooke M, Tait A, Thomas C and Selwood R (1983) The effect of counselling on physical disability and social recovery after mastectomy. *Clinical Oncology,* **9**: 319–324.

Mangen S (1982) *Sociology and Mental Health.* Edinburgh: Churchill Livingstone.

Marcia J (1982) Identity in adolescence. In: *Handbook of Adolescent Psychology,* ed. Anderson J. Chichester: John Wiley.

Meredith Davies B (1991) *Community Health and Social Services.* London: Edward Arnold.

Miles A (1981) *The Mentally Ill in Contemporary Society.* Oxford: Martin Robertson.

Mosak H (1976) Subjective criteria of normality. In: *Readings in Abnormal Psychology: Contemporary Perspectives*, eds Allman L P and Jaffe D T. New York: Harper and Row.

Parkes C (1977) *The Use of Community Care in Prevention.* Oxford: Mental Health Research Trust, Pergamon Press.

Paton D and Brown R (1991) *Lifespan Health Psychology Nursing Problems and Interventions.* London: HarperCollins Nursing.

Paykel E (1974) Recent life events and clinical depression. In: *Life Stress and Illness*, eds Gunderson E and Rahe R. Illinois: Charles Thomas.

Peplau H (1952) *Interpersonal Relations in Nursing.* New York: G P Putnam's Sons.

Platz C and Kumar R (1991) Management of post-natal depression. *Maternal and Child Health*, January 1991, 29–32.

Pound A and Mills M (1983) *The Impact of Maternal Depression on Young Children.* Paper presented at the Tavistock Centre Scientific Meeting, London, 10 January 1983.

Ramshorn M and Pearlmutter D (1982) Social, cultural and historical aspects of mental health. In: *Comprehensive Psychiatric Nursing*, eds Haber J *et al.* New York: McGraw-Hill.

Richards D (1973) Depression after hysterectomy. *Lancet* ii: 430–433.

Richman N, Stevenson J and Graham P (1982) *Pre-School to School.* London: Academic Press.

Roberts B (1990) Nursing research in geriatric mental health. *Journal of Advanced Nursing*, **15**: 1030–1035.

Robertson J (1970) *Young Children in Hospital.* London: Tavistock.

Rutter M (1981) *Maternal Deprivation Reassessed.* Harmondsworth: Penguin.

Rutter M, Graham P, Chadwick O and Yule W (1976) Adolescent turmoil: fact or fiction? *Journal of Child Psychology and Psychiatry*, **17**: 35–56.

Schaffer H (1964) The too-cohesive family: a form of group pathology. *International Journal of Social Psychiatry*, **10**: 266–275.

Schoolcraft V (1984) *Nursing in the Community.* New York: John Wiley and Sons.

Seeman T and Berkman L (1983) Structural characteristics of social networks and their relationships with social support in the elderly: who provides support. *Social Science and Medicine*, **26**: 737–748.

Sheehey G (1976) *Passages.* New York: Dutton.

Sluckin W, Herbert M and Sluckin A (1983) *Maternal Bonding.* Oxford: Blackwell.

Snow R and Crapo L (1982) Emotional bondedness, subjective well-being and health in elderly medical patients, *Journal of Gerontology*, **37**: 609–615.

Szasz T (1972) *The Myth of Mental Illness.* New York: Harper Row.

Tizard B (1979) Early experience and later social behaviour. In: *The First Year of Life*, eds Schaffer H and Dunn J. Chichester: Wiley & Sons.

Trevarthen C (1977) Descriptive analyses of infant communicative behaviour. In: *Studies in Mother–Infant Interaction*, ed. Schaffer, H. New York: Academic Press.

Weissman M and Klerman G (1977) Sexual differences and the epidemiology of depression. *Archives of General Psychiatry*, **34**, 98–111.

Wolfer J and Visintainer M (1979) Pre-hospital psychological preparation for tonsillectomy patients: effects on children's and parent's adjustment. *Pediatrics*, **64**: 646–655.

World Health Organisation (1973) *Evaluation of Mental Health Education Programmes*. Report of Working group. Copenhagen: WHO.

2 Nursing Process
Peggy Martin

The nursing process is a systematic approach to care, consisting of four phases: Assessment, Planning, Implementation and Evaluation. Some theorists include an additional stage which follows Assessment, that of Nursing Diagnosis. The nursing process was adopted from the United States in the 1970s, at a time when there was considerable discontent within British nursing. Not only were nurses unhappy about systems of task-orientated care, they were also concerned about their professional status and autonomy. De la Cuestra (1983) suggests that the nursing process presents nurses with a means of furthering their professional status and autonomy, while Dickinson (1982) argues that the nursing process offers nurses a means of recovering the only territory they can claim as their own, in the hope that they will gain a share of the benefits accruing from the professional status enjoyed by doctors with whom they work.

It is important to state here that the nursing process on its own does not *do* anything. Some writers have expressed concern about the way in which it is being used. According to Lawler (1991) the nursing process is promoted as a tool to enhance holistic and humanistic practice. She suggests that it is positivist, reductive and mechanistic to the extent that the patient can be reduced (at least on paper) to a set of problems, needs or diagnoses. Henderson (1982) feared that the nursing process was being used as a substitute for nursing because, as it leans so heavily towards the scientific side, it seems to belittle the intuitive, artistic side of nursing. There has been much debate about nursing and whether it is an art, or science, or a combination of both. Lawler (1991) argues that nursing is none of these. She remarks 'I think we should get on with the business of articulating what a rich and interesting discipline it is and just call it nursing'. Lawler feels strongly that what separates the 'proper' nurse from those who are technically competent to perform nursing care is not *what* is done, but rather *how* it is done. She suggests that nursing is a social entity rather than anything else.

ASSESSMENT, PLANNING AND IMPLEMENTATION

Assessment marks the beginning of an ongoing series of events and concerns the collection of data. Barker (1986) gave a particularly apt description of assessment when he wrote 'In assessment we begin to write the story of someone's life'. The patient's life story is of particular significance in mental health nursing and whenever possible the patient should be the main source of information. However, there may be times when a patient may be unable to give an accurate account of himself, and in these circumstances information may be sought from the patient's family or people who know him well.

When taking a history from a patient, therapeutic concern should be paramount; idle curiosity should never govern the collection of data (Kratz, 1979). Each individual has a unique background, home environment, support system, needs and problems. Therefore, each person requires an individualised approach and plan of care. The nurse needs to have a special faculty for objectivity, so that she can accept what she hears from another person without passing judgment. Even when a person's beliefs and values differ greatly from her own views, she must treat that person in the same way as she would treat any other person. Such objectivity can be quite hard to sustain, but it is vital to the nurse as a professional carer (Cooper, 1981). Observation will add significantly to the overall picture of the patient and forms an important part of data collection. Brown and Fowler (1971) describe three functions of the nurse as an observer: as spectator, as participant and as introspectionist. As a spectator the nurse 'looks in' on a situation; as a participant the nurse engages in some function or activity with the patient. Through introspection, the nurse observes herself and learns to recognise and understand her own reactions in the situation. Understanding the patient as a unique individual and assessing his needs is dependent on the nurse's receptiveness to his non-verbal messages and the ability to validate their meaning. There are significant cultural differences in the way in which people use their bodies. Tschudin (1982) suggests that the message a person gives through his body language is probably nearer to the truth, in some instances, than actual words.

Collecting data from a patient requires the nurse to have certain levels of skill and knowledge. The nurse who grows in self-knowledge can use this self-knowledge in her relationships with patients. This will enable her to understand the patient from his own point of view and in the light of his own unique experiences.

Peplau (1952) emphasises the importance of the nurse viewing the patient as a stranger; otherwise preconceived ideas could influence the relationship in a way that could be detrimental to the patient. Peplau's book, *Interpersonal Relations in Nursing* (1952), provided the first theoretical framework for psychiatric nursing and focused on the nurse–patient relationship. Peplau defined nursing as 'A significant therapeutic, interpersonal process that aims to promote a patient's health in the direction of creative, constructive, productive, personal and community living'. Peplau described a number of therapeutic roles for nurses as they pass through the developmental phases of the nurse–patient relationship: leader, counsellor, resource person, surrogate, teacher, technical expert and stranger. The phases of Peplau's Developmental Model (Orientation, Identification, Exploitation and Resolution) are overlapping and interlocking.

Nurses rarely work in isolation; most nurses are part of a team and work with professionals from other disciplines. Like all professionals, nurses will differ in the specialist knowledge and skills they have to offer; for example, while one nurse may specialise in family therapy or counselling, another may have a specialised knowledge concerning the application of behavioural techniques. A study by Brunning and Huffington (1985) examined roles within the multidisciplinary team by setting up a workshop to explore how health care workers viewed each other. They found that some nurses did not have a constructive view of their role and felt 'put upon' by other disciplines. They felt that a conscious effort was needed to define professional roles within a team, and in relation to particular patients, they emphasised the need for professionals to work co-operatively with each other in bringing their different skills to the patient.

Groups, as well as individuals, may strive to establish their identity by establishing boundaries. One professional group may fear that other professionals may encroach upon their area of practice. Ruch (1984) stresses the importance of clear discipline boundaries as part of team functioning, but suggests that these boundaries should be based on individual areas of expertise.

The aspects of self that the nurse as a person brings to her various roles can actually enhance the performance of such roles. Downie (1985) suggests that duties can be performed with cheerfulness, courtesy and compassion. These qualities are not part of the role, but what a person brings to the role.

Farrell (1991) points out that there is an enormous proliferation of assessment tools which aid nursing assessment. Many of these guide the needs to be assessed and the observations to be made. However, assessment packages are only as good as the expertise of the person collecting the data. Skilled interviewing within the nursing context requires that nurses establish more than a surface rapport with patients. Assessment requires a commitment of time; the patient's story will only unfold as a trust relationship is established. The problems and needs presented by a patient may be complex; not all problems will be amenable to nursing care and the nurse will need a sound knowledge of other available resources.

The care plan is based on the data gathered during assessment and will focus on the patient's psychological, physical, sociological and spiritual needs. The plan of care acts as a communication tool between nurses and other disciplines, and should be regularly updated and available. Once a plan of care is formulated all staff should adhere to that plan. Inconsistencies in approach to a patient can have a detrimental effect on patient care. Whenever possible the patient should be involved in formulating his own plan of care. Goals are unlikely to be met if the patient is unaware of the aims of his treatment and nursing care.

Implementation is the actual delivery of nursing care, and something which many nurses have difficulty in documenting. Instrumental or physical activities are readily documented, but low visibility actions are less easily described and recorded. Such nursing interventions are highly valued by patients, and form the focus of mental health nursing.

EVALUATION

Finally, evaluation enables nurses to determine the effectiveness of nursing care, by asking if the plan of care and the prescribed nursing actions have assisted the patient to achieve his goals. Evaluation is an ongoing process and not something which occurs only at the time of discharge. Evaluation may occur at predetermined dates when both the nurse and the patient can make judgments about the achievement of outcomes.

REFERENCES

Barker P (1986) Mechanical faults, mental health nursing. *Nursing Times*, **82**(39): 55–56.

Brown M M and Fowler G R (1971) *Psychodynamic Nursing*. Philadelphia: W B Saunders.

Brunning H and Huffington C (1985) Altered images. *Nursing Times*, **81**(31): 24–27.

Cooper S (1981) What is nursing? Occasional Paper, *Nursing Times*, **77**(34): 136.

de La Cuestra C (1983) The nursing process from development to implementation. *Journal of Advanced Nursing*, **8**: 365–371.

Dickinson S (1982) The nursing process and the professional status of nursing. Occasional Paper, *Nursing Times*, **78**(16): 61–64.

Downie R (1985) Telling the truth. *Nursing Mirror*, **160**(23): 43.

Farrell G A (1991) How accurately do nurses perceive patients needs? A comparison of general and psychiatric settings. *Journal of Advanced Nursing*, **16**: 1062–1070.

Henderson V (1982) The nursing process: is the title right? *Journal of Advanced Nursing*, **7**: 103–109.

Kratz C, ed. (1979) *The Nursing Process*. London: Baillière Tindall.

Lawler J (1991) *Behind the Screens*. Edinburgh: Churchill Livingstone.

Peplau H E (1952) *Interpersonal Relations in Nursing*. New York: G P Putnam's Sons.

Ruch M D (1984) The multidisciplinary approach: when too many is too much. *Journal of Psychosocial Nursing*, **22**(9): 18–23.

Tschudin V (1982) *Counselling Skills for Nurses*. London: Baillière Tindall.

3 Ethics and Education in Psychiatric Nursing
Phil Clegg

INTRODUCTION

The Mental Health scene in the UK in the 1990s is one dominated by contradiction. On one hand, we have commitment to Community Health, together with a growing emphasis on mental health promotion and illness prevention, and on the other hand a scenario of shrinking resources, especially for the elderly. We have continuing managerial euphoria about structural changes in service provision coupled with a sense of crisis generated by increasing demand on short-stay provision. We have patients whose lives are often dominated by problems resulting from poverty and inequality, and an NHS dominated by entrepreneurial and consumerist values. We have patients, whose lives may challenge middle class notions of appropriate behaviour, and a health care system that has been growing increasingly secretive and conformist. Increasingly, the nurse, whether involved in acute psychiatry or related fields, such as drug dependency and learning difficulties, may find that she is required to travel between two different and sometimes opposing value systems, especially where patients exist outside the dominant culture. This situation may be potentially compromising, since she may well be forced to collude with her patients in what she could not condone to her managers (e.g. knowledge of crimes). Alternatively, she may feel that she is being drawn into acting as an agent of social control (e.g. in relation to illegal drug use). Such situations can occur with the best of therapeutic intentions, and may sorely test the nurse's negotiation skills and skills of self-awareness.

In this chapter, I will argue that self-awareness training, although valuable, is not enough to equip the modern psychiatric nurse to face the political and ethical realities of her therapeutic task, that nurse educators need to link such training to an examination of the political issues in nursing care, and that Critical Theory offers a solution to the problem of how

27

nurses can help the oppressed without themselves oppressing those they wish to help.

THE IMPORTANCE OF SELF-AWARENESS TRAINING

Rawlinson (1990) states that acceptance of the term 'self-awareness' is now widespread in nursing. It is, for example, the first item in the 1982 Syllabus for Psychiatric Nurses (ENB, 1987), and is being included in some of the proposed common foundation programmes for all nurses. In these programmes, the 'self' is seen as a tool of effective nursing care. Thus the ENB (1987), in its syllabus for part 3 of the register, states that:

> Self awareness skills are vital for all therapeutic interaction and the development of such skills should be built into the training programme at the earliest stage possible (ENB, 1987, p.1).

The importance of these skills is stressed by Burnard (1985, 1989a) as enabling the nurse to help others intentionally. Williams (1986, cited by Rawlinson, 1990) using a repertory grid, identified self-awareness as a primary attribute of the 'good' psychiatric nurse role model. The contribution of self-awareness is not limited to psychiatric nursing. Interactional models of nursing such as that of Imogene King (see Evans, 1991) emphasise the perception, judgment and action of the nurse, and the inter-relationship with the corresponding aspects in the patient in communication and interaction. This process is seen as the essence of nursing (Chapman, 1985, cited by Rawlinson, 1990). Self-awareness enables the nurse to appreciate the origin of each aspect, and differentiate between patient- and nurse-centred perspectives, appreciating when subjective observations are being made. The self-aware nurse seeks to know her own beliefs, values and attitudes in order to enable her to counteract, for example, the influence of prejudice and stereotyping (Rawlinson, 1990).

THE LIMITS OF SELF-AWARENESS TRAINING

The above changes in the content of nurse training curricula have caused many tutors to rethink their educational practices. However, these have not gone unchallenged. Thus Burnard (1986) questions whether or not all these changes are 'theoretically sound and predicated on rational thought'. Wadeson (1992) accuses nurse tutors of 'introspection that borders on self-indulgence' while Fielding and Llewelyn (1987) argue that the time has come for a critical appraisal of the limitations of communications skills training theory and practice. It is thus necessary to probe the beliefs which underlie 'self-awareness' training.

Burnard (1986) points out that it is common among the new generation of tutors to talk of the need for 'personal growth', a concept difficult to define, but apparently linked in some way to the concept of 'self-actualisation' (Maslow, 1972, p.150). But what is 'self-actualisation'? As Burnard (1986) points out, Maslow himself was hard put to describe what he meant by the term, and borrowed Nietzsche's contradictory and enigmatic exhortation 'Become what thou art!' as a means of conveying the essence of the idea. One might ask, then, what is the meaning of the concept of 'self'? Here it is interesting that the concept of self, accepted recently so eagerly and unquestioningly by nurse educators as a main focus of concern, has caused philosophers much difficulty. Thus Hume (1711–1776) conceded ironically that there may be some philosophers who can perceive their selves:

> but setting aside some metaphysicians of this kind, I may venture to affirm of the rest of mankind, that they are nothing but a bundle of different perceptions, which succeed each other with inconceivable rapidity, and are in perpetual flux and movement (Hume, cited by Russell, 1961, p.636).

In other words, in Hume's view (and also in Russell's) the self as an operational concept does not exist.

The purpose of self-awareness training is to help others, and has as its goal 'a reflective nurse who considers her actions and who chooses appropriate strategies for care' (Burnard, 1986). I would not wish to reject the insights which such an approach can offer. The concept of self does, however, have its limits, and it might be inadvisable to construct one's philosophy of nurse education entirely on the concept of self-awareness alone, since if taken to its limit all knowledge and experience is seen as primarily subjective from this viewpoint. Thus Ogata (1959) writing about the state of 'enlightenment' known in Japanese as *satori* or *kensho*, meaning 'seeing into self-nature', states:

> In the satori state of mind one sees the world, including oneself, from a new viewpoint; that is to say one transcends oneself. All discriminative ideas, such as mind, body, death, time and space, which are intellectual analyses of life as a whole and of reality, cease to disturb your peace of mind in its natural state. It is perfect emancipation from everything; it is that passivity of mind which in Buddhism is called Nirvana (Ogata, 1959, p.50).

Doubtless this statement contains a special truth, albeit one of metaphysical dimension. Perfect emancipation from everything, however, is a goal somewhat difficult for the western mind to grasp, since the occidental concept of emancipation is one of material and political emancipation rather than emancipation in the spiritual dimension. As the poet Gary Snyder expressed it:

The mercy of the west has been rebellion; the mercy of the east has been insight into the basic self (Snyder, 1964, p.256).

THE DEVELOPMENT OF A 'NEW PARADIGM' WITHIN NURSING

Currently our conception of emancipation is encapsulated by the term 'empowerment'. This is defined by Gibson (1991) as 'a process of helping people to assert control over the factors which affect their lives' (Gibson, 1991, p.354). The term forms part of the language of holistic care, and in this context it may be that it captures something of both the spiritual and material dimensions of emancipation. Thus Lister (1991) states that concepts such as holistic care and the empowerment of people to influence their own health status form part of a 'new paradigm' which is becoming apparent in nursing, mainly through the influence of ideas and attitudes from humanistic psychology, feminism and non-western philosophies (Lister, 1991, p.211). According to the philosopher of science Kuhn, 'paradigms' are differing systems of prejudice about what constitutes useful and respectable data, what forms theories should take, what sort of language scientists should use, how they should go about their business and so on (Ingleby, 1981).

Gibson (1991) argues that such a 'paradigm shift' will radically alter both the practice and education requirements of nursing. Nurses will need to develop new skills and specialisations in enabling and empowering people for self-care, self-help and environmental improvement as well as in promoting positive health behaviours of people to maintain health (Magiacas, 1988, cited by Gibson, 1991). Gibson (1991) argues that although sidetracked into providing illness-orientated services, nursing's unique contribution has always been health promotion, with efforts directed at improving health potential and maintaining health balance. She argues that nurses, today and in the future, will need knowledge of the structural and functional interrelations of the health care system as well as an awareness of social, political, economic and demographic conditions (Gibson, 1991). Indeed, political activities must be seen as a mode of nursing practice and nurses will need to be provided with theoretical frameworks in which social, economic and political forces are given equal weight with the interpersonal aspects of nursing (Magiacas, 1988, cited by Gibson, 1991). Shifting professional boundaries in health promotion (Beattie, 1991), and the development of patterns of health care provision which emphasise spending on community and primary services rather than acute care hospitals (Mohan, 1991; Land, 1991; Brindle, 1992c) are examples of trends which are likely to make demands of nurses' political skills as different disciplines and interest groups fight for their 'share of the cake'. The concept of empowerment then, captures not only the individual's responsibility in achieving health (the emphasis in 'self-awareness' work) but also the effect of the social and political environment on personal health (the emphasis in our western concept of emancipation).

EMANCIPATORY ACTIONS IN NURSING CARE

Poverty, education and social problems are inextricably linked to problems of mental health (Monahan and Vaux, 1980; Blackburn, 1991). However, as poverty and inequality increase in our society, nurses are faced with the dilemma, outlined by Reverby (1987), of how to care for people in a society that does not value caring. Moccia (1988) asks if nurses should focus on helping people adapt to poverty or focus on how to help people learn how to influence the environment that has contributed to their situations. Clearly taking the latter view, Moccia (1988) claims that, in the past, nursing has been involved with the traditional aims of helping people adapt to their oppression, maintaining the current social system, rather than helping people to change their situation. Building on this work, Kendall (1992) argues that nurses should promote 'emancipatory nursing actions', the goal of which would be to help oppressed and disenfranchised people gain freedom from the people, ideology or situation that keeps them oppressed:

> Instead of helping people cope with poverty, should not nurses be helping people fight back against the forces that maintain their homelessness, hopelessness and hunger? (Kendall, 1992, p.2).

Psychiatry and psychiatric nursing abound with other examples of people being helped to adapt to their oppression, many arising from the medicalisation of social phenomena. Thus, just as people may be required to 'adapt' to homelessness and poverty, women with oppressive domestic situations may be treated with tranquillisers and antidepressants rather than be encouraged to become aware of and challenge their oppression (Callaghan and O'Carroll, 1993). Similarly, the mental casualties of racism may be treated with medications, and/or culturally incongruent therapies rather than by specific therapies and activities that generate cultural pride and solidarity, or challenge paternalistic views of ethnic minorities (Sidran, 1971; Leiniger, 1988; Lake, 1991).

Questions arising here are:

1. What are the characteristics of emancipatory actions?
2. How do they differ from actions that are oppressive or non-emancipatory?

3. What theoretical frameworks need to inform and underpin emancipatory actions?
4. What ethical issues can arise in relation to emancipatory nursing actions, and how can these be resolved?
5. What education do nurses need to participate in emancipatory nursing care?

One potential ethical dilemma is that an act of emancipation would appear to imply a challenge to one value system by another. For the nurse to take such an adversarial position may render the patient open to an abuse of power and privilege by the nurse unless some specific contract is obtained, even if this is only tacit. However, this is no different from the use of challenging interventions in counselling situations. Key questions here are how can nurses engage in political discourse without imposing a particular value system on patients? And how can nurses help to liberate the oppressed without themselves behaving in a manner which itself may be deemed oppressive? Before answering these questions, we need to look at nurses' own oppression and need for emancipation, since it is unlikely that those who are themselves oppressed can contribute to the emancipation of others without confronting their own oppression. It should also be borne in mind that psychiatrists and psychiatric nurses are sometimes implicated not only as being agents of adaptation to oppression but also as being the outright agents of oppression. Examples include: instances when containment strategies such as restraint, seclusion and 'time-out' have been used with punitive rather than therapeutic intent, the use of high dosages of psychotropic medicines for the comfort of the staff rather than the well-being of the patient, and the misuse of behaviour modification as a form of social control and even social retribution (Wilson, 1993).

It is acknowledged that the strategies and techniques referred to in the latter examples may be considered controversial even when the intent behind them is not punitive but therapeutic. However, it would go beyond the scope of this chapter to discuss them in detail since the intention is to focus on issues of power and empowerment in the nurse–patient relationship, rather than on the use of individual treatment regimes.

THE EMANCIPATION OF NURSES

The question of how nurses can contribute to the empowerment of patients is made more complicated by the fact that nurses are themselves an oppressed group requiring political emancipation (Hedin, 1986; Thompson, 1987). This situation has developed and been maintained because of:

- Historical factors in nursing associated with institutionalised passivity, conformity and the existence of the nursing 'hierarchy'.
- Alienation of nurses at the sharp end of the health care system from the decision-making centres of that system.
- The current atmosphere of 'fear and despondency' within the National Health Service.

Freire (1970) defines oppression as the prescription of one person's or group's behaviour by another, that is the imposition of the choice of one person or group on that of another. He also describes it as any situation in which one person hinders another's pursuit of self-affirmation as a responsible person. The issue of oppression thus appears to be closely linked to the apparently endless debate in nursing about the issue of 'autonomy' (defined by Lewis and Batey (1982) as 'the freedom to make discretionary decisions consistent within one's scope of practice and freedom to act on those decisions'), particularly in relation to how such autonomy is constrained by the organisational structures within which nursing takes place.

THE ORGANISATION OF NURSING

Since its inception, the main organisational framework on the nursing profession has been essentially one of 'bureaucracy', defined by Max Weber as being 'a hierarchical organisation designed rationally to coordinate the work of many individuals in the pursuit of large-scale administrative tasks and goals' (Max Weber in Gerth and Mills, 1948). Bureaucracy in nursing existed until recently in the form of a pyramid from the top level of nursing organisation down to ward level. Here it tends to stop and the picture changes to that of a web-like structure with the ward manager (that is, until recently, the 'Ward Sister') at the centre of a complex communication network (Chapman, 1977). The latter form of organisation provides an 'organic' structure which contrasts with the vertical lines of the classical bureaucratic model.

Although Max Weber thought bureaucracy provided a high degree of efficiency and that the system was the 'most rational known means' of organisational control, bureaucracies have been criticised for being cold and impersonal and for discouraging innovation and autonomy of decision-making (Haralambos, 1985). Bureaucracies are thus, almost by definition, instruments of oppression.

Recently however, government policy has been to reorganise bureaucratic organisations since these are seen nowadays as wasteful and inefficient. It is, perhaps, too soon to say whether recent organisational changes have reduced or increased the amount of bureaucracy in the NHS (this would make an interesting project for further research). Certainly, the structures have become more complex, and the old nursing 'pyramid' appears to have been broken up with nurses now managerially accountable to non-nurses in many instances. However, it is difficult to say that there has been a weakening of 'hierarchy' within the health care system. Indeed, recent instances of restrictions imposed on nurses' freedom of speech (Turner, 1992; Cassidy, 1994), and the acknowledgement of former NHS Chief Executive Duncan Nichol that a 'macho management' had spread 'fear and despondency' in the NHS (Brindle, 1992a) do not give an impression of a climate where professional autonomy is likely to flourish (see Footnote).

PRIMARY NURSING – A TROJAN HORSE?

A further recent development in British nursing organisation has been the introduction of the system of care delivery known as 'Primary Nursing', defined by Marran *et al* (1974) as 'the distribution of nursing so that the total care of an individual patient is the responsibility of one nurse, not many'. This system apparently provides an 'organic' structure for care delivery and aims to give nurses greater autonomy and accountability within a 'flattened hierarchy'. However, again it is difficult to comment on the success of this venture, mainly because of the lack of research data, although some preliminary studies indicate that in the UK at least, wards espousing primary nursing also show many features of other systems of care delivery (Thomas and Bond, 1990).

In commenting on the problems of the latter research, Thomas and Bond (1990) state:

Footnote: This situation is acknowledged by NHS managers themselves. Thus Pamela Charlwood, Director of the Institute of Health Services Managers, admitted to that organisation's conference that: 'Many feel that the climate in the NHS in the last couple of years had positively discouraged questioning and challenge of any kind' (Brindle, 1992b). Similarly, in a recent *Nursing Times* article, Rowden (1992) states: 'We still inculcate rigid respect for hierarchy and place an unhealthy regard for adherence to inflexible and outmoded rules. This is all equated, in a nonsensical manner with 'being a good nurse' (Rowden, 1992, p. 31). In the same article, Rowden (1992) made an indictment of nurse education for doing little to overcome such compliant passivity, stating:

> We will increasingly require the professional nurse to be a creative, assertive and questioning self-starter. I see no great evidence that we are really prepared to take this on board in nursing education (Rowden, 1992, p. 21).

Operational definitions of primary nursing, essential to provide replicable research into the organisation of nursing care are lacking in available research literature (Thomas and Bond, 1990, p. 1106).

Given such poverty of data, one might wonder what the basis is for the popularity of primary nursing for NHS managers. Bowers (1989) suggests that the attraction is that 'the clear lines of accountability provided by primary nursing' create 'tools' for providing 'objective' information on the performance of individual nurses. In other words, rather than being an efficient system of care delivery, which is as yet unproven, it is an efficient system of managerial control.

This is not to deny the therapeutic value of patients being able to identify a nurse within the system with whom they can have a therapeutic encounter, but to point out that while primary nursing may free the nurse from the mind-deadening burden of task allocation, it also locks her into a managerial framework that may be oppressive if nurses are to be held accountable for all aspects of the patient's care.

Thus Salvage (1985) criticises the concept of individual accountability as applied to nursing. She argues that if individual nurses are to be held accountable for the care they give 'at the bedside' (i.e. in close contact with clients), this is in some respects grossly unfair. The 'bedside' nurse has little control over her work situation, for example, resource allocation, staffing levels, etc. How could a nurse be held accountable for poor quality care if she has too many patients to care for adequately? Salvage also argues that the autonomous nurse is inevitably locked in conflict with the medical staff as their commands limit what she may do with her patient. Bowers (1989) states that these arguments might lead to the somewhat dismal conclusion that nurses are not accountable for anything they do, but also points out that an alternative conclusion is that nurses can make some decisions but need to be very clear about the exact limits of their responsibility, and the risks that they take within hierarchical organisational structures whose goals may sometimes be in conflict with their professional judgments. They also require political strategies for their professional survival (witness the cases of 'whistle-blowers' such as Graham Pink (Turner, 1992)) within these structures. Nurse training, however, rarely acknowledges the need for nurses to understand the structures of the health care system, or the need to examine the political significance of such structures for nursing. Possibly this is because nurse training institutions have traditionally had a 'hidden curriculum of social control' (Holloway and Penson, 1987) requiring that nurses learn 'good' behaviours (such as punctuality, speed and 'busyness') rather than develop insight into their social situation. Yet without a thorough grasp of the social and political realities within which they operate, nurses are unlikely to be able to offer more than a limited and essentially technically orientated service.

THE NURSING FUNCTION – A SYSTEMS VIEW

In a study redefining nursing in terms of social systems theory, Lees (1980) defines the nursing function as 'managing the patient "on behalf of" the family, managing his condition "on behalf of" the medical staff, and managing the daily transactions across the hospital–family boundary' (that is to say, managing whatever it is that determines the image of the hospital in the eyes of the public). Lees (1980) suggests that there is a tendency in traditional thinking to suggest that if a conflict occurs between an organisation and its substantive environment, the effects of this are felt mainly by those whose task it is to manage the organisation. It is their task to minimise the effects on those further down the organisation so that internal equilibrium is maintained. Lees (1980) argues, however, that it is those at the sharp end of the boundary between the organisation and its environment who will experience the greatest conflict. In the NHS it is the nurses who live at the sharp end, being unable to distance themselves from the expectations, anxieties and demands of the public in the ways that are open, for instance, to hospital managers. Thus the medical staff may define a patient in terms of his condition, the administrative staff may define him as a unit of cost, but the nurse's task is to define the patient as closely as possible in terms of a whole person. In doing this the full impact of managing what Lees calls the 'hospital–family boundary' is experienced, 'boundary' meaning the dividing line between different components of the system being analysed. Thus Lees (1980) states:

> To accept a patient and manage him 'on behalf of' the family can be likened, in Bion's (1962) term, to a 'container' not just for all the family's anxieties about coping with the patient, but also for their demand, indeed the demand of society at large, which says 'we want the best'. Likewise on the other side of the boundary (of the system), to accept the management of his condition 'on behalf of' the hospital [and by extension the health care system as a whole – author's comment] can be likened to being a 'container' for all the anxieties caused by an organisation with limited resources saying, in effect, 'all you get is this' (Lees, 1980, p.334).

Nursing, of course, takes place in a wide variety of environments. In some of these, the treatment model is one of cure. The sick are made well and the knowledge that patients may be returned to the community as convalescents allows for a general optimism to prevail. Although it is the nurses who bear the anxiety of managing the 'hospital–family boundary' they can, to some extent, project their hopes and fears onto the medical staff, who possess the appropriate technology to fulfil the hopes, allay the fears, and despite occasional failures, maintain the overall sense that things will eventually come right for the patients in their care.

Nevertheless, anxiety and role conflict inevitably occur as the nurse struggles to meet the demands of the different components of the system, while being at the same time distanced from the decision-making centres of that system. Lacking any form of democratic structure or model of mature professional practice, the tendency must be ever-present to revert to the bureaucratic decision-making that diminishes professional judgment (McDonagh *et al*, 1989). Recent developments in the NHS, such as the growth of free-market ideology, the devolution of budgetary decision-making and the replacement of a caring discourse by calculative thinking and consumerism, have done nothing to improve this situation. Thus, in a recent television documentary (cited by Darbyshire, 1993 in a *Journal of Advanced Nursing* Editorial) on the growth of autonomous trust hospitals, a ward sister describes how as a budget holder she now found herself asking whether particular nursing interventions would be 'worth it' for a patient: 'As she herself realized', states the *Journal of Advanced Nursing*, 'this is the point of no return, the point at which something elemental in the nurse's caring relationship is corrupted'.

In other environments, particularly those affecting the mentally ill and handicapped, the situation is rendered more complex by the fact that a far smaller proportion of patients may be treated in the belief that a cure is to be effected. Here the goal is not cure but 'containment' of 'the madness, the disability, the deformity, and some of the violence which the community wishes to disown and keep out of sight' (Lees, 1980, p.335). With these patients, medical staff do not claim the technical skills to make the sick well. Although resources may be meagre nurses still have to cope only with the demands of society, which says 'we want the best' for patients. However, in addition comes the realisation that, in stark contradiction to its demand for the best, society also says: 'we are prepared, in some instances, to write people off – as long as they are hidden away either in institutions or in parts of the community we can afford to ignore'. Such a contradictory state of affairs can only lead to disillusion and despair.

The community thus offloads its contradictory hopes and fears concerning the seriously mentally ill onto nurses, but in this case the nurses cannot unload their emotions onto the medical staff since prognoses are poor and expectations low. The nurses are left to cope with patients who may be incapable, violent or suicidal in the depressing knowledge that, in the absence of the technical means of cure, they will have to help maintain these patients at a subsistence level of existence either on long-stay wards or through an endless series of readmissions until death.

Left to care in a society that does not value caring, nurses of the severely and long-term mentally ill appear to be in the grip of a vicious double bind, which says something like 'you must look after these people well but since little can be expected of them, we will give you few resources to do the job, and even take away the resources you already have. If you cannot cope with this, you will be blamed and probably punished in some way'. This is certain to create anomic feelings of helplessness for nurses and little sense of purpose other than to fulfil the demands of a spurious institutional efficiency. In this is the psychiatric nurse's true oppression.

PSYCHIATRIC NURSING AND THE MEDICAL MODEL

In anxiety-provoking situations, self-awareness training is no doubt of great value in helping the nurses to cope with their own physiological responses to stress as well as feeding back to their patients a role model of calm and security. In situations of acute distress such role modelling can be crucial in preventing anxiety and other disorganising emotions from spilling over into overt aggression and other chaotic behaviours.

However, there is another side to the coin. This consists of the nurse being sufficiently self-aware to manage their own anxiety in potential emergency situations but insufficiently socially or politically aware to comprehend the role conflicts imposed on them by the contradictory expectations of society and the health care system of which they are a part. Flanagan (1986) states that generally the nurse is not politically minded, nor is she aware of the art of politics or the strategies of using power. She has extensive theoretical and practical training in patient care, but none at all in the skills and insights needed for coping with life in a complex bureaucratic organisation. This means that despite the large part that institutional politics plays in her life, the nurse is poorly placed to hold her own within the health care team or to represent the patient's interests, either within the health care system or outside it. Thus, in describing the work of the Mental Health Commission, Brown (1991) says: 'Although we often hear talk of nurses being patients' advocates, all too often no action is taken to protect individuals' (Brown, 1991, p.65). Similarly, Walsh (1985) says: 'Within today's health service, nurses, both on a collective and an individual level have extreme difficulty in representing their own interests and protecting their own position, let alone that of their patients' (Walsh, 1985).

Such statements indicate that nurses are insufficiently aware of social realities and of the role contradictions inherent in their nursing function.

The result of this failure to comprehend social realities and hence to develop a coherent ideology of psychiatric nursing is to hide behind the parapets of the medical model, whose primarily drug-centred orthodoxy continues to rule nursing concerns. In this connection, Clarke (1991) states:

Nurses rarely (if ever) question their relationship to the administration of drugs. Rather they continue to be given to patients simply because they are prescribed (the ongoing battle with junior medical personnel is seen as the expressed annoyance at 'too low' dosages of drugs prescribed by the junior) (Clarke, 1991, p.31).

The dominance of the medical model, of course, does little or nothing to clarify social realities for the nurses who are 'perennially bewildered', to use Louis Flanagan's choice phrase, by the medical profession's 'multitudinous models of madness' (Flanagan, 1986), and therefore ideologically disarmed and alienated from those it is their duty to help and nurture (Barber, 1988).

Against the view that psychiatric nurses are too closely tied to the medical profession, it may be argued that many users of psychiatric services are suffering from illnesses that are real, incapacitating and in need of chemotherapeutic or other medical intervention (the controversial treatment, ECT, is an example of such an intervention), and that the link with psychiatry remains central to mental health nursing services. Thus the report *Working in Partnership: A Collaborative Approach to Care* (Department of Health (DoH), 1994a) recommends that:

> The essential focus for the work of mental health nurses lies in working with people with serious or enduring illness in secondary and tertiary care, regardless of setting (DoH, 1994a).

Morris (1994) notes that this emphasis on mental illness comes at a time when there is concern that 'psychiatric nurses have drifted too far from (their) roots' (in psychiatry, presumably), a view echoed by Professor Patrick Darcy in a review of the Government's Consultation paper *Guidance on the Discharge of Mentally Disordered People and their Continuing Care in the Community* (Department of Health, 1994b). Professor Darcy states:

> Future provision of mental health care must not be based on the ideological baggage of the 1960s. The anti-psychiatry lobby needs to be balanced by the fears and concerns of patients and families. The prevailing ideologies that tried to convince society that there was no such thing as schizophrenia and that mentally ill people who commit crimes are criminals who should be put in prison are outdated. Today, such views would get little sympathy from Ben Silcock or Jayne Zito or the countless relatives of those mentally ill patients seeking admission to hospital or relief from prison (Darcy, 1994).

However, the need to review the ideology of mental health and the need to resource mental illness services adequately should not obscure the fact that nurses are often rendered helpless by the organisations that employ them. Apathy, frustration and 'burn-out' appear to be endemic (McKenna, 1993). Unsupported and under-resourced, nurses do their best teaching 'self-care' and 'activities of daily living', although these are mostly bleak substitutes for a meaningful existence.

Nursing needs to develop as a discipline in its own right. Central to this discipline should be a consideration of the ethics of care (i.e. as opposed to those of cure). The focus of such discourse needs to be on the relationship of patients and carers to the people who make decisions about their health and to the power structures within which these decisions are made. The report *Working in Partnership: A Collaborative Approach to Care* recommends that:

> The principle of choice for people who use services and their carers needs to be fully established as a basis for the practice of Mental Health Nursing (DoH, 1994a).

That nurses and doctors should collaborate to provide such choice stands to reason. However, the existence of physical and social constraints on the freedom of psychiatric patients, coercive treatments, lack of access to information, failure to recognise racial and ethnic needs, insensitivity to a range of gender issues (including the need to provide for women's safety within in-patient facilities) and the bureaucratic nature of the health care system means that the issue of choice cannot be addressed independently of the ways in which health professionals conduct themselves in relation to issues of patients' rights. With respect to this latter issue, it is a matter of urgency that nurses put their house in order. A description by Martin Brown of a typical visit of the Mental Health Act Commission amply illustrates this point:

> Regrettably eight years after the enactment of the Mental Health Act (in 1983) and despite a plethora of study days, most nurses are still uncertain about crucial parts of the act. Topics such as consent to treatment, nurses' holding powers and rights to appeal too often cause consternation. Most nurses express surprise that they are liable to sanctions if they administer medicine without obtaining proper consent after three months; many nurses adopt a cavalier approach to obtaining consent and regard patients as fair game for every type of treatment (Brown, 1991, p.64).

In resolving the ethical problems of care, the nurse cannot hide behind the doctor or, indeed, any other person. Nurses must debate and form their own particular perspective based on a duty to protect the patient from the excesses of the medical model and from the bureaucratic ineptitudes of health care institutions. If nurses are to collaborate with doctors they must also learn to assert their own interests, since collaboration only deserves the name when it can be achieved from a position of freedom, of social independence, and of being 'equal but different'. Otherwise it is collusion.

Nursing's failure to challenge medical orthodoxy is not confined to the hospital setting. Clarke (1991) states that despite the therapeutic networks open to community nurses, the literature on Community Psychiatric Nurses reveals the existence of a 'lip-service approach to psycho-social nursing' together with a 'peculiar inability among nurses to achieve more than a moderate articulation of the growing desperation of the socially-deprived, discharged hospital clients' (Clarke, 1991, p.31). 'With very few exceptions', states Clarke, 'the community nursing literature reveals the apolitical stance endemic to classical British psychiatry' (Clarke, 1991, p.31).

Thus, despite the fact that a central concern in health work is the need to challenge and change the many forms of disadvantage, oppression and discrimination that people face and that may adversely affect their health (Wallenstein and Bernstein, 1988; Ewles and Simnett, 1992), psychiatric nurses appear to be powerless to do so themselves and are themselves an oppressed group. Playing safe by associating themselves with the 'biological deficit' ideology of mental illness (Clarke, 1991), acceptance of the status quo by which medical staff dictate the agenda of care, lack of a clear nursing ideology, and passive acceptance of clients' social and personal situations are all examples of nurses adopting what Freire terms 'adopting oppressor group behaviour patterns', and this in turn is a classic example of what he calls 'oppressed group behaviour'. The conformity and collusion that this implies presents psychiatric nursing with the moral challenge of liberating itself from its traditional passivity in relation to the politics of mental health care.

THE CRITICAL PARADIGM

Both to prepare them for the changes that are currently happening in health care and to make sense of and counter their own oppression within the present structures of the health care system, it seems that nurses need a large injection of political knowledge and skills. The theoretical frameworks of Jürgen Habermas and Paolo Freire, which together form part of the 'critical paradigm' that has been gaining ground in nurse education and health education over recent years, mainly in Australia and the USA, are particularly relevant here (Hedin, 1987; Crane 1991; Embden, 1991; Kendall, 1992; Taylor, 1993).

Habermas, in his development of 'Critical Theory', exhorts individuals to examine critically the reality around them and expose those relationships and traditions within society which are unnecessarily constraining and to replace these with something more 'freeing' (Habermas, 1968). Freire (1970), in his experiences of teaching illiterate adults in Third World countries, has developed a model of oppressed group behaviour and pedagogy of the oppressed which leads to the development of 'Critical Consciousness'.

Critical consciousness is characterised by the attitude of practising depth in the interpretation of problems; being receptive to the new, with the good sense not to reject the old just because it is old; having no pre-conceived notions towards analysis and avoiding distortion when seeing problems; rejecting a passive position; testing findings and having an openness to revision; and having a soundness of argumentation (Freire, 1973).

Freire states that the roots of a 'freeing education' are characterised by 'dialogical' relations. As described by Freire (1970), such relations are based on love, humility, faith and a horizontal (non-hierarchical) relation-ship of trust. The identification of the world for what it is, as a first step toward transforming it, is a task that cannot be done *for* others but only *with* others (Hedin, 1986). As such, freeing education is incompatible with actions that prescribe, oppress, exploit or alienate individuals (Hedin, 1986).

There is nothing here, of course, that is incompatible with self-aware-ness training but there is an added emphasis on social context. Thus Habermas (1968) is very concerned with the question of the relationship between socioeconomic interest groups and knowledge. He argues that so long as there are conflicts of interest in human societies knowledge will remain infected by them and distorted. Habermas is particularly concerned with the distortions produced as a result of class conflict in the sphere of human economic activity. When people stand in relation-ships to each other which are characterised by economic exploitation and political oppression, they will inevitably develop one-sided view-points (Glover and Strawbridge, 1985). From this perspective, the oppres-sion of nurses and their clients can be seen as part of a much broader system of social control. Such a system is characterised by Habermas as a 'self-regulated system of purposive-rational action and adaptive beha-viour' (Habermas, 1971, p.117). Habermas' concept of this system differs from the classic Marxist model of 'forces of production' and 'relations of production' in that it is based on a more abstract understanding of work and human interaction.

In Habermas' view, it is only as conflicts of interest are overcome, and relationships of exploitation and oppression are replaced by relationships based on mutual interests and the common good, that knowledge undis-torted by conflicting interests will become possible. Undistorted or com-petent communication, which is necessary for the development of undistorted knowledge, is linked with the development of societies free from class conflict, and for that matter any other fundamental conflict of interest, such as race, nation, religion or gender (Glover and Strawbridge, 1985).

Porter (1994) argues that the ideas of Habermas are relevant to the 'New Nursing Paradigm' discussed earlier, since attempts to reduce the power differentials that exist between nurses and patients encourage rational rather than distorted communication between lay and professional participants in health care encounters. However, Porter cautions that the central position of language in Habermas' argument leads him to a naïve rationalism of which nurse reformers should be wary. Thus Porter argues that it is not only distortions in language and communication but structural and material constraints that provide barriers to human action. Against this however, one could argue that understanding is a necessary antecedent to action and that it is precisely through language that our understanding of barriers to human potential is revealed.

Critical theory, then, points beyond the relativity of viewpoints linked to conflicting interests by looking forward to a society free of such conflicts. This is a position which echoes a conception developed by Marx of human beings as beings capable of becoming 'species-beings'. In other words, they are capable of realising themselves as members of the human species as a whole and of developing the potential of the species (Glover and Strawbridge, 1985).

Doubtless, there are affinities here with the 'cosmic consciousness' of some of the more mystically orientated proponents of self-awareness training, the adherents for example of 'New Age' thinking (Bonewitz, 1989; Gawain, 1982). Both attempt to see the world holistically and both see reality in terms of processes rather than as static definitive forms. Both have goals of human liberation. However, there are also differences.

Thus, in the mystic view, the universe is seen as harmonious and 'unfolding perfectly' (Gawain, 1982). Critical theory makes no such idealistic assumptions of perfection. The adherents of mysticism see the forces of nature as 'flowing' and visualise the way to higher consciousness as 'going with the flow' of such forces (Gawain, 1982) – an ancient idea associated primarily with Taoism, a philosophy which advocated the renunciation of the world and a return to 'natural simplicity', to the harmony of nature (Hookham, 1969). Critical consciousness also incorporates the idea of transformation of consciousness but poses a world that is dialectical, where change takes place through the interaction of forces which are by no means harmonious, and where 'truth' (based on common consensus) involves overcoming one-sided interests (Hedin, 1986; Glover and Strawbridge, 1985).

Freire's premise is thus that it is through education (formal and informal) that the consciousness of a people can be changed. When individuals are enabled to 'see through' the consciousness imposed by the oppressor group and judge it for what it is, they can visualise other possibilities (Hedin, 1986). An education that is 'freeing' is needed to do this. Such an education is a freeing from a prescribed consciousness and a freeing to be fully human, to be fully a participating subject in the world (Hedin, 1986).

Applying such principles within the work of the psychiatric nurse would focus on the needs of disadvantaged and oppressed groups, including women, cultural and ethnic minorities, clients who are affected by the stigma of mental illness, and clients who experience powerlessness and inequality in their lives either within or outside hospital settings. Such work is by no means easy, and like all other 'therapies' carries with it potential 'side-effects' and risks. Thus Kendall (1992) discussing the use of an 'emancipatory' model in work with battered women points out:

> The risks are enormous for battered women, for they, as well as many oppressed groups have utilised much of their energy and will to learn to adapt to and survive the violence and oppression forced on them (Kendall, 1992, p.14).

Issues of physical and emotional safety lie at the heart of such work and present the 'emancipatory nurse' with ethical dilemmas, since for battered women the danger of violence increases as their awareness and freedom advance. Thus the more the client proceeds along the path of self-determination, the greater may be her danger. The nurse must consider how to support her client should she decide upon a challenge to the status quo while at the same time ensuring that nursing interventions are always in her best interests and safety. Politics and ethics are thus intertwined, and at each stage of the client's self-discovery and growth the essential question for the nurse will be: 'In whose interests am I working, the client's or my own?'

IMPLICATIONS FOR THE EDUCATION AND TRAINING OF NURSES

The implications of this discussion for the education and training of nurses are as follows.

First, the teacher needs to abandon any position that can be expressed in terms of being the 'fount of all knowledge'. Students should be encouraged to find their own 'truths' and sources (Hedin, 1986). This means an emphasis on the 'process' of learning (i.e. 'how we learn') rather than the product of learning ('what we learn'). In the process model of learning, outcomes are conceived in terms of the development of certain desirable processes and potentialities, or in other words, ways of thinking, acting and feeling that the student is able to use for his own purposes (Further Education Curriculum Review and Development Unit (FEU) cited by Sheehan, 1986). In addition the teacher should abandon any presumption of superior values (examples of apparently 'superior' values currently fashionable are the 'individualist values' of 'self-reliance' and 'independence', said to be gaining ground at present in nursing, at the expense of the bureaucratic values of the old NHS (Bowers, 1989; Clarke, 1981). Alternatively, the 'humanistic' and 'collectivist' values of 'care' and 'service', associated with the past might be contrasted with the apparently self-serving 'individualist' values of the 'New Right' (George and Wilding, 1985 cited by Bowers, 1989). The function of the teacher thus becomes to help students explore and clarify their own value systems, and also to question the values of the organisation, and even of society as a whole rather than to 'inculcate' any particular 'professional' or institutional values.

The concept of a 'freeing education' has much in common with the concepts of 'androgogy' (Burnard, 1989b) and 'learner-centred' education (Sweeney, 1986). Democratic participation in curriculum planning is encouraged. Programmes and timetables may be negotiated, and time may be set aside for students to deliberate on what they want to study, what they feel they need to study, and how they feel they should go about their studies, both as individuals and as a group. They are thus encouraged to take control of their learning at all points, and may also take over administrative tasks (Hedin, 1986).

The development of critical consciousness may be facilitated by setting aside time for students to examine incidents arising from their work situation and to explore, with their peers, alternative ways of dealing with these. At a hospital in the South of England, I was able to observe such a situation at first hand: a student described how she had been labelled 'idealistic' by trained staff for objecting to an approach taken to a particular patient, which seemed to curtail certain of the patient's rights (details omitted for reasons of confidentiality). The trained staff apparently thus managed to undermine the student, marginalise her and trivialise her contribution to the patient's care. During discussion of this incident, the student's peers gave her support and ventilated their feelings of anger and frustration about the ward staff, who were seen as 'punitive'. A lecturer present made links with theory and psychiatric knowledge (e.g. 'negative reinforcement' of the patient, and 'projective/introjective mechanisms' among the staff were suggested as possible 'operators'). At the same time, she validated the student's feelings and right to assert herself. Out of this discussion came not only a new view of the 'punitive' nurses as being themselves in need of support and care, but also the suggestion that a new and potentially important member of the team might make a 'useful ally'.

With careful guidance, then, a problem which initially seemed 'personal' was being transformed into one where a political strategy (through the formation of an alliance) and a perspective of unification (through support and reconciliation) could be envisaged. The possibility of thus transforming the relationships of all the staff concerned was born. However, just as with violence against battered women, the 'oppressor' group (in this case the trained nurses) will be unlikely to give up its domination easily, and careful attention to the safety of the alliance and, in this instance, to the process of reconciliation, will be needed.

In a freeing education, history, tradition and the past are examined, not for their own sakes, but to determine the formative influence they have had on individuals, institutions and cultures (Hedin, 1986). Thus in the above example there was a discussion of how certain details of the case described was likely to have reawakened anxieties connected with early childhood and how these might relate to the confrontative atmosphere on the ward.

Similarly, whenever possible, linkages are made between problems, topics, themes of discussion and theoretical perspectives (Hedin, 1986). Students are also encouraged to follow up their own theoretical leanings and affinities. This does not mean that all aspects of the curriculum are under student control or that a 'freeing education' is impossible where nurses need to work to a prescribed syllabus. The principle of mutuality means that programmes emerge from the perceived needs of both students and tutors, and that the need of the faculty to meet course objectives is taken into account as well as the students' perceptions of their own needs (Hedin, 1986; Burnard, 1989b).

EPILOGUE

Further research needs to be done on how nurses experience and deal with situations of oppression. Self-awareness needs to be taught alongside and within the context of developing social awareness, and a broad knowledge base.

According to Habermas (1968), knowledge is pursued in a 'technical interest' for the desire for prediction and control; knowledge pursued in a 'practical interest is for the development of self and mutual understanding; and knowledge pursued in an 'emancipatory interest' is for liberation from outmoded relations and structures. All types of knowledge are necessary for the development of the fully human person and no one type is presumed superior to another (Hedin, 1986). All types of knowledge are also necessary for the development of the discipline of nursing which has only recently begun to develop its potential as a separate entity in its own right with its own defined body of knowledge (Bennett, 1991). The central concerns emerging currently within this discipline relate to the use of 'reflection' as a means of practice development and integration with theory, the use of research paradigms based on study 'with' rather than 'on' people, the need to understand and treat health problems within their socio-cultural context, the empowerment of people to make informed health choices, the nature of caring as both art and science, the clarification of professional values in nursing, and a growing critique of the phenomenon of domination in nursing (Embden, 1991; Lorenson, 1988; Lumby, 1991; Thomspon, 1987). Critical Theory is emerging as an appropriate foundation for the study of these disciplinary concerns (Birx, 1993; Embden, 1991; Holter, 1988).

However, the creation of such a foundation will meet many obstacles. In reviewing the recent history of psychiatric nursing, Dr Hildegard Peplau warns that the resurgence of the biomedical model, and the return of the nature–nurture debate represent a major challenge to psychiatric mental health nurses in relation to the future patterns of their nursing practices (Peplau, 1994). In addition, the fragmentation of services and weakening of nurses' organisations represent powerful factors forming barriers to change.

Finally, emancipation (the goal of critical theory) is not possible without the support of the participants themselves for such a programme. People can invest heavily in their own oppression and it can be painful and risky to give it up. Better simply to take orders than risk the responsibility of acting on one's own behalf. In this regard, Hedin (1987) states that change will not come in nursing until nurses can be made aware of the potential of their healing powers in the many areas of society. I would add that the realisation of this potential will itself occur only with the development of a greater social engagement than is presently the case in nursing. This relationship, between the potential to heal and social engagement, was expressed rather more poetically by the 16th century explorer Alva Nuñez Cabeza da Vacha who, according to Haniel Long, the author of Alva's fictional biography, stated in his final letter to King Ferdinand I of Spain:

> If one lives where all suffer and starve, one acts on one's own impulse to help. But where plenty abounds, we surrender our generosity, believing that our country replaces us each and several. This is not so, and indeed a delusion. On the contrary the power of maintaining life in others, lives within each of us, and from each of us does it recede when unused. It is a concentrated power. If you are not acquainted with it, your Majesty can have no inkling of what it is like, what it portends, or the ways in which it slips from one . . . (Long, 1939, p.35).

The power that Alva refers to is, of course, the power of love . . .

REFERENCES

Barber P (1988) The psychiatric nurse's failure therapeutically to nurture. *Nursing Practice*, **1**(3): 138–141.

Beattie A (1991) Knowledge and control in health promotion: a test case for social policy and social theory. In: *The Sociology of the Health Service*, eds Gabe J *et al.* London: Routledge.

Bennett M (1991) Foreword. In: Gray G and Pratt R (eds) *Towards a Discipline of Nursing*. Melbourne: Churchill Livingstone.

Bion W R (1962) *Learning From Experience*. London: Heinemann.

Birx E C (1993) Critical thinking and theory-based practice. *Holistic Nurse Practice*, **7**(3): 21–27.

Blackburn C (1991) *Poverty and Health: Working with Families*. Milton Keynes: Oxford University Press.

Bonewitz R (1989) *The Crystal Heart – A Practical Guide to Healing the Heart Centre with Crystals*. Wellingborough: The Aquarian Press.

Bowers L (1989) The significance of primary nursing. *Journal of Advanced Nursing*, **14**: 13–19.

Brindle D (1992a) NHS bosses told to stop macho sackings. *Guardian*, 12 June, p.2.

Brindle D (1992b) NHS staff to get code on speaking out. *Guardian*, 13 June, p.4.

Brindle (1992c) Task force urged to end London health care 'time warp'. *Guardian*, 24 June, p.6.

Brown M (1991) Watching the detentions. *Nursing Times*, 3 July: 64–65.

Burnard P (1985) *Learning Human Skills: an experiential guide for nurses*, 2nd edn. Oxford: Butterworth Heinemann.

Burnard P (1986) Psychiatric nurse education: a question of balance. *Nurse Education Today*, **6**: 215–218.

Burnard P (1989a) *Teaching Interpersonal Skills: A handbook of experiential learning for health professionals* (Therapy in Practice 10). London: Chapman and Hall.

Burnard P (1989b) Experiential learning and androgogy – negotiated learning in nurse education: a critical appraisal. *Nurse Education Today*, **9**: 300–306.

Callaghan P and O'Carroll M (1993) Making women mad. *Nursing Times*, 27 July: 27–29.

Cassidy J (1994) Report urges free speech for NHS staff. *Nursing Times*. 19 Jan: p.6.

Chapman C (1977) *Sociology for Nurses*, London: Baillière Tindall.

Clarke L (1991) Ideological themes in mental health nursing. In: *Ethical Issues in Mental Health*, eds Barker P J and Baldwin S. London: Chapman Hall.

Clarke M (1981) Two aspects of psychology and their application to nursing. In: *Nursing Science in Nursing Practice*, ed. Smith J P. London: Butterworths.

Coxon T (1990) Ritualised repression. *Nursing Times*, **86**: 35–37.

Crane S (1991) Implications of the critical paradigm. In: *Towards a Discipline of Nursing*, eds Gray G and Pratt R. Melbourne: Churchill Livingstone.

Darbyshire P (1993) Guest editorial: preserving nurse caring in a destitute time. *Journal of Advanced Nursing*, **18**: 507–508.

Darcy P (1994) Accountability and the mental health services. *British Journal of Nursing*, **3**(6): 254–255.

Department of Health (1994a) *Working in Partnership: A Collaborative Approach to Care.* London: HMSO.

Department of Health (1994b) *Guidance on the Discharge of Mentally Disordered People and their Continuing Care in the Community: A Consultative Document.* London: HMSO.

Embden C (1991) Becoming a reflective practitioner. In: *Towards a Discipline of Nursing*, eds Gray G and Pratt R. Melbourne: Churchill Livingstone.

English National Board 1987 (reprinted from GNC 1982) *Syllabus of Training – 1982 Professional Register, Part 3.* ENB London and WNB Cardiff.

Evans C L S (1991) *Imogene King: A Conceptual Framework for Nursing.* Newbury Park: Sage.

Ewles L and Simnett I (1992) *Promoting Health: A Practical Guide*, 2nd edn. London: Scutari Press.

Fielding R G and Llewelyn S P (1987) Communication training in nursing may damage your health and enthusiasm: some warnings. *Journal of Advanced Nursing*, **12**: 281–290.

Flanagan L (1986) A question of ethics. *Nursing Times*, 27 Aug: 9–41.

Freire P (1970) *Pedagogy of the Oppressed.* New York: Continuum.

Freire P (1973) *Education for Critical Consciousness.* New York: Continuum.

Gawain S (1982) *Creative Visualisastion.* New York: Bantam (New Age).

George V and Wilding P (1985) *Ideology and Social Welfare.* London: Routledge and Kegan Paul.

Gerth H H and Mills C W (eds) (1948) *From Max Weber: Essays in Sociology.* London: Routledge and Kegan Paul.

Gibson C H (1991) A concept analysis of empowerment. *Journal of Advanced Nursing*, **16**: 354–361.

Glover D and Strawbridge S (1985) The sociology of knowledge. In: *Sociology: New Directions*, ed. Haralambos M. Ormskirk: Causeway.

Habermas J (1968) *Knowledge and Human Interests.* Boston: Beacon Press.

Habermas J (1971) *Towards a Rational Society: Student Protest, Science, and Politics.* London: Heinemann.

Haralambos M (1985) *Sociology: Themes and Perspectives*, 2nd edn. London: Unwin Hyman.

Hedin B A (1986) A case study of oppressed group behavior in nurses. *IMAGE: Journal of Nursing Scholarship*, **18**(2): 53–55.

Hedin B A (1987) Nursing education and social constraints: an indepth analysis. *International Journal of Nursing Studies*, **24**(3): 261–270.

Holloway I and Penson J (1987) Nurse education as social control. *Nurse Education Today*, **7**: 235–241.

Holter I N (1988) Critical theory: A foundation for the development of nursing theories. *Scholarly Inquiry for Nursing Practice: An International Journal*, **2**(3): 223–232.

Hookham H (1969) *A Short History of China.* London: Longmans.

Ingleby D (1981) Understanding 'mental illness'. In: _Critical Psychiatry: The Politics of Mental Health_, ed. Ingleby D. Harmondsworth: Penguin.

Kendall J (1992) Fighting back: promoting emancipatory nursing actions. _Advanced Nursing Science_, 15(2): 1–15.

Lake Medicine Grizzlybear (1991) _Native Healer: Initiation into an Ancient Art_. Wheaton, Illinois: Quest Books.

Land H (1991) The confused boundaries of community care. In: _The Sociology of the Health Service_, eds Gabe J _et al_. London: Routledge.

Lees S (1980) Developing effective institutional managers in the 1980s – part 2: some new directions. _Journal of Advanced Nursing_, 5: 329–339.

Leininger M (1988) Leininger's theory of nursing: cultural care diversity and universality. _Nursing Science Quarterly_, August: 152–160.

Lewis F M and Batey M V (1982) 'Clarifying autonomy and accountability' in nursing service. _Journal of Nursing Administration_, 12(10): 10–15.

Lister P (1991) Approaching models of nursing from a postmodernist perspective. _Journal of Advanced Nursing_, 16: 206–212.

Long H (1939) _The Marvellous Adventure of Cabeza de Vaca_. London: Souvenir.

Lorensen M (1988) Response to 'Critical Theory: A Foundation for the Development of Nursing Theories'. _Scholarly Inquiry for Nursing Practice: An International Journal_, 2(3): 235–236.

Lumby J (1991) Threads of an emerging discipline: praxis, reflection, rhetoric and research. In: Gray G and Pratt R (eds) _Towards a Discipline of Nursing_. Melbourne: Churchill Livingstone.

Magiacas A (1988) Health for all: nursing's role. _Nursing Outlook_, 36(2): 66–71.

Marran G D _et al_ (1974) _Primary Nursing – a model for individualised care_. London: C V Mosby.

Marx and Engels (1972) Critique of materialism. In: _Karl Marx: The Essential Writings_, ed. Bender F L. New York: Harper.

Maslow A H (1972) _Motivation and Change_, New York: Harper and Row.

McCarney J (1990) _Social Theory and the Crisis of Marxism_. London: Verso.

McDonagh K J _et al_ (1989) Shared governance at Saint Joseph's Hospital of Atlanta: a mature professional practice model. _Nursing Administration Quarterly_. 13(4): 17–28.

McKenna H (1993) A long-term view. _Nursing Times_, 13 Oct: 50–53.

Moccia P (1988) At the faultline: social activism and caring. _Nursing Outlook_, 36(1): 30–33.

Mohan J (1991) Privatization in the British health sector: a challenge to the NHS. In: _The Sociology of the Health Service_, eds Gabe J _et al_. London: Routledge.

Monahan J and Vaux A (1980) Task Force report: the macro-environment and community mental health. _Community Mental Health Journal_, 16: 14–26.

Morris M (1994) Working in partnership report signals a pivotal role for mental health nurses. _British Journal of Nursing_, 3(6): 253–254.

Ogata S (1959) _Zen for the West_. London: Rider.

Peplau H E (1994) Psychiatric Mental Health nursing: Challenge and change. *Journal of Psychiatric and Mental Health Nursing*, **1**: 3–7.

Porter S (1994) New Nursing: The road to freedom?'. *Journal of Advanced Nursing*, **20**: 269–274.

Rawlinson J W (1990) Self-awareness: conceptual influences, contribution to nursing, and approaches to attainment. *Nurse Education Today*, **10**: 111–117.

Reverby S (1987) A caring dilemma: womanhood and nursing in historical perspective. *Nursing Research*, **36**: 5–11.

Rowden R (1992) Self-imposed silence. *Nursing Times*, **88**: 31.

Russell B (1961) *A Short History of Western Philosophy*, 2nd edn. London: George Allen and Unwin.

Salvage J (1985) *The Politics of Nursing*. London: Heinemann.

Sheehan J (1986) Curriculum models: product versus process. *Journal of Advanced Nursing*. **11**: 671–678.

Sidran B (1971) *Black Talk*. New York: Da Capo.

Snyder G (1964) Buddhist anarchism. *Anarchy* **4**(8): 254–256.

Sweeney J F (1986) Nurse education: learner-centred or teacher-centred. *Nurse Education Today*, **6**: 257–262.

Taylor J (1993) Education can never be neutral – only subversive. *Nurse Education Today*, **13**: 69–72.

Thomas L H and Bond S (1990) Towards defining the organisation of nursing care in hospital wards: an empirical study. *Journal of Advanced Nursing*, **15**: 1106–1112.

Thompson J L (1987) Critical scholarship: the critique of domination in nursing. *Advances in Nursing Science*, **10**(1): 27–38.

Turner T (1992) The indomitable Mr Pink. *Nursing Times*, **88**: 26–28.

Wadeson B (1992) We don't do mad people now. *Nursing Standard*, **6**(33): 56.

Wallerstein N and Bernstein E (1988) Empowerment education: Freire's ideas adapted to health education. *Health Education Quarterly*, **15**(4): 379–394.

Walsh P (1985) Speaking up for the patient. *Nursing Times*, 1 May: 24–26.

Williams M (1986) *Identification of Psychiatric Nursing Skills*. Unpublished Thesis, Bristol Polytechnic/Frenchay Health Authority.

Wilson M (1993) Seclusion practice in psychiatric nursing. *Nursing Standard*, 2 April: 28–29.

FURTHER READING

Altschul A T (1978) A systems approach to the nursing process. *Journal of Advanced Nursing*, **3**: 333–340.

Burnard P and Chapman C (1990) *Nurse Education: The Way Forward*. London: Scutari Press.

Freire P and Shor I (1987) *A Pedagogy for Liberation: Dialogues on Transforming Education*. Houndmills: Macmillan Education.

McCarthy T (1984) *The Critical Theory of Jürgen Habermas*. Cambridge: Polity.

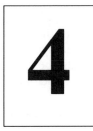

4 | Family Therapy
Gwynneth Down

INTRODUCTION

Nurses, in common with other mental health workers, often become involved with families when a crisis occurs with one of their members. This person (who becomes identified as the client or patient) is usually then offered treatment or therapy, based on an assessment of their individual need. Support and advice may be given to relatives, but this has traditionally been seen as an adjunct to the major therapeutic work with the individual.

This chapter addresses a different treatment approach which considers problems in the context of the relationship network in which they occur. The theory and concepts which underpin this approach are discussed here and the particular relevance to mental health nursing will be highlighted, with reference both to relevant literature and case examples.

FAMILY THERAPY

As with individual and group therapies, the field of family therapy is rich and varied. The *Handbook of Family Therapy* (Gurman and Kniskern 1991) offers no fewer than 12 major models of family therapy, including the psychoanalytical, structural, strategic and behavioural approaches. As it would be impossible to do justice to this diverse field in one chapter general concepts and applications of theory are illustrated, by focusing mainly on one model of family therapy – Milan Systemic Therapy (Jones, 1993).

Models of family therapy may differ in a number of respects – in their emphasis on beliefs, or structure and hierarchy, in their view of dysfunction or health, or in the types of interventions used. All models of family therapy can, however, be described as 'systemic', in that they recognise the interconnections between individuals, families and social networks.

Therapists using a systemic approach aim to promote change by intervening in a broader network or system, rather than with an individual alone. The network of intimate relationships that is most usually considered is that contained in a family; however, problems may also be viewed within friendship, work, organisational and indeed the wider sociopolitical contexts.

Whereas individual therapies attend to an individual's intrapsychic processes, family therapy focuses mainly on the interpersonal connections, patterns and relationships between people as the area for change. This conceptual difference between an individual and a relationship focus has major implications for the way in which nurses might intervene in particular circumstances. If a person's distress is viewed as intrapsychic the nurse will approach that individual alone.

If however, the meaning, maintenance and resolution of individuals' distressed feelings or actions are seen as connected to their relationships with others, it begins to make sense to involve them in the therapeutic process (Burnham 1986).

FAMILY THERAPY IN THE FIELD OF MENTAL HEALTH

The family therapy movement grew out of the general field of psychiatry, with developments taking place independently in both the USA and the UK during the 1950s. Prior to this, the most influential approaches to psychotherapy were Freudian psychoanalysis and Rogerian client-centred therapy (Nichols, 1984). These individual-orientated therapies were seen by some as contributing to the bias held by clinicians to avoid and even discourage contact with patients' relatives (Nichols, 1984).

Some clinicians (e.g. John Bowlby, John Bell, Nathan Ackerman), however, became frustrated with the limitations of individual therapies and began experimenting with seeing whole families rather than an identified patient alone. The development of family therapy was also accelerated by the vast amount of research done in the 1950s and 1960s on links between schizophrenia and family dynamics. An extremely influential paper of this time, *Toward a Theory of Schizophrenia* (Bateson *et al*, 1956), introduced the concept of the 'double bind'. This was seen as a dysfunctional communication style between family members which might lead to schizophrenic symptomatology.

While this concept has now been discredited, modern-day therapists and researchers have also focused on family therapy approaches to treating people with schizophrenia. Over the last decade, six important research trials have demonstrated that the efficacy of family treatment, in combination with maintenance neuroleptic drugs, in preventing relapse of schizophrenia (Goldstein *et al*, 1978; Leff *et al*, 1982, 1989; Falloon *et al*, 1982; Hogarty *et al*, 1986; Tarrier *et al*, 1988).

Original research in this area developed from the work of Brown and colleagues, who found that relapse was related to the family environment to which the person with schizophrenia was discharged (Brown and Rutter, 1966). Further research by Leff and Vaughn (1981) showed that high relapse rates were related both to high levels of expressed emotion (EE) and high face-to-face contact with relatives. (Expressed emotion is defined as criticism, hostility and over-involvement.) Psychosocial intervention packages for families (described more fully later) have been found to reduce relapse rates significantly by reducing rates of expressed emotion. In one study by Leff and colleagues (1990) the 2-year relapse rate was 40 per cent where family social intervention was offered, compared to 75 per cent where families were offered no help. This has obvious implications for mental health service providers.

Family therapy has been used in many other areas of the mental health field, some of which will now be described in more detail.

In the field of adult mental health, family therapy has been used for a variety of difficulties, including alcoholism and depression (Bennun, 1986), sexual abuse (Jones, 1991), manic depressive disorder (Moltz, 1993), relationship difficulties and a variety of other problems described by adults who attended a family therapy clinic in a psychiatric department (Chase and Holmes, 1990).

Anorexia nervosa has been treated with family therapy for many years (Minuchin, 1978). It appears to be the treatment of choice for some groups; a study comparing individual supportive psychotherapy with family therapy found that the latter was markedly more effective in achieving improvement in patients who developed anorexia before the age of 18 years and who had been ill for less than 3 years (Dare *et al*, 1990).

Despite growing evidence of the family's importance in this area however, Cottrell's (1989) review of the case notes of adult psychiatric patients appeared to show that psychiatrists did not think family issues (or indeed contact with relatives) were relevant in 'patient management', despite evidence that family events were thought to have precipitated crises for at least a quarter of the sample.

In child mental health settings, however, family therapy is often the primary treatment approach, with research showing that while it can be at least as effective as other treatments in symptom change, it can also achieve more changes for other family members and take less time (Simpson, 1990).

The following section addresses the involvement of nurses in family therapy practice and research.

NURSES AND FAMILY THERAPY

Nurses seem to be in an ideal position to work in a systemic way with families. Whether in the client's home, hospital, hostels, clinics or other settings, nurses are often the professionals closest to the client and having most contact with relatives on a regular basis. Traditionally nurses have offered support, information and advice to families, while continuing to view the individual as the 'identified patient'. This type of intervention has been described as 'family-focused' nursing (Friedemann, 1989). Here the nurse directs her actions mainly towards individuals in a family and towards individual and family goal achievement through the interpersonal process.

Family-focused nursing is distinct from the approach primarily described in this chapter, which sees the family system as the unit for change. Friedemann (1989) describes this as 'family systems nursing'. Wright and Leahey (1990) also make the distinction between approaches, clarifying their view that either is valid: 'The practice of family (focused) nursing as compared to family systems nursing is no less inferior, no less important, only different'.

Reviewing current literature in this field highlights that American nurses seem far more likely to be involved in family therapy or family systems nursing than their British counterparts. While references within British journals and textbooks are somewhat sparse, this does not appear to be the case in American literature, with textbooks wholly devoted to family systems nursing (Clements and Buchanan, 1982; Friedman, 1986; Leahey and Wright, 1987).

Tennant (1993) found an enormous international literature base pertaining to families and nursing overall. This included the work of intensive care nurses with patients' relatives (Krozek 1991), and a variety of approaches for relatives where a family member has experienced physical trauma of some kind (Killen, 1990; Schlum-Urquhart, 1990; Solursh, 1990). While Tennant also found some important contributions by mental health nurses, his major conclusion was that 'the importance of the family system has . . . been de-emphasised in the planning and delivery of mental health services' and that this was reflected in the paucity of literature concerning families and psychiatric nursing practice.

The context in which nurses work and their position in the hierarchy may determine how able nurses feel to intervene with families. It is interesting that other professionals have seen nurses as a resistant force, rather than holding the possibility that nurses may actually practise family therapy themselves. Dungworth (1988) discusses contexts for setting up family therapy practice thus:

Psychiatric hospitals are hierarchically structured but this should not mislead us into believing that we can, or should ignore nursing staff and others in favour of the professions with more prestige. Forming an alliance with a 'friendly' psychiatrist can lead to resentment and resistance amongst other staff groups (Dungworth, 1988).

Despite this rather gloomy picture, there is some evidence that mental health nurses are successfully using systemic family therapy ideas and interventions in a variety of settings.

Examples include community psychiatric nurses offering family therapy to treat (successfully) a young woman with anorexia nervosa (Moores and Dunne, 1988) and help a heroin addict and family to deal with the problem (Blank, 1987). Staff in a short-term rehabilitation centre have used an amended version of a behavioural family therapy approach to improve the communication skills of a group of people with schizophrenia. This example is particularly interesting in that it uses the milieu of the centre, the residents and staff as 'family', thus illustrating the wide applications of this approach (Elliot *et al*, 1991).

The majority of mental health nursing and family therapy literature focuses on work with people who have a diagnosis of schizophrenia and their families. The approaches which are most commonly used are the psychoeducation or psychosocial programmes. As these developments are extremely important to mental health nursing, more detail will be given here.

Psychoeducational and psychosocial approaches

Nurses can be at the forefront of good practice in this area. Brooker and Butterworth (1991a) have described Department of Health-commissioned research into outcome in families, after Community Psychiatric Nurses (CPNs) have received training in psychosocial intervention strategies. The early results have shown encouraging improvements both in the clients' symptomatology and social functioning and in relatives' satisfaction and minor psychiatric morbidity. Families caring for a mentally ill relative can face a number of adverse consequences, including reduction in income and social activities and significantly more stress (Grad and Sainsbury, 1963).

The psychosocial programme of care is based on the work of social psychiatrists, discussed earlier, which has shown convincing evidence that relapse in schizophrenia can be improved if families receive a detailed package of care. The package is based on the belief that having a serious mental illness makes patients sensitive to stress ('stress vulnerability'). One source of stress may be the 'expressed emotion' (EE) within the family, which has been shown to be a good predictor of relapse. Families are not held responsible for causing their relative's illness, but are seen as an extremely important resource in helping to reduce stress for their relative, to their mutual benefit.

Detailed assessments of individual and family need are the first step in the psychosocial programme offered. These often include some measure of the expressed emotion within the family. The major aims of intervention will then be to reduce relatives' expression of criticism, hostility and overprotection, particularly towards the ill person. One of the ways in which this is achieved is through a health education programme.

Research by Vaughn and Leff (1976) showed that while relatives with low expressed emotion are more likely to see any bizarre or odd behaviour in their relative as a symptom of genuine illness, high expressed emotion relatives believed that the behaviour was deliberate and within control. This led them to be more critical of the sufferer. Up to 70 per cent of critical comments by relatives have been shown to refer to the negative symptoms of schizophrenia (Kuipers *et al*, 1992).

The health education programme is then aimed at teaching family members about the nature and possible course of schizophrenia. Families can be helped to see negative symptoms as part of an illness, thus reducing their expressed emotion. Brooker (1991) also points out that this programme addresses relatives' needs for information, usually not met by professionals.

Psychosocial interventions may take different forms depending on the assessment. It is important that nurses acknowledge the range of strong emotions that families are likely to feel when a diagnosis of schizophrenia is given to one of their members. They may feel bereaved at the loss of the person that existed before the illness, or terrible guilt which can underlie an overinvolvement with the ill person. These issues need to be addressed, to reduce family stress and help them to deal with their situation as constructively as possible.

Families can be helped to cope by offering carers' and users' groups to provide support and a peer group who have some experience of the problems encountered. By offering this support alongside structured (individual) family sessions, nurses will be aiming to improve communication between all family members.

A behavioural problem-solving approach will also be taught to the family to enable them all to prioritise problems, negotiate and identify solutions. Problems may initially seem all-encompassing – 'he's so lazy' can be reframed as 'he doesn't get up till lunch' – daily expectations can then be negotiated and small manageable goals set (Kuipers *et al*, 1992). Current training courses in this approach for nurses, completed after 6 months, will enable nurses to work with families in a very specialised (but limited) area.

WHO CAN BE A FAMILY THERAPIST?

In a survey of professionals' attitudes to family therapy for older adults, nearly half of the district nurse group questioned reported that they practised family therapy (Gilleard *et al*, 1992). This, of course, raises questions about the nurse's understanding of what family therapy is and is not. It seems unlikely that the district nurses surveyed would have either undertaken family therapy training or be using systemic thinking in their understanding of the problem presented. It may be more likely that their important intervention with relatives would perhaps be recognised as 'family nursing' (Friedemann, 1989) rather than family therapy.

Friedemann (1989) proposes that family nursing could and should be practised by all nurses. However, she suggests that family systems nursing (family therapy) requires 'holistic understanding of the intricate relationships between family system components and the skills of clinical specialists'. By what route would nurses gain the proficiency and qualifications needed to change from novice to advanced nurse, and on to becoming an expert nurse (Benner, 1984) in this specialised area?

Many centres of nurse education are now introducing systemic/family therapy concepts to training, providing an alternative view to the individual models most traditionally used. Nurses may also undertake one of the many multidisciplinary foundation courses on offer which will enable them to use family therapy concepts and skills within their work contexts. In order to become clinical specialists, more advanced training will be required.

In order to become a qualified family therapist, eligible to be registered by the United Kingdom Conference for Psychotherapy, the nurse will need to undertake foundation level family therapy training (e.g. 2 years' part-time study to certification level), followed by an advanced level training (with a minimum of 320 hours of therapeutic practice and 320 hours of academic study).

CLINICAL APPLICATIONS

What is a Family?

Before moving on, the reader is invited to consider their own response to this question. If this question could be asked of your grandparents, how do you imagine their description would differ? Did your description of 'family' contain lists of people to be included, or a description of what a family does? The answers given will vary greatly according to the reader's own experience of family, which will have been shaped by their culture, gender and current societal mores.

Wide-ranging changes have taken place in family life over recent years, yet some sections of the media continue to represent the 'family' as a group containing two parents (male and female) holding traditional roles. The father is seen as the 'breadwinner', out at work, the mother as the housewife and carer of their 2.4 children. Research has shown, however, that significantly large numbers of people do not live in traditionally structured households at all (Kiely and Richardson, 1991).

In England today, family structures also include single parents, lesbian or gay couples (with or without children), serial cohabiting or married heterosexual couples and step-families. Individuals will differ greatly in whom they would include in their description of family, and this will be influenced by their ethnicity and culture. For some, family may indeed be 'nuclear', for others it may include an extended network of aunts, uncles, cousins and grandparents, or a wide informal network of kin and community including long-time friends (Carter and McGoldrick, 1989).

It is very important that we as nurses can recognise our own beliefs about families *as beliefs*, constructed from our own experience, and shaped by our culture, gender and the current societal mores. If this is not recognised, nurses will be in danger of conveying to our clients a message that our view of family is the norm.

Family Life-Cycle

Many individual therapies (e.g. psychoanalytical) have at their base a view about the importance of an individual's progression through various stages of development. The family therapy field also places importance on developmental stages, but in this case those taking place within a family network. This approach acknowledges both an individual's development, the effect of this on other relationships, and the development of the family as an entity.

It is important to recognise that a person's development is both dependent on, and has an influence on, their family relationships. Transition points for an individual (birth, adolescence, leaving home, living with a partner) are also transitions for parents, siblings and grandparents. Families have to change to allow and accommodate change in one of their members. A family life-cycle will include expected additions or leavings such as the birth of a child or the death of grandparents in old age. Adolescence, leaving home, marriage and retirement may all entail changes in the roles, boundaries and rules of a family. Whether transitions are around joyful or sorrowful events, family stress will often be at its greatest at these times.

In many differing cultures, life-cycle events are marked by rituals or ceremonies, such as christening, marriage ceremony, bar mitzvah, cremation or burial services. These rituals can aid family transition and acceptance of change providing 'a safe and manageable context for the expression of strong emotions' (Imber-Black, 1989).

The pace of social change currently taking place in England has been such that structures and rituals which might aid some family transitions have not yet been created. Separation, divorce and the formation of step-families are life-cycle stages negotiated by increasing numbers of families, without 'rites of passage' (Friedman, 1989) to help them. 'Divorce parties' are one such development, marking a change in family roles and relationships.

For the most part, the high degree of flexibility required to negotiate family change is taken for granted, and the individual and family develop well with few problems. In some circumstances, however, these transitions are not negotiated appropriately, leading to difficulties. Individual and family ability to accommodate, for example, may be stretched thin if several life events occur within a short space of time. Equally problematic may be the negotiation of a life-cycle stage which has presented difficulties in the previous generation:

Case 1

The Brown family presented to a child mental health service with concerns about their 15-year-old daughter who was seen as 'going off the rails' by her parents. She was staying out late with her friends, drinking and then lying in late and missing school. When at home she had 'terrible' rows with her mother.

In therapy, discussion took place about what rules and expectations the parents had for their daughter. Both said they lacked confidence in their ability to negotiate their daughter's adolescence, while disagreeing with each other's approach to limit-setting. As they wavered, their daughter, unsure about expectations, proceeded to push them.

Exploring life-cycle issues was very important in understanding their situation. Mrs Brown's mother had died when she was 12 years old, and she went to live with her elderly grandparents. Her memory of this time was that although she received much love and attention, she was the carer for her grandparents as they became older and more frail. She said 'while the other girls at school were going out with boyfriends and having fun, I was at home making cocoa!'.

Mr Brown's experience of adolescence was somewhat different – one of a large family, he felt he was given plenty of freedom to do as he wished. Perhaps this freedom was too great, and he didn't get the guidance and support that he wanted, as he became involved in petty crime with his peers, only stopping after a spell in a remand centre.

For this couple, then, their experience was of extremes – at one end of the spectrum too much freedom, without appropriate responsibility, guidance or support and at the other, too much responsibility and not enough independence. Negotiating the life-cycle stage of adolescence was difficult because of issues arising at the same stage, in the parents' own family of origin.

The importance of considering a developmental view of family life needs to be stressed. While nurses and other professionals will be aware that a life event such as relationship breakdown can be the trigger for an *individual's* distress or disturbance, Carter and McGoldrick (1989) also highlight that 'symptoms are most likely to appear when there is an interruption or dislocation in the unfolding *family* life cycle'. They suggest that where this occurs, therapeutic efforts will often need to be directed towards helping family members to reorganise so that they can proceed developmentally.

SYSTEMS

Earlier in this chapter I suggested that there were significant differences between an individual and systemic view of the problems that people may face. To understand the systemic concepts that underpin most models of family therapy, a visual image may be helpful.

Think of a decorative mobile, the type that might hang over a baby's cot or near a doorway to catch the draught. The ornaments (for example, sheep) on the mobile all hang and move in relation to each other, even though the threads that connect them are less easy to see. The mobile represents a system: *a set of elements that stand in some consistent relationship with each other and which can be seen as more than the sum of their parts.* In families those elements are people, and although we cannot see the threads that connect them (e.g. emotional ties) we know they are there, because family members hold particular relationships with each other. Just as a mobile is more than a group of sheep, a family is more than just a group of individuals related by birth or marriage.

If we consider now what happens to a mobile when one of the sheep is pushed, the sheep and threads move and the whole mobile moves into a different constellation. Similarly, if a sheep is either added or taken away, the balance of the mobile is completely changed. Compare this to a family – when a son gets married, he and his wife begin new couple and new in-law relationships. His parents (and other family members) also have to adjust to different roles and relationships with each other. Thus, change in one part of the 'system' also affects other parts.

Change can, of course, occur in people's beliefs, behaviour or relationships without actual losses or additions to a family. As mental health professionals, nurses will often be attempting to help people to change, and will need to have regard both for how change is supported or hindered by their relationship network, and the effect of any change on the network.

Case 2

Mrs Thomas, a 35-year-old woman, was referred to a psychiatrist by her GP, who described her as depressed and anxious. As part of a package of care, she was offered a place in a women's group held at the local psychiatric day hospital. After some time in this group, Mrs Thomas was able to disclose for the first time that she had been sexually abused by her father from the age of 8 years until she had finally left home at 16 years.

Initially, the nurses facilitating the group felt she made good use of it, offering and gaining a great deal of support from the other women. They thought she had gained confidence, appeared happier and had become more assertive. After some time, however, the nurses noticed that she had become quieter, appearing subdued and preoccupied.

When this was commented upon, she said that she was concerned about her husband: 'We just don't seem to get on any more – he follows me around and wants to know about everything I do. If I tell him to leave me alone it just starts an argument'.

It was decided to offer Mrs Thomas and her husband an opportunity to talk together with a family therapist, and both readily agreed to this. In this session it became apparent that a balance in the couple's relationship had also changed when Mrs Thomas began to change her behaviour. Whereas Mr Thomas had previously perceived his wife to be emotionally somewhat fragile, and in need of looking after, his wife was now challenging this view. She no longer felt she needed him to accompany her on trips out of the house, or to make decisions for her.

Mr Thomas was upset that his wife had not told him about the abuse before telling 'outsiders'. He was frightened that she no longer needed him and might leave; hence he tried to hold on to his familiar role with her. Work with the couple then focused on helping them to find new ways of relating. The therapy needed to acknowledge the losses involved in changing roles (particularly, in this case, for Mr Thomas), as well as the gains for them both. The therapist also helped them to communicate directly about the sexual abuse and its effects on their relationship.

From Linear to Circular

This is an example of a conversation between Mr and Mrs Thomas, the couple discussed above:

Mr T: (reading paper): There's a good film on this evening.

Mrs T: (quietly): I'm going out later.

Mr T: You don't normally go out, where are you going?

Mrs T: I'm just going out with one of the girls from the group.

Mr T: Yeah, but where are you going? Why didn't you tell me?

Mrs T: Look I'm only going to Sheila's house, I won't be back late.

Mr T: I'll give you a lift, it'll be dark soon, better than waiting for a bus.

Mrs T: I wish you'd stop fussing, I'm quite capable of going out by myself.

Mr T: (angrily): Don't you dare tell me I'm fussing, you used to want me to drive you everywhere till you went to this bloody group.

Readers may like to consider how this conversation became an argument, and whose 'side' they would place themselves on.

If this situation was viewed from Mr Thomas's perspective, one might say that his wife is being secretive, withholding information from her husband, information that might reassure him about her evening out. Because of this he is worried and concerned about what is going on. From Mrs Thomas's perspective, however, one might consider that Mr Thomas is trying to control his wife, wanting her to remain in a dependent role. Little wonder she keeps things to herself, one might say, if that's his reaction. These uni-directional views of this interaction illustrate what is known as 'linear causality', where **A** causes **B** to happen:

Mrs Thomas is secretive about her   ——▶   Mr Thomas becomes worried, tries to
evening out   find out more

                           A   **B**

or

Mr Thomas acts intrusively   ————▶   Mrs T is wary about telling him about her
                                               activities

                           A   **B**

In family therapy terms, attempts to describe what happens in an interaction, from the viewpoint of a particular participant, is called 'punctuation' and is something that most of us do in everyday conversation, for example: 'she doesn't let him get a word in edgeways', 'he's always fighting with his sister', and so on.

These individual ('linear') viewpoints may organise both family members and professional teams into debating which is the correct interpretation and may also lead them into a blaming stance against one of the participants.

It is clear, however, that to describe the behaviour of one person as having a direct causal effect on the other's behaviour may ignore how both behaviours interact with each other *and* miss important information about the couple's relationship. 'A systemic view would see each view as an arc of a circular sequence or a partial explanation of the event' (Burnham, 1986). Taking a 'circular' view will help the therapist and couple to focus attention on the patterns that have developed *between* the couple and avoid apportioning blame to either person.

Focusing on the circular interaction between the couple highlights a pattern of behaviour that occurs between them: it can be seen that Mrs Thomas is initially reticent in talking to her husband about her evening out with friends, and only gives him the barest of details. He responds to this by trying to elicit more information from her, as he feels left out and perhaps a little suspicious about this change in her behaviour. She in turn may then perceive him as trying to control her and becomes more reticent, and so on.

Of course, the couple's behaviour does not occur randomly, but rather in response, both to the other's behaviour and to *the meaning that they ascribe to that behaviour*. In order for their behaviour and the meaning that they ascribe to it to make sense, we need to understand the different contexts in which they occur.

MEANING IN CONTEXT

Individuals and families both hold premises, presuppositions and beliefs that constitute their 'maps of the world'. These maps of how life is seen act as the contexts within which we create meaning out of events and relationships.

Our beliefs themselves need to be seen in context. We will have been influenced by our families of origin, the societal and cultural contexts, and other experiences of life (which for nurses may include their professional training and work settings). The beliefs and ideas that we hold are extremely important, because we *act* according to these beliefs. If a mother believes her child is having a tantrum deliberately to spite her, she may act to punish it. If she believes, however, that this is a normal developmental stage for a 2-year-old she may ignore the behaviour or try to distract the child.

While therapists using Milan systemic therapy focus on people's beliefs as an area for change, they are also aware that beliefs are influenced by the societal context. To view any couple, family or individual, without attending to the cultural context, will at the very least lessen the effectiveness of interventions but may also pathologise individuals for problems caused by social inequalities.

To illustrate these concepts further, let us consider again Mr and Mrs Thomas. Their relationship needs to be considered in relation to gender norms, which shape the way in which men and women are expected to behave. Thus, beliefs that they may hold about themselves and each other (e.g. men should be protective, women need looking after) may be commonly held in society. If I now specified that Mr and Mrs Thomas were black, we would also have to consider the societal context of racism and its effect on the couple. Is there a greater need to protect in this context?

It is crucial, therefore, that nurses are able to identify their own beliefs and views and those of their clients as deriving from the different cultural contexts in which they live. Nurses should explore the meaning of difficulties and distress within this framework.

Case 3

An 8-year-old child was referred to a child mental health clinic by his schoolteacher. Assim had some specific learning difficulty around reading, which the teacher had discussed with his parents. The teacher was concerned that this had resulted in the parents putting undue pressure on Assim, expecting him to do 2 hours' homework every night. (This referral raises the issue: for whom is this a problem? Whereas the teacher was concerned, there was no information about the responses of Assim or his parents.)

The therapist decided in the first instance to meet with Assim's parents and schoolteacher. At this meeting the following information was obtained: Assim's parents originated from Pakistan, coming to England in 1970. His father had been made redundant from his engineering job 2 years previously, his mother worked part-time as a secretary. They explained that they were worried that their son would not be able to get a job when he grew up, if he could not overcome his difficulty in reading. They did not want him to suffer the financial hardship that they were currently encountering.

As black people are disadvantaged and discriminated against in the employment market, as in other areas, the meaning of Assim's learning difficulty for his parents could be understood in this context. This understanding helped the teacher to stop seeing them as 'pushy' parents. Instead, it was possible for her to empathise with their worries and arrange for extra tuition within the school setting.

The meaning of the problems and distress that clients show us can only be looked at in context. As nurses, the meaning that we ascribe to clients' problems will also be affected by our own contexts, including our own family background and culture, training, theoretical frameworks and work contexts.

INTERVENING IN SYSTEMS

Therapeutic context

The original 'Milan Team' was made up of four therapists (Palazzoli, Boscolo, Cecchin and Prata) who set up the first centre for family therapy in Italy. They developed a way of working with families where a therapist interviewed the family while team colleagues supervised from behind a one-way screen. This commonly used approach allows the therapist in the room to become involved with the family and the process of interaction, while the team held a different perspective – a double description (Bateson, 1979). The team may call the therapist out of the room or 'phone in' to share their ideas and hypotheses with the therapist, who may then share the ideas with the family or use them to explore further.

Each family therapy session is classically organised into five parts, a pre-session discussion for discussing information about the family and forming hypotheses, the interview with family, the in-session consultation where the therapist joins her colleagues to discuss ideas, the final part of the session where the therapist returns to the family to give them a message or intervention from the team and a post-session discussion between therapist and team.

While this is a typical family therapy structure, many nurses do not have the freedom or equipment to pursue this. Many practitioners have found ways of adapting and using systemic practice in their work-place, and it is hoped that the interventions suggested here have wider applications.

Hypothesising

Whenever we meet with a patient or client we come to the meeting with ideas and assumptions based either on information we have been given or from our previous meetings with other clients. In family therapy it is often helpful to formulate hypotheses about the family to be seen, to explain why it is the way it is now. Hypotheses are often attempts at linking people's beliefs, behaviours and relationships with the problem they have presented with. Hypotheses are not 'the truth', but simply act as a guide for the nurse/therapist in talking with the family. They may also make explicit the prejudices and beliefs that the nurse herself holds.

Circular Questioning

As described earlier, families have a 'map of the world' or world view. Within this, they will hold beliefs about what constitutes a problem for them (which may not be a problem for other families), and what solutions are available to them.

The aim of the therapist (using Milan systemic family therapy) is to introduce new information and connections, between behaviours and beliefs and between behaviours, beliefs and relationships. This allows individuals to alter some of their present beliefs and to consider new solutions.

To achieve this the therapist uses 'circular questions'. The therapist asks a question, then builds on the feedback to ask new questions which challenge beliefs held by the interviewees. Feedback may be verbal or non-verbal or may relate to discrepancies between the two. The interviewer takes a stance of 'curiosity' or naive enquiry, not taking sides with any family member. She aims to help families to become curious about themselves, their own beliefs and how they developed. By becoming 'observers' to themselves, they may achieve a way of perceiving themselves differently. For example:

Therapist (to son): Why do you think your father is so worried about your mother?
Son: Well she gets very depressed.
Therapist: How does she show that she is depressed?
Son: Well, she shouts at us a lot.
Therapist (to father): Who would your wife shout at the most?
Father: Me, mostly!

The above example illustrates several points. The therapist listens to what people say and uses this to formulate different questions, in a way that may introduce differences into their perception of how things are. The therapist is seeking views from various people, who may not share the same perceptions, thus highlighting connections between beliefs (about depression), behaviour (shouting) and possibly relationships (the mother shouts at her husband the most). The therapist is also asking the son to be specific about what he understands his father to mean by 'depressed'. Individuals are often given labels: 'he is spiteful, stubborn, lazy', etc. These descriptions actually give little information and are just one person's view of reality. Families and therapists may unhelpfully 'fall in love with the verb "to be"' (Mason, 1989). Alternative, more helpful questions may be 'how does it show?', or 'what does she do or say that makes you think she is mad?'

Readers may also have noticed that the therapist asks the son to comment about his father and mother. This may appear quite strange, but can actually be engaging, allowing family members to listen to how others perceive them. To ensure that each person speaks for themselves, the therapist will preface their questions with phrases such as 'in your opinion' or 'from your point of view' (Burnham and Harris, 1988).

Circular questions are, in themselves, seen as interventions for change. The skills and techniques involved could be used and developed by nurses in many contexts to good advantage. An interesting example is given by Mason (1991), who has written about the use of systemic principles and circular questioning in nursing 'handovers' (Mason, 1991). This process helps nurses in hospital or residential settings to become 'observers' to themselves in relation to their clients, develops new skills and ideas and enables them to be more effective 'helpers'.

CONCLUSION

This chapter has attempted to give an overview of family therapy within the field of mental health and more specifically to address its relevance to mental health nurses. While some of the major theoretical concepts underpinning family therapy have also been introduced, it has only been possible to focus on one model in more detail. It is hoped that readers will take away some relevant ideas and perhaps some enthusiasm for discovering more about this exciting field.

REFERENCES

Bateson G, Jackson D D, Haley J and Weakland J H (1956) Toward a theory of schizophrenia. *Behavioural Science*, **1**: 251–264.

Bateson G (1979) *Mind and Nature; A necessary unity.* New York: E P Dutton.

Benner P (1984) *From Novice to Expert; Excellence and power in clinical nursing practice.* Menlo Park, CA: Addison Wesley.

Bennun I (1986) Evaluating family therapy: a comparison of the Milan and problem solving approaches. *Journal of Family Therapy*, **8**: 225–242.

Blank M (1987) Hannah's family. *Nursing Times and Nursing Mirror*, **83**: 61–62.

Brooker C (1991) Meeting the needs of families. *Nursing*, **4**(29): 13–16.

Brooker C and Butterworth C (1991) Working with families caring for a relative with schizophrenia: the evolving role of the psychiatric nurse. *International Journal of Nursing Studies*, **28**(2): 189–200.

Brown G and Rutter M (1966) The measurement of family activities and relationships: a methodological study. *Human Relations*, **19**: 241–263.

Burnham J (1986) *Family Therapy.* London: Routledge.

Burnham J and Harris Q (1988) Systemic family therapy: the Milan approach, Chapter 3. In: *Family Therapy in Britain*, eds Street E and Dryden W. Milton Keynes: Open University Press.

Carter B and McGoldrick M (eds) (1989) *The Changing Family Life Cycle.* London: Allyn and Bacon.

Chase J and Holmes J (1990) A two year audit of a family therapy audit in adult psychiatry. *Journal of Family Therapy*, **12**(3): 229–243.

Clements I W and Buchanan D M (eds) (1982) *Family Therapy: A Nursing Perspective*. New York: Wiley.

Cottrell D (1989) Family therapy influences on general adult psychiatry. *British Journal of Psychiatry*, **154**: 473–477.

Dare C, Eisler I, Russell G and Szmuckler G (1990) The clinical and theoretical impact of a controlled trial of family therapy in anorexia nervosa. *Journal of Marital and Family Therapy*, **1**: 39–57.

Dungworth D (1988) Context and the construction of family therapy practice. In: *Family Therapy in Britain*, eds Street E and Dryden W. Milton Keynes: Open University Press.

Elliot H, Stockwell C and Metcalfe M (1991) Family therapy in a rehabilitation hostel. *Nursing Standard*, **5**: 29–31.

Falloon I, Boyd J, McGill C *et al* (1982) Family management in the prevention of exacerbations of schizophrenia. *New England Journal of Medicine*, **306**: 1437–1440.

Leff J P and Vaughn C (1981) The role of maintenance therapy and relatives' expressed emotion in relapse of schizophrenia: A two-year follow-up. *British Journal of Psychiatry*, **139**: 102–104.

Friedemann M (1989) The concept of family nursing. *Journal of Advanced Nursing*, **14**: 211–216.

Friedman E (1986) *Family Nursing: Theory and Assessment*. New York: Appleton Century Crofts.

Friedman E (1989) Systems and Ceremonies: A Family View of Rites of Passage. Chapter 6 in: Carter B and McGoldrick M (1989) *The Changing Family Life Cycle*. Boston: Allyn and Bacon.

Gilleard C, Lieberman S and Peeler R (1992) Family therapy for older adults: a survey of professional attitudes. *Journal of Family Therapy*, **40**: 413–422.

Goldstein M, Rodnick E, Evans J *et al* (1978) Drug and family therapy in the aftercare treatment of acute schizophrenia. *Archives of General Psychiatry*, **42**: 887–896.

Grad J and Sainsbury P (1963) Mental illness and the family. *Lancet* **1**: 544–547.

Gurman A and Kniskern D (1991) *Handbook of Family Therapy Vol II*. New York: Bruner/Mazel.

Hogarty G, Anderson C, Reiss D *et al* (1986) Family psychoeducation, social skills training, and maintenance chemotherapy in the aftercare treatment if schizophrenia. *Archives of General Psychiatry*, **43**: 633–642.

Imber-Black E (1989) Idiosyncratic life cycle transitions and therapeutic rituals. Chapter 7 in: *The Changing Family Life Cycle*, eds Carter B and McGoldrick M. London: Allyn and Bacon.

Jones E (1991) *Working with Adult Survivors of Child Sexual Abuse*. London: Kamac Books.

Jones E (1993) *Family Systems Therapy. Developments in the Milan-Systemic Therapies.* New York: Wiley.

Kiely G and Richardson V (1991) *Family Policy: European Perspectives.* Dublin: Dublin Family Studies Centre.

Killen J (1990) Role stabilization in families after spinal cord injury. *Rehabilitation Nursing,* **15**(1): 19–21.

Krozek C (1991) Helping stressed families on an ICU. *Nursing,* **21**(1): 52–57.

Kuiper L, Leff J and Lam D (1992) *Family Work for Schizophrenia.* London: Gaskell.

Leahey M and Wright L (1987) *Families and Psychosocial Problems.* Springhouse, Pa: Springhouse Corporation.

Leff J P, Kuipers L, Berkowitz R *et al* (1982) A controlled trial of intervention in the families of schizophrenic patients. *British Journal of Psychiatry,* **141**: 121–134.

Leff J P, Berkowitz R, Shavit N *et al* (1989) A trial of family therapy v. a relatives group for schizophrenia. *British Journal of Psychiatry,* **154**: 594–600.

Mason S (1989) Handing over. *Developing Consistency Across Shifts in Residential and Health Settings.* London: Karnac Books.

Minuchin S, Rosman B and Baker L (1978) *Psychosomatic Families: Anorexia Nervosa in Context.* Cambridge: Harvard University Press.

Moltz D (1993) Bipolar disorder and the family: An integrative model. *Family Process,* **32**: 409–425.

Moores A and Dunne G (1988) Unhappy families. *Nursing Times,* **84**: 67–68.

Nichols M (1984) *Family Therapy: Concepts and Methods.* New York: Gardner Press.

Schlump-Urquhart S (1990) Families experiencing a traumatic accident: implications and nursing management. *Clinical Issues in Critical Care Nursing,* **1**(3): 522–534.

Simpson L (1990) The comparative efficacy of Milan family therapy for disturbed children and their families. *Journal of Family Therapy,* **13**: 267–284.

Solursh D (1990) The family of the trauma victim. *Nursing Clinics of North America,* **25**(1): 155–162.

Tarrier N, Barrowclough C, Vaughn C *et al* (1988) The community management of schizophrenia: a controlled trial of behavioural intervention with families to reduce relapse. *British Journal of Psychiatry,* **153**: 532–542.

Tennant D (1993) The place of the family in mental health nursing: past, present and future. *Journal of Advanced Nursing,* **180**: 752–758.

Vaughn C and Leff J (1976) The influence of family and social factors on the course of psychiatric illness. *British Journal of Psychiatry,* **129**: 125–137.

Wright L and Leahey M (1990) Trends in nursing of families. *Journal of Advanced Nursing,* **15**: 148–154.

Perspectives on Therapeutic Community Practice
Bill McGowan

5

APPROACHES TO TREATMENT IN PSYCHIATRY

In psychiatry we use the word 'therapeutic' rather glibly and often without much serious thought or consideration as to what it actually means.

If we administer a prescribed drug for consumption, enter purposefully into a conversation or provide a series of social activities for a client we are making an intervention which we refer to as 'treatment'. The intention is to treat the individual and by so doing help to resolve the difficulties which the individual is experiencing. If the intervention or range of interventions generate effects which are of a beneficial, healing, recuperative or rehabilitative nature then the outcome for the individual is considered to be 'therapeutic'.

It is a widely held belief within the professions in psychiatry that therapeutic outcomes may be effected at three different levels:

1. *Pharmacological*: at a biological level the pharmacological approach is assumed to work through physiological mechanisms within the body.
2. *Psychological*: at the level of the individual, therapeutic effects are assumed to work through psychological mechanisms within the psyche. This may involve affective, cognitive or behavioural components.
3. *Social*: at the level of the social, effects are assumed to work through 'sociotherapeutic' mechanisms or processes operating between 'self and others' as a result of engagement and participation in social interactions.

The therapeutic community as a treatment method tends to focus upon both the psychological and social levels of intervention as the dominant treatment mode and although pharmacology may be used as an adjunct, it is never the mainstay of treatment.

THE CONCEPT OF COMMUNITY

The term 'community' is much used but little understood and poorly conceptualised. Sociologists have and indeed still do spend much time in discussion and debate regarding the concept. Hillery (1955), in a quest for a definitive definition of this elusive concept, unearthed no less than 94 definitions. There appears, however, to be two major themes which are central to the concept of 'community'. The first theme emphasises *community as a collectivity* or social group and implies the presence of cohesion. The second theme emphasises *community as a type of social relationship*, sentiment or attitude.

From a sociological viewpoint, the idea of community as a collectivity refers to:

- A social group sharing a defined physical or geographical space, e.g. a neighbourhood, village, etc.
- A social group sharing common traits which is characterised by a sense of belonging and which is held together by social ties and mutually reciprocal interactions which help to shape it into a distinct social identity, e.g., ethnic, religious, professional community.
- All the daily activities (both work and non-work) take place within particular geographic areas.

Toennies' (1957) concept of *Gemeinschaft* encapsulates the idea of community as both a collectivity and a social relationship. This term implies a spontaneous taken-for-granted relationship. Fellowship ties (*bunds*) are consciously sought and are emotionally laden. He suggests that these latter features are particularly true of religious sects and ideological groups.

Rather than over-concern ourselves with the academic debate, it is sufficient to say that a central feature of social life is that individuals have a strong tendency or valency (Bion, 1955) to come together or affiliate in social groups. This coming together leads to the colonisation of physical space and the conscious organisation of social and interpersonal relations over time. In the claiming of territory and the act of identification with the declared aims and purpose of the group, investment in time and emotional energy occurs and attachments or bonds are formed. These bonds represent the 'social glue' which helps to hold the social group together and maintain group cohesion.

That a community may be viewed as potentially 'therapeutic' suggests that all communities have latent therapeutic properties which in normal everyday life are beneficial to the well-being of the individual member. After all, we grow up and continue to develop our unique personalities as a consequence of our immersion and participation in the day to day life experience of our immediate social group, whether it is our family of origin, family of destination, our peer group, work group or the wider community beyond our immediate social group.

Shenker (1985) compared a number of known therapeutic communities with a number of other organisations, sects and religious communities. He suggests that therapeutic communities are 'intentional communities' which share certain features with organisations, sects and religious groups but yet are different. He describes 'intentional communities' as a small group of individuals who create a new 'way of life' for the attainment of a set of goals. They are 'intentional' in that they are consciously and deliberately designed. They are not left to develop spontaneously in a *laissez-faire* fashion. They are communities in that they attempt to create an entire 'way of life' – unlike organisations. He also points out that they are characterised by face to face communications and embrace communalism as an end in itself.

The term community in the sense of the Therapeutic Community implies a certain informality, closeness or intimacy within relationships, coupled with a strong sense of identity and bonding within the context of a social group. It is these 'low visibility' affective ingredients which are considered important for the provision of a healing matrix, an issue which we shall return to later in the chapter.

THE CONCEPT OF THE THERAPEUTIC COMMUNITY

The term 'therapeutic community' was coined by Tom Main in 1946 following his experiences and those of a number of his contemporaries, Bridger (1946), Jones (1956) and Bion (1961) at the Northfield Military Hospital and Mill Hill during and after the Second World War. The term is synonymous with 'Therapeutic Milieu', 'Milieu Therapy', 'Socio-Therapy', 'Social Therapy' and 'Planned Environmental Therapy'.

In the mental health field it developed as part of the wider movement of social psychiatry. This movement concerned itself with an exploration of the role of psychosocial factors in the genesis, development, maintenance and treatment of mental disorder.

In this context the therapeutic community movement can be seen as a reaction against the anti-therapeutic effects of custodial practices within mainstream psychiatric hospitals and as part of a search for alternatives. The idea of the therapeutic community developed from the premise that if the social environment of the psychiatric hospital could do so much harm to the individual (Barton, 1959; Goffman, 1968), it could also be used to liberate and benefit the individual. The view was held that the deliberate manipulation and modification of the social environment could be used to harness and mobilise the social processes involved to reverse and prevent the damaging effects of stigmatisation and institutionalisation, so prevalent within mainstream psychiatry at the time.

It is important to note, however, that the idea has a longer lineage in the mental health field since it goes back to the 'moral treatment' era, which began with the establishment of The Retreat at York by William Tuke in 1792. The approach also developed separately but in a parallel fashion in other fields, such as education and youth work (Whiteley *et al*, 1972). It emerged in psychiatry at Mill Hill and Northfield because of the general social upheaval which followed the end of the Second World War. This led to a loosening of formal social structures and role specifications, and created a climate within which experimentation could occur, which in turn led to the development and application of psychoanalytic techniques to the social residential group.

The therapeutic community movement was, and still is, characterised by the following.

- Liberal humanitarian values.
- A view which asserts that mental disorder is the product of social/interpersonal forces and is amenable to psychodynamic interpretations and interventions.
- A strong preference for group and communal therapies over physical methods of treatment although they may co-exist side by side (Cain and Smail, 1969).

Whiteley (1987) identifies three stages in the development of the therapeutic community, starting with its origins in the military neurosis camps in the UK and in similar settings in the USA, following similar problems. The second stage was a period of 'incorporation' of the ideology in the 1950s and 1960s. (For a discussion of the reasons which led to the widespread dissemination and influence of the ideas see Cain and Smail, 1969 and Whiteley and Collis, 1987.) This latter stage was a period of implementation and testing-out of ideas which also led to an awareness of the limitations and obstacles to therapeutic community work. The third stage from the mid 1960s onwards has led to further analysis and refinement of therapeutic community practice and to a clarification of the concept.

The term 'therapeutic community' is probably one of the most misused and misunderstood concepts in modern psychiatry. It suffers because of a lack of clarity in its definition and because of its global appeal and broad application to all sorts of treatment/education/rehabilitation settings. In an attempt to clarify and tighten the definition, Clark (1965) drew a distinction between the 'therapeutic community approach' and the 'therapeutic community proper'. Clark suggested that therapeutic community ideas applied to a large psychiatric hospital helped to 'liberalise' such regimes and could be seen as the 'therapeutic community approach'. The 'therapeutic community proper' occurred as the result of a small self-contained unit, ward or hospital being intentionally designed so as to make the social environment the main therapeutic tool. A similar distinction has been made by Crockett (1966) between the general therapeutic community, in which individual treatments (including physical treatments) were supported by group and community methods, and the 'psychotherapeutic' community in which community and group methods were the main treatment methods. Manning (1975) sought empirical support for this distinction between the two types and his results confirmed the existence of both the 'therapeutic community approach' and the 'therapeutic community proper' operating as distinct forms within the UK. Indeed, he went further and identified the characteristics which served to distinguish the two types (see Table 5.1).

Table 5.1 Types of therapeutic community

Therapeutic community approach	Therapeutic community proper
Acute admissions service	No acute admissions service
Catchment area from which most patients are drawn	No catchment area
Do not specialise in certain disorders/ problems	Do specialise – favour neurotics/ personality disorders over psychotics
Majority of patients are non-residential	Majority of patients are residential
Patients generally older (40 years+)	Patients generally younger (most in their 20s)
Most referrals from GPs	Most referrals from psychiatrists, special units, social services, etc.
Most referrers have no alternative place to refer	Most referrers could have referred elsewhere
Number of referrals per year is higher (400–600+)	Number of referrals is lower (200–300)
Do not encourage or discourage referrals	Do tend to encourage (and sometimes discourage) referrals

Source: Manning (1989).

Having considered the origins and historical development of the concept and its definition, we must now consider some of the features which characterise the therapeutic community.

Features of the Therapeutic Community

Any organisation or social group which intentionally sets itself up as a therapeutic community has certain features which are common to all institutions.

- It is a social system within a wider super-system.
- It has an explicit function or purpose; to educate, treat, rehabilitate, etc.
- It erects a social structure designed to enable it to channel energy and provide direction, thus enabling it to achieve its goal.
- The structure which is erected is determined by, among other factors, a philosophy or a set of values, beliefs and ideals which underpin and inform the way in which things are done. In short – it has a culture.

In his review of therapeutic community practice, Wilson (1979) developed a conceptual framework which modelled aspects of the therapeutic community along an organisational dimension. This model highlights four perspectives which, he believes, help illuminate key features of the therapeutic community. These perspectives may be used to view the therapeutic community alternately as either a social system, or an organisational function, structure or culture.

A SYSTEMS PERSPECTIVE

Systems theory is a global theory of how systems in general operate and has been applied to both the physical and social sciences. It deals with the universal features of systems, the relationships between systems and the structures within systems. By so doing it helps to illuminate features of systems functioning.

A system may be defined as a whole with interrelated parts in which the parts have a function and the system as a whole has a function. This is expressed in the *Gestalt* principle, 'the function of the whole is more than the sum of the parts'. Systems operate in relation to, and within the context of, an environment through the processes of input, throughput, output and feedback. The environment surrounding a system may be defined as those elements external to the boundary of the system. A system therefore is delineated by its boundary with the environment (see Figure 5.1).

A boundary may be defined as a line forming a circle around the system and where there is a greater exchange of energy within the circle (system) than on the outside (environment). This boundary gives shape or form and provides an invisible but identifiable structure. In a sense, it contains the system and determines or defines where the system begins and ends. It differentiates between system identity (that which is within the boundary) and non-system (that which is outside in the environment).

A second function of the boundary is to regulate the relationship between the system and its environment. It is helpful to visualise the boundary as a filter or as a flexible structure which permits or restricts

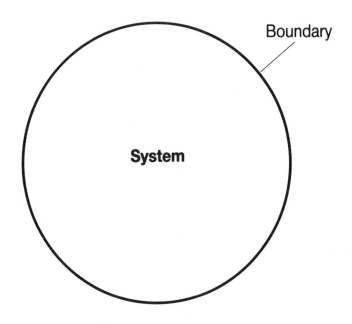

Figure 5.1 External environment (supra-system).

the exchange of elements, information or energy between the system and its environment. The filter may alter its character according to its degree of 'porosity' possibly in response to feedback from the outer environment or the inner state of the system. Three types of alteration are possible. The boundary may become permeable, semi-permeable or impermeable. A permeable filter will allow for a wide range of materials to cross between the system and environment. A semi-permeable filter is 'selective' and will allow a restricted range of materials to pass between the two. An impermeable filter will create a barrier to the passage of elements between the two. The function of this selective filter can be seen in terms of system maintenance. The boundaries which regulate the relationship between system and environment are dynamic: they are in a constant state of flux and tend towards change over time in accordance with the needs of the system.

It is possible to characterise systems on the basis of their degree of inter-action with the surrounding environment. Systems may be categorised as 'open' or 'closed' depending on the degree of porosity of the boundary maintaining mechanisms, with the more open systems resulting in greater contact with the surrounding environment. All living systems are open systems but it is nevertheless helpful to visualise social systems along a system continuum with open systems and closed systems at either end. There is, of course, no possibility of a completely closed system remaining viable, since in biological terms this leads to death and in social systems terms represents a level of functioning which is repressive, restrictive and possibly inefficient. The closest approximation to a closed system in this sense would be a prison, or some other form of 'total' institution. Equally, a fully open system is not possible since this also represents system dysfunction and could lead to system exhaustion and collapse. It is helpful, nevertheless, to plot systems in terms of their degree of boundary flexibility or rigidity along an open/closed continuum, the balance between rigidity and flexibility being determined by the boundaries which give the system shape and which play a crucial role in determining its level of functioning.

Systems operate within systems. A system which operates within a larger system is called a sub-system and the larger system or environment within which the sub-system is located is called the supra-system. Systems therefore are arranged and organised within a hierarchical structure.

A therapeutic community may be conceived of as a system which is a sub-system within a wider social system, e.g. a large psychiatric hospital or a social services department which are in turn sub-systems within a wide range of socioeconomic-polical supra-systems.

Using Millard and Kirk's (1979) concept of levels of resolution, the hierarchy of systems within a therapeutic community may be illuminated and clarified as follows (see Figure 5.2).

1. *Level 1* The community as a total entity.
2. *Level 2* Community parts, e.g. large group meetings, small group meetings, work groups, etc.
3. *Level 3* Interactions between individual participants within groups and during community activities.
4. *Level 4* Individual behaviour – cognitive, affective, perceptual, communicative and other psychic processes.
5. *Level 5* Part function of individuals in terms of intra-psychic pathology, e.g. splitting, denial, projection, sublimation, dissociation, etc.

A system therefore occupies geographic space within the supra-system in which it is embedded and has a physical boundary and, in the case of the therapeutic community, an ideological boundary with which it may be identified. It also has internal structures, the function of which is to ensure the effective transformation of materials from the outside environment into materials which are useful for the survival of the system and of the supra-system upon which the system is dependent.

Within a therapeutic community itself there is a structuring of time and social space. Time may be structured according to the work to be done; or,

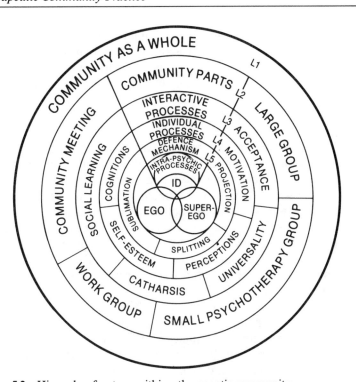

Figure 5.2 Hierarchy of systems within a therapeutic community.

as Kennedy (1987) puts it, 'the work of the day', into numerous personal, group, social, domestic and recreational activities. Social space will be differentiated in that geographic areas may be boundaried or set aside and sanctioned as the area for certain activities, e.g. groupwork, art therapy, music therapy; specific functions, e.g. games room, utility room, time out room; or identified with certain individuals or groups of individuals, e.g. doctor's office, nursing office, community dormitories, etc.

As part of the process of system transformation time boundaries are operative in that patients are admitted, affiliated and become assimilated within the community; they engage in work, prepare for disengagement, disengage and leave. In systems terms this is input, throughput and output.

There are other examples of internal structuring. Certain criteria will be applied to determine who may or may not enter the community boundary. Once accepted into the community and throughout the 'transformation process' criteria will be continually applied to determine the individual's continued access to different parts or aspects of community life, e.g. work groups, roles within community, community meetings, etc. In a sense a continuous internal filtering process is in operation.

Thus we can conclude that a therapeutic community, like all social systems, has an identity, a goal or a function, internal structures which facilitate and contain the internal processes, all of which operate in the interest of goal achievement and ultimately to system survival.

A FUNCTIONAL PERSPECTIVE

As we have already noted, a community is a group of people who share particular expectations of each other in order to achieve a particular goal. This goal will determine the *modus operandi* of the group. The group therefore will have a purpose, much of which may be clear (conscious), but some of which may not be so clear (unconscious).

A community aspires to be 'therapeutic' if it intentionally defines its goal to be so and with this in mind erects a social structure, the purpose of which is to provide a social environment which will achieve, as far as is possible, therapeutic outcomes on behalf of its members.

A range of variations on this theme is possible in that a number of goals or combination of goals may be possible. A therapeutic community may aspire to provide an environment, the function of which is to provide a sociotherapeutic experience (Whiteley and Gordon, 1979), psychotherapeutic experience (Crockett, 1966), rehabilitative experience (Hull and Pullen, 1988), or an educational experience (Rose, 1986; Neil, 1968). It is possible therefore to have a variety of therapeutic community environments distinguished by their functional goals and structured accordingly (Wilson, 1979).

Traur (1984), in his review of the status of the therapeutic community, supports the above proposition. He argues that the most successful and convincing applications of therapeutic community practice have occurred with patient groups homogeneous for primary disorder. In support of this position he points out that Maxwell Jones's original work was with individuals suffering from 'effort syndrome'; the Henderson unit went on to specialise with personality-disordered individuals (Whiteley *et al*, 1972); the unit studied by Caine and Smail (1969) accepted only patients with neurotic problems and the Cassell treats families and adolescents (Kennedy, 1986).

Edelson (1964) suggests a number of reasons why this might be so. First, he argues that there are destructive aspects of the interaction between individuals with different kinds of disorder, which would get in the way of productive therapeutic work. Secondly, he suggests that the creation of a social environment which is helpful to patients with different degrees of ego-impairment is problematic. What might be helpful to one may be contraindicated for another. Methodological problems aside, there is a small number of empirical research studies which help to illuminate this issue and, to a large extent, support Edelson's view (Myers and Clark, 1972; Letemendia *et al*, 1967; Miles, 1972; Cain and Smail, 1969). Finally, he suggests that there are difficulties in recruiting staff who are equally skilful in working with all types of patients. In short, the 'design of atmosphere' (Rose, 1986) has to be matched with the type of patient target group which ideally should be homogeneous for primary disorder. Units which admit patients with widely varying disorders may not be able to provide a sufficiently well-tuned environment and may be less than therapeutically effective as a result (Kennard, 1979). For a comprehensive review of these issues see Karterud (1989). In particular he suggests that a cluster of milieu characteristics may be emerging which could be expected to constitute a more optimal therapeutic environment for individuals diagnosed as suffering from schizophrenia. He cites such features as a high level of order and organisation, practical orientation with support and a low level of anger and aggression and highlights the conditions under which such a milieu could be maintained and developed.

Traur (1984) also points out that district general hospital psychiatric units are unsuited to functioning as a therapeutically effective 'milieu' within which growth and personal change might be effected. He argues that this is so because district general hospital units have a catchment area-wide responsibility (see Table 5.1), and must therefore admit patients who are heterogeneous for primary disorder. This unsuitability is compounded by the trend in acute units to shorter in-patient stays. This precludes the patients from staying long enough to enable them to make an investment in the community (White, 1972), since a certain minimum length of time is necessary to enable the psychological and social changes necessary for personal growth to take place (Kennard, 1979).

Ideally, therefore, an optimum social structure should be erected which would facilitate maximally a given function for a particular group of individuals in pursuit of a common goal over a specified period of time.

A STRUCTURAL PERSPECTIVE

Weber (1947), in his concept of the 'rational bureaucratic organisation', argued that organisations required a clear hierarchy of offices (roles and responsibilities), clear functional specifications of each office (job description), impersonal duties (administrative responsibilities) and a system of control and discipline based on an agreed set of rules (procedures). This rationalisation (standardisation) serves an important function in that it enables the application of general rules to particular cases. It saves effort and reduces confusion by eliminating the need to develop a new solution for every problem. It creates safe, predictable structures which encourage, or indeed demand, rule-bound behaviour from the individuals operating within its structure.

Bureaucracy, however, as a mode of organisation, has certain limitations when it comes to the unique treatment of individual cases according to individual needs. A careful look at the historical development of the 'asylum movement' in mental health illustrates only too well how the increased bureaucratisation of the asylums led to the creation of a 'warehousing' culture. This culture was custodial, repressive, stigmatising and institutional, the effects of which have been well documented (Barton, 1959; Goffman, 1968; Caudill, 1958; Stanton and Schwartz, 1954). As we have already seen, the therapeutic community model was developed as the result of a search for an alternative social structure to replace the bureaucratic model which tended to standardise and alienate the individual, see Table 5.2. Therefore it follows that if the bureaucratic model when applied to care settings tends to produce the total institution, an alternative model might then produce the minimal institution or mobilise the community or relational aspects of the organisation to produce the therapeutic community. This is not to suggest that 'anarchy' should rule, but that structure should be seen as a means to an end and not an end in itself.

Table 5.2 Differences between the characteristics of a bureaucratic model and a therapeutic model

Bureaucracy	Therapeutic Community
1. Clear hierarchy of offices	Blurring of hierarchical roles
2. Impersonal duties and professional distance	Reduction of social distance and increase in personal involvement
3. Written documentation specifying roles and individual behaviour	Situations dealt with on an *ad hoc* basis
4. Rule-bound behaviour	Spontaneous behaviour
5. Standardisation of individual response	Variability of individual response
6. Communication guarded	Open communication

Weber's view of formal bureaucracy is an 'ideal type' and does not occur in practice as a fixed entity, but rather represents an approximation of what might or could occur. Organisations are living, dynamic entities and the rigidity or flexibility of their structures will shift one way or another over time.

In the therapeutic community the goal or aim is to provide a social environment which will facilitate therapeutic, educational and rehabilitative experiences for the individual. This requires a clear structure for the creation of living/learning experiences (Jones, 1952; Clark, 1965), but one which is sufficiently loose to create 'space' for reflection and which will facilitate the exploration and analysis of social and interpersonal relations between individuals. This relatively permissive approach to the examination of behaviour is the lynchpin of the therapeutic community, the life and work of which is organised or structured around a series of social events or group meetings. Some of these (small groups, large groups) are unstructured to allow for the exploration and analysis of spontaneous (emotionally structured) interpersonal relationships between the participants, while others are structured. The structured events tend to take the form of business/community meetings or work groups and tend to have a practical orientation, in that in any community or organisation there are important practical tasks to be done to ensure the maintenance and survival of the community or organisation, e.g. washing-up, tidying-up, cooking rotas to be negotiated, menus to be agreed, the food budgeted, bought, prepared, cooked and served, etc.

A balance has to be struck between the need to allow the community to reflect on internal events in an atmosphere of relative psychological safety and the need for the community to service itself and maintain a realistic perspective in relation to the outside world.

In any organisation, beneath the formal structure there are naturally, spontaneously occurring patterns of relationships. These are emotionally structured, tend to be hidden and represent the 'latent' aspect of organisational life (Chinoy, 1967). This is an aspect which is informal and exists alongside the legitimate formal structure. It does not form part of the organisation's conscious view of itself. It is ignored, denied, repressed and relegated to the organisational unconscious. It nevertheless has an important part to play in influencing the overall level of organisational function.

The formal structure, on the other hand, represents the manifest aspect of organisational life, it is legitimate and is consciously erected in order to achieve the goals of the organisation. Overall, the latent aspect could be said to serve an expressive function and the manifest aspect, an instrumental function, and it is important for the stability and cohesion of the organisation that there is a balance between the two.

However, organisations over time are not static. Tensions develop and dynamic shifts occur in the balance between the latent and manifest aspects which often lead to movement along both ends of a positive/negative continuum. At the positive end this leads to enfunction (Levy, 1952) whereby stability, cohesion and efficiency are enhanced and conversely at the negative end to dysfunction (Levy, 1952), leading to instability, goal displacement and reduced efficiency.

The therapeutic community structure is deliberately loose so as to facilitate the disclosure, exploration and analysis of latent material. This occurs at an individual, interpersonal and organisational level, which renders it vulnerable to wide variations in organisational drift along both ends of a positive/negative continuum. Roberts (1980) puts it succinctly when he suggests that:

destructive processes occur in all human groups and the therapeutic community is a group situation which acts as a magnifying glass through which much that is normally concealed or seems irrelevant can be seen with a new and frightening clarity.

Other writers have also drawn attention to similar phenomenon. Main (1977), during wartime experience, observed that two units in the army, despite having a similar social structure, had quite different levels of morale and experience of psychological disturbances. He concluded that despite the similarity in structure, each unit had its own 'system' for operating the structure, the crucial point being that something 'hidden' entered the structure – what he called the 'human folkways by which the structure is operated'.

Hinselwood (1987) also proposes that organisations can be infiltrated by 'psychologically determined disruptions'. Because of the unconscious nature of these disruptions, they evade correction by conscious means. He talks in terms of the 'neurotic organisation' where the 'grit' which gets in between the cogwheels is the pain and defensiveness of individuals within the system. There is now substantial literature on a wide range of aspects pertaining to organisational and therapeutic community dysfuntion (Menzies-Leith, 1988; Bion, 1955; Rapaport, 1960; De Board, 1978; Hinselwood, 1987; Hobson, 1979; Savalle and Wagenborg, 1980; Baron, 1987; Jacques, 1953).

The history of psychiatry is littered with examples of public scandals and enquiries (Beardshaw, 1981), many of which might easily have been avoided or prevented if the teams and authorities concerned had paid more attention to the dynamic tensions between the latent (unconscious) and manifest (conscious) aspects of their work-place.

Therapeutic community practitioners are respectful of the latent aspects of organisational life and conscious of the need to manage the cyclic tensions between these two powerful forces. They are constantly on the alert in seeking to secure the most effective combination at any one point in time to achieve a dynamic equilibrium which ideally provides the optimum therapeutic effect for the maximum number of individuals (Wilson, 1979).

Ideally, then, the therapeutic community should be sufficiently self-regulating over time to provide a 'good enough' social environment (Winnicot, 1965), to enable the growth-generating features of community life to be optimised within the structural overlay of the organisation.

A CULTURAL PERSPECTIVE

All societies and social groups reflect a 'way of life' or a culture which defines the appropriate or required modes of thinking, acting and feeling. A culture prescribes a way of 'doing things' and through the socialisation processes we are socialised into an acceptance of our cultural inheritance from birth through childhood and throughout adulthood. Individuals become socialised in order to 'fit' into society; culture therefore performs an integrative function for the social system, it influences and shapes the individual through the mechanism of social learning (Bandura and Walters, 1963), and by so doing it maintains social cohesion and ensures system survival.

Chinoy (1967) suggests that culture may be analysed and broken down into a number of component parts.

● *Institutions*: these are norms or rules which govern behaviour.
● *Ideas*: these are non-material or abstract products like varieties of knowledge and belief, e.g. religious, theological, moral, scientific, technical, philosophical, historical, etc., which influence and underpin the institutions.
● *Material products*: these are artefacts which all human groups produce and use in the course of their lives, e.g. houses, utensils, tools, etc.

Culture therefore has both an 'expressive' function, in that it enables us 'to be', and an instrumental function, in that it ensures that 'things get done'.

In organisations, culture gives rise to shared beliefs and assumptions. These provide meaning for individual tasks and the goals which organisations aspire to pursue. It also reflects the fundamental values and philosophy which define the organisation's perception of itself and its mission. It provides an expressive and highly symbolic framework by which members of the organisation can interpret the situations they encounter and defines the boundaries of appropriate behavioural responses. Through the formal and informal networks individuals learn the values, attitudes, expected behaviours and knowledge which enable them to become culture carriers and to participate appropriately and effectively in organisational life (Hughes, 1990; Dill, 1981; Tierney, 1988; Louis, 1980). As with social structure, organisational culture is both implicit (unconscious) and explicit (conscious). The shared values and beliefs are 'taken for granted' and are not always consciously verbalised.

The therapeutic community requires a social structure which is sufficient to 'contain' anxiety (Menzies-Leith, 1988; Bion, 1955) and provide stability and direction, but sufficiently loose to enable a culture of acceptance, exploration and analysis of everyday social events (Clark, 1965) to take root and develop. Against this sympathetic background an understanding of the individual's normal pattern of relating or behaving is sought. These are not judged as either good or bad but as either useful or less than useful in terms of the acceptability or otherwise of the individual's relationships with significant others, in particular, and the community or society, in general.

The first major research study of a leading therapeutic commuity was undertaken in the mid 1950s and published in 1960 (Rapaport, 1960). Rapaport identified six core features or beliefs underlying therapeutic community practice which include the following:

- The total social organisation in which the patient is involved is perceived as affecting the therapeutic outcome.
- The social organisation is regarded as a vital force for creating a 'milieu' which will maximise therapeutic effort.
- There is provision of opportunities for patients to take an active part in the affairs of the organisation.
- All relationships within the organisation are potentially therapeutic.
- The quality of the social climate is of utmost importance.
- Communication *per se* is central to the therapeutic process.

Rapaport also identified four cultural themes which constituted an ideology. This ideology or value system underlay and informed the practice of the unit studied. They are outlined as follows.

- *Permissiveness*: this relates to the belief that all members of the community should tolerate in one another a wide range of behaviour which would otherwise be considered deviant or destructive if measured against the standards or norms in society.
- *Democratisation*: this relates to the view that individuals have the right to participate in sharing power and in decision making about community affairs.
- *Communalism*: this refers to the belief that the therapeutic community's functioning should be characterised by tight-knit, intercommunicative and intimate sets of relationships, e.g. sharing amenities, use of first names, etc.
- *Reality confrontation*: this refers to the view that patients should be continually presented with interpretations of their behaviour as it is perceived by other community members.

Note that the first three themes relate to a 'loosening' of boundaries, whereas the last theme relates to 'firming' up or strengthening of boundaries. For a critique of Rapaport's study see Manning (1989) and Sharp (1975).

We can conclude that social structures in and of themselves have no curative power; rather, they represent the framework within which a healing matrix might develop (Tosquelles, 1964). This healing matrix derives its power from the highly symbolic and expressive framework of the community culture.

THE MANAGEMENT OF THERAPEUTIC COMMUNITY PROCESSES

I would now like to deal with some of the challenges of managing therapeutic community processes in practice and to do this it will be helpful if we focus our discussion at the level of:

1. The social system as a whole.
2. The staff community.
3. The patient community.

The Social System

Social systems have to be managed in relation to the supra-systems upon which they are dependent. Therapeutic communities obtain their patients from referral agents or agencies in the wider professional field and must therefore provide a good enough service to remain viable and credible. To remain viable the public relations exchanges between a therapeutic community and the agencies of the supra-system, e.g. GPs, social workers, voluntary agencies, etc., have to be developed, maintained and managed astutely and sensitively, often in the face of difficulty.

A relatively 'open system' within a relatively 'closed' supra-system may well be perceived as a threat. Hostility may be directed towards the community and antagonism felt towards its particular ethos. This may raise a number of problems for the leaders of the community. On one hand, the community must encourage an exchange of elements, e.g. information, influence, staff, patients, etc., from the wider professonal network. On the other hand, it must protect and insulate itself from potential and actual hostility, and the possibility of being overwhelmed by the influence of the environment external to its boundaries.

The community leaders may have to 'straddle' this boundary and mediate between the needs and demands of the two systems. Within the community the leaders may be expected to take a low profile, facilitate open communication, share and delegate responsibilities and decison-making functions and operate in a democratic leadership mode. Outside the community and in relation to the supra-system the community leaders are expected to liaise with external agencies in order to compete for resources, develop mutually reciprocal alliances, make decisions unilaterally, take a high profile, be authoritative and appear authoritarian if necessary to defend, support and protect the interests of the community.

The leadership task is to ensure that the boundaries of the community are sufficiently semi-permeable and receptive to outside influences, but sufficiently firm to contain and insulate the community from being overwhelmed and collapsing in on itself as a result of excessive influence from the wider environment. A shift to the extreme in either direction may cause problems. Roberts (1980) has identified a number of variations on this theme. Blurring of boundaries may lead to loss of identity and direction (autolysis), and boundary rigidity may prevent exchange between the two systems and lead to insularity and institutionalisation (encapsulation).

The community itself may require good leadership in order to effectively manage some of its own negative energy. This may be thrown up or let loose by the permissive orientation facilitated by its social structure and may occur particularly if the community is under threat and where there may be some degree of uncertainty regarding the future of the community or its place within the supra-system. Under these conditions disruption of the social structure (container) may occur because the problems to be contained exceed the capacity of the social structure's ability to cope (Bion, 1977). This phenomenon has been known to occur in waves of cycles over a long period of time and has been identified by a number of systems observers. Rapaport (1956) referred to these cyclic system variations as 'oscillations'.

Threats to the system may be real or imagined but nevertheless, under these conditions, in order to preserve its integrity, level of morale and cohesion the community may well resort to the collective use of primitive defence mechanisms. 'Splitting' may occur which will result in unwanted 'bad bits' of the collective community psyche being denied and projected onto external agencies within the supra-system. This may function (temporarily at least) to preserve the illusory perception that all is well and harmonious within, while everything on the outside is nasty and bad (Roberts, 1980; Hinselwood, 1987). Alongside this, idealisation of the community by its members may lead to smugness and complacency, a state of lowered self-criticism and massive levels of denial, all of which function to maintain some sense of illusory equilibrium and system stability.

The leadership task therefore is to mediate between the often conflicting needs and demands of the two systems; to ensure the effective regulation of the internal structures and processes and to manage such tension and conflict as may arise between the community and the wider social environment.

The Staff Community

Within the community, staff members may have to mediate between patients as some of the tensions which occur between patients may be left unresolved. These may be left for staff to contain and defuse. Staff therefore need to be mindful of the boundaries which govern such interventions.

It is widely accepted that a prerequisite for admission to any therapeutic community is an acceptance by patients that they have a responsibility towards each other and will be expected to assist with the examination, analysis and interpretation of behaviour. As a result of their stay within the community, many patients become very skilled and play a productive part in facilitating growth and change. One of the problems for staff may well arise from knowing how and when to step in and use their authority and skill without undermining the authority and role of the effective patient therapist (or community). This is a particularly important boundary issue, since it involves the 'contracting out' of professional responsibility and authority. In other words, the staff's responsibility and authority are handed over to the community or to representatives of it (Main, 1946). This arrangement needs to be handled with care and integrity so that it does not become an opportunity for 'hiving off' important but less socially valued and less rewarding responsibilities upon the community.

The issue of staff/patient boundary maintenance is a complex and potentially problematic area. Therapeutic communities tend to perpetuate the 'we are all the same' myth. The sharing of roles, blurring of boundaries and absence of clear rules may lead to staff over-identification with patients and may result in staff 'taking on board too much of the other' across the professional boundary. Naïve, idealistic, enthusiastic but inexperienced staff may be, for reasons of their own, only too ready to relinquish important parental, containing or limit-setting aspects of their role and fail to discharge their responsibilities adequately. The reverse may also be true. Out of anxiety or personal insecurity, over-reaction of an authoritarian nature may inhibit and suppress potentially therapeutic interactions from taking place, thus leading to a build-up of anger, resentment and tension. Lack of experience and poor supervision arrangements may cause inappropriate timing of otherwise appropriate responses, thereby rendering them less than effective.

In a permissive setting there is always the possibility that patients with stronger ego-strength, forceful personalities and high social status may attempt to dominate less forceful individuals. The challenge for staff in this context is to know when and how to assert their authority and expertise in order to set limits on behalf of the individual or community without undermining the authority invested in either. This is particularly important since the arena where staff–patient boundary issues are most readily exposed to public scrutiny is in the large community group. Great skill and experience are required to handle these potentially difficult situations and balance the interventions so that the community retains its authority and credibility.

The Patient Community

For the individual patient exposure to permissive unstructured situations may cause regression. Under these circumstances fantasies and primitive anxieties may be released. This may lead to individuals recreating situations and experiences in the 'here and now' which belong in their past. Such responses from the past may well have been invested with personal security in the 'there and then' but over time, and carried over into new social contexts may prove to be socially maladaptive. This public exposure and subsequent obligation to reconsider and examine the personal effectiveness of such behaviour in the light of feedback and confrontation from others, may, in the case of individuals with weak ego-defences, lead to confusion, trauma and a sense of personal devastation. A great deal of support must be mobilised in order to assist the individual to re-orientate, work towards and internalise a more appropriate self-image.

The act of self-disclosure itself, to share hitherto private personal confidences to a group of strangers, represents a crossing of personal boundaries. Some patients may be reluctant to do so and may need to be encouraged and supported. Others might be only too ready to 'strip' inappropriately and 'declare all' before the community is ready to receive it and may need to be protected and supported by the judicious use of limit-setting interventions by either the staff or fellow patients. Similarly, some patients may be overly impulsive and too readily 'act out' their impulsive fantasies within the community in response to the minimum provocation. These individuals may have to be encouraged to develop firmer boundaries, and improve impulse control by holding in (containing) their urges. This may be achieved as a result of feedback and confrontation designed to contract and 'firm up' or strengthen personal boundaries.

Exposure to a permissive, loosely structured communal environment, where living arrangements provide an important opportunity for social learning (Bandura, 1963; Jones, 1982), may highlight the difficulties of daily living among individuals, some of whom may have weak or extended domestic/organisational boundaries and who present with a sloppy, untidy, chaotic life-style, while others may be neat, tidy, immaculate and punctual. Within this closely knit social, physical and interactional space, tensions will invariably arise and require exploration, analysis and appropriate intervention.

There is a tendency for individual patients within the therapeutic community to 'pair off' with 'another'. Where the 'other' is a staff member, care must be taken. Rapaport (1960), in his study, observed that those patients who improved substantially often tended to identify with high status staff. This finding clashed with the belief (shared by many staff at that time) that identification and transference should be directed towards and invested in the community. One-to-one relationships were discouraged on the grounds that they divert energy and detract from the therapeutic group-work programme. Such 'pairing' may lead to a situation whereby the 'special' relationship may cause a 'split' within the staff group (Main, 1957; Roberts, 1980; Hinselwood, 1987). In this case patients may project positive aspects of their 'self' onto certain staff and negative aspects of their 'self' onto others. Those staff who experience the positive projections may collude, idealise and place an inappropriate investment on the patient doing well (halo effect), while denying the patient's negative aspects. The resulting split among staff may lead to failure of communications and hostility (often veiled) within the staff group. This invariably leads to a rise in tension, resulting in 'acting-out' and behavioural disturbance within the patient community (Stanton and Schwartz, 1954).

In summary, not only does the therapeutic community need to manage and regulate its boundary relations with the external environment, it also needs to pay attention to the management of its internal boundaries and the structuring of interactions between the two main sub-systems within – the staff and patient community.

THEORETICAL PERSPECTIVES ON THE THERAPEUTIC COMMUNITY

Therapeutic community practice appears to be influenced by two separate but mutually compatible approaches, the psychological and the social.

The Psychological Approach

This approach is directed towards the individual and may be defined as: 'All measures by legitimate personnel which have as their principal aim, the alteration of personality towards better intra-psychic integration' (Rapaport, 1960). The dominant psychological model which prevails within therapeutic community practice is the psychoanalytic model, whereby psychodynamic principles commonly applied to the individual are applied to the social group and to the community as a whole. There are numerous, useful examples of this approach in the literature (Main, 1977; Crockett, 1966; Hinselwood, 1979, 1987).

The 'permissive orientation' in therapeutic community practice is the lynchpin upon which this model rests. The term 'permissiveness' has been a familiar part of the contemporary social scene since the 1960s and is now an accepted part of our everyday language. In this broad context it is taken to imply a relaxed attitude to sex, social deviance, violence or drug abuse and often conjures up hedonistic fantasies of narcissistic, indulgent pleasure-seekers laying aside all social and moral restraints in pursuit of pleasure and gratification. This reflects an exaggerated view – a popular stereotype!

Permissiveness within the context of the therapeutic community has a more precise meaning. It refers, as we have already seen, to the ideology or belief that the community should function with its members tolerating from one another a wide range of behaviour which may well prove to be distressing, anxiety-provoking, embarrassing or deviant according to the ordinary norms of behaviour as stipulated in society, outside of the confines of the community context.

Ideally, the orientation or ethos should allow the individuals to relax their guard and to expose freely their normative patterns of relating so that they may be observed, experienced, examined, discussed and so that community members may react openly and spontaneously to these patterns. In this way community members may place before the individual the consequences of his/her actions (confrontation).

Permissiveness not only lightens negative sanctions upon behaviour in order to further understanding; it also ensures a lessening of bureaucratic impositions (democratisation). Alongside this, the tensions and difficulties generated as a consequence of living together in a tight, close-knit community (communalism), under permissive conditions produces highly emotionally charged material for exploration and examination. This is not to say that anything goes! Permissiveness is intended to expose the individual to a fairly unstructured situation which is designed to provide 'space' to enable the individual to 'act out' their difficulties; to transfer carry-over behaviour from the past to the 'here and now'; to re-examine fantasies of what may have happened in the past, or indeed feelings about what did not happen. In this way previously repressed, traumatic experiences can be relived, re-examined and new ways of relating developed with the support of the community.

The therapeutic rationale for this stance is drawn from the belief widely held in psychoanalytic circles in the value of the 'permissive orientation' otherwise known as the 'opaque stance'. Within the context of an empathetic, non-directive relationship, the analyst gives permission for the analysand to 'free associate'. The analyst represents a blank screen onto which the analysand spontaneously projects emotionally charged thoughts, feelings and fantasies. By doing so the analysand externalises personally significant features of his/her internal world. This transference relationship provides the analyst with the material for analysis. The analyst attends to both the manifest (conscious) and latent (unconscious) content of the transference experience; gathers it in; 'unpacks' it in terms of its meaning and significance and hands it back to the analysand in the form of an interpretation.

Often the mere ventilation or catharsis of emotionally charged affects may, of itself, bring immediate benefit. Over time this approach is believed to lead to increased self-understanding, ego-restructuring, ego-integration and overall improvement in self-image and general well-being. This approach has as its aim the exploration of the analysand's feelings and the reconstruction of his/her internal world through the use of interpretation. This is assumed to lead to the facilitation of corrective emotional experiences; the development of cognitive insights; cognitive restructuring and ultimately to perceptual and behavioural change (Alexander and French, 1946).

In summary, the community functions as the analyst, develops a 'therapeutic alliance' with the community member (analysand) within an empathetic community relationship. The permissive stance facilitates the open disclosure of affects, thoughts and behaviours to be commented upon by the community (analyst) for the benefit of the individual community member (analysand).

The Social Approach

This approach emphasises the social situation of the individual and the need to explore the individual's patterning of social relationships in the 'here and now'. It seeks to bring about change and foster personal growth within the individual as a result of the mobilisation of social factors. It is often associated with rehabilitation and may be defined as: 'those measures which have as their aim, the fitting of the personality to the demands of the on-going social system' (Rapaport, 1960). This involves the facilitation of social role adaptation and an improvement in the individual's overall level of social functioning, by which we mean their ability to adopt a variety of appropriate role sets (worker, parent, wife, etc.), and discharge the responsibilities commensurate with adult roles (parenting, companionship, civil obligations, etc.).

Whiteley and Gordon (1979) argue that the way an individual behaves in a social situation will be seen as a lead into understanding why he/she reacts in such a way; that the social process leads to psychological awareness and personality change is effected through social interaction. As a result of his experience at the Henderson Unit, he identifies three principles underlying a sociodynamic approach.

1. *Social interaction is promoted* and all matters of community life are fed back through community meetings. The community members living closely together are mutually dependent on each other for emotional, social and material support and co-operation. Interaction is maximised in a way that allows little personal space or privacy – 'all that happens is treatment'.

2. *Exploration of observed social behaviour* is essential to the understanding of it. This is facilitated through the repetitive cycle of group

meetings or social events, all of which have different structures, compositions, settings and tasks. This provides for the individual member a rich source of feedback from a wide range of perspectives.

3. *Experimentation of new modes of social behaviour* must then follow if existing behavioural repertoires, having been examined and found wanting, are to be replaced. A therapeutic community can provide a range of role opportunities and role models which would enable individuals to adopt certain roles and assume certain responsibilities based, not on their existing abilities, but on their treatment needs. This is based on the in role/out of role concept. Thus an individual who is shy and reticent may be allocated a role within the community which requires that he/she make an effort to communicate and interact with other members in order to fulfil his responsibility to the community. This would be designed deliberately to ensure that some degree of support was inbuilt and the pressures controlled so that he/she would not be overwhelmed by the role demands. This would provide a living/learning situation whereby the individual would progressively, over time, graduate from an 'out of role' position to a confident 'in role' position, characterised by a sense of mastery, improved self-confidence, social functioning and enhanced social status and prestige within the community. The emphasis here is on the process of social learning.

Jones (1952), in his concept of living/learning situations, viewed therapy as a form of social learning. By social learning he meant a two-way communication in a social situation which produces interaction motivated by inner needs or stress, leading to the covert or overt expression of feeling. This leads to a change in the individual's attitudes or beliefs which are incorporated into a changed self-image. He suggests that all routine social situations which confront us in life provide potential living/learning situations. He points out that often we meet challenging situations in a stereotyped way often by withdrawal or denial. While this tactic may help to alleviate anxiety in the short term, in the longer term nothing is learned and we may be faced with the same challenge in the future. If, however, we reflect on the experience, listen to feedback from others and examine our behaviour, we may be able to modify our behavioural repertoire and develop more effective ways of responding to such situations in the future. Thus learning is a more or less permanent change in behaviour which occurs as a result of social experience.

As a result of a 10-year study of eight different therapeutic communities within the UK, Bloor *et al* (1988) conclude that re-socialisation of the individual is the core of therapeutic community treatment. Underlying this belief is the perception that the individual entering any therapeutic community is inducted into a new social world emphatically different from the individual's familiar world. The individual encounters not just a new physical environment but adopts new ways of perceiving and of construing social life and is forced to re-evaluate his/her place within it. As a result of re-socialisation within the community 'social reconstruction' takes place leading to modification of the individual's subjective reality, self-image, social conduct and ways of relating to others. They identify two broad approaches to re-socialisation. Where socialisation proceeds through the deliberate creation of a controlled environment, the supervision of individual task performance and where behavioural change is brought about by the impact of the social structure of the community upon the individual, Bloor and colleagues refer to this as 'instrumentalism'. Where it proceeds through the continuous portrayal to individuals of certain aspects of their conduct as unacceptable and by repeated appeals for a conscious change of conduct they refer to this as 'reality confrontation'. There is much common ground here between Bloor and colleagues' conclusions, Whiteley's and Gordon's (1979) description of the sociodynamic approach and Bandura's social learning theory.

In summary, the sociological approach emphasises the way in which the individual's inner subjective reality is socially reconstructed by the complex interaction of external factors operating within the individual's social field.

Integration of the Social and Psychological Approaches

Edelson (1970), in an attempt to distinguish between psychotherapy and sociotherapy, emphasises the role of the large group as the medium for the exploration of interpersonal relations and interactions between community members. It is in this arena, he suggests, that the social therapist (as opposed to the psychotherapist) directs his/her attention to the social dynamics of the group and seeks to clarify the way in which the internal or intrapsychic dynamics of the individual play themselves out in the social arena. He argues that both are important but distinctive aspects of community work and suggests that both approaches may give rise to conflict over the interpretation of events and priorities for work. This is a criticism which has also been made by Rapaport (1960), and to a lesser extent by Manning (1989). Edelson suggests, however, that their careful interrelation 'in phase' could produce optimum results.

Manning (1989), while critical of the lack of clarity and theoretical justification for the social approach, argues that integration of the psychological and the social approach is achieved through the incorporation of group psychotherapy into therapeutic community work. He refers to the small psychotherapy group as representing the 'symbolic heart' of the therapeutic community and argues that this is the area where the social and the psychological converge to achieve some degree of integration.

The relevance of group psychotherapy to the therapeutic community has been well illustrated by the extension and application of early research into curative or therapeutic factors (Yalom, 1979; Bloch and Crouch, 1985) to the therapeutic community by Whiteley and Collis (1987). This early research identified 10 therapeutic factors central to effective psythotherapy groups.

1. *Acceptance* relates to a feeling of being accepted by other group members or a sense of belonging.
2. *Universality* relates to the realisation that other members have similar problems.
3. *Altruism* relates to the sense of feeling good about helping others in the group.
4. *Instillation of hope* relates to the fostering of a sense of optimism or faith about the benefit of the group experience.
5. *Guidance* relates to the provision of information or advice and explanation.
6. *Vicarious learning* relates to the way in which members learn vicariously by being there and observing others in the group.
7. *Self-understanding* relates to the development of insights about oneself brought about by feedback within the group.
8. *Learning from interpersonal actions* relates to the way in which members make an effort to relate to a constructive way within the group either by initiating a behaviour or by responding to other group members' overtures.
9. *Self-disclosure* relates to the way in which previously hidden, private, personal information is revealed to the group.
10. *Catharsis* relates to the ventilation of highly charged, emotional feelings within the group.

Whiteley and Collis (1987) replicated this research within an established therapeutic community and their findings concur with the earlier research. They point out, however, that in addition to the therapeutic factors occurring in the small psychotherapy group programme, 50% of the events identified also occurred within the wider community context and outside the formal group psychotherapy programme. They conclude that the therapeutic community has the advantage over formal psychotherapy in that it provides an opportunity to put into practice insights or realisations gained in therapy and to experiment with new roles and modes of coping in accepting and understanding the demands of the social system. The therapeutic community provides an ongoing, corrective, emotional experience which, because of its concern with the realities of living together and dealing with real life situations as they occur, facilitate a carry-over of learning and coping skills from the community treatment situation to outside life.

In summary the psychological approach is concerned with how the internal world of the individual has been constructed. There is an emphasis on the exploration of the individual's past or 'there and then' through interpretation. The social approach is concerned with how the internal world of the individual is externalised in the 'here and now' or how the intrapsychic dynamics are played out in the social arena. The emphasis is on the exploration of social relations through confrontation. Ideally, a skilful blend of psychosocial interventions is necessary in order to ensure the optimum therapeutic effect.

THE TRANSFORMATION PROCESS AND THE HEALING EFFECT

Thus far we have discussed the therapeutic community in terms of its general systems features: boundaries and internal structures. To complete the picture we must now consider the issue of what happens to the material which enters the system and is exposed to the internal system processes, and consider what modification occurs as a result of its passage through the system before leaving to return to the external environment (see Figure 5.3).

Manning (1989) notes that the therapeutic community as a social system must have a boundary which demarcates the community from the outside world and orders or structures the internal life of the community so that therapeutic work can take place. We must now turn from these aspects of boundaries and internal structures to discuss the dynamic process of transformation which they facilitate; in other words, we move from the issue of the potential healing matrix to the actual 'healing effect'.

Whiteley and Gordon (1979) provide us with a clear picture of the transformation process in a leading therapeutic community. Drawing on his extensive experience at the Henderson Unit he has charted the passage of patients through the therapeutic community. He points out that, once in, patients very quickly settle down to display patterns of relating with which they are familiar and feel safe. The community provides little in the way of diversionary 'hospital treatment' with which they can become preoccupied or diverted. Furthermore, the minimal social structure ensures that the individual's customary pattern of relating (for which they have been referred) soon emerges.

He suggests that these early days are the most difficult for the community, which must tolerate defensive ploys, acting-out, avoidance tactics and the general manipulation of others within the newcomer's immediate social group. However, the community must persevere and maintain a permissive stance in order to tolerate this while at the same time attempt to confront and curtail such behaviour. The relationship between the

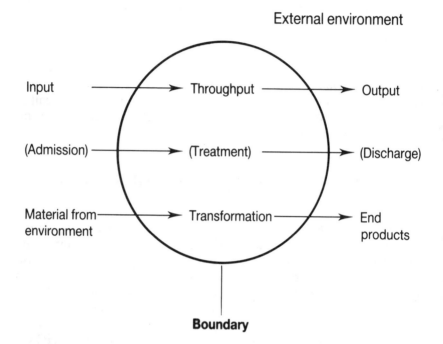

Figure 5.3   Progress entering, passing through and leaving the system.

patient and the community reaches a point whereby it soon becomes clear that he/she must change or leave the community.

Whiteley suggests that at this point, 20–30% of patients leave for a variety of reasons. Some 'take flight' into health, others may begin to change but family or marital partners pressure them into leaving because the status quo of the family/marital relationship is under threat. Most, he suggests, will leave because they see that the commitment to change is too much for them, the direction of change too uncertain and the rewards poor, relative to the effort and risks involved. Whatever their reasons, motivation is poor, attachment and identification with the community are weak. They cling to familiar perceptions of themselves, retain customary patterns of relating to others and when their manoeuvering and manipulations of the community fail, they depart.

Those who remain develop a positive attachment (transference) to the community which promises much (idealisation). They engage enthusiastically in the activities of daily life within the unit and take community responsibilities seriously. Under increased stress, however, 'acting-out' continues as a defence against revealing latent emotional responses. Gradually, over time, firmer bonds are established and reach a stage whereby the patient feels safe enough to experience and disclose such feelings and within 2–3 months will often complain that they are worse than on admission and that they feel depressed, hopeless and inadequate. This is the stage of negative transference (disillusionment) in which the patient experiences the community as hurtful. At the same time, this 'feeling' individual is most active in helping newcomers to the unit. The individual 'works through' this stage and gradually the 'good' and 'bad' aspects of the community experience are brought into perspective; reality is substituted for fantasy and a more mature, balanced personality emerges.

Whiteley's observations suggest that the community provides a 'healing' matrix (Foulkes, 1975) in which the individual may make an investment. This may provide a 'secure base' (Winnicot, 1974) from which the individual might take risks and explore alternative models of relating. This engagement with the community brings about internal change within the individual. This extends to the social arena and translates into change in relationships with significant others. It is important, therefore, to consider what might be the nature of this 'healing' effect.

A number of writers (Almond, 1974; Lear, 1987; Frank, 1989) have observations to make which help to shed some light on this very complex issue. Lear (1987) suggests that 'healing' in psychological terms may be equated with a wound where there is a breach in body tissue. This leads to a breakdown of existing tissue and the development of new growth. This is the healing process which finally joins the edges together. Similarly, a hurt mind may lead to dismay, confusion, disorganisation, anger, depression, etc. and may be remedied by an understanding of the disjointed feelings and the meaning or personal significance of the experience for the individual. The significance or meaning of the experience (neither right nor wrong – but heavily invested with emotional charge) is (like dislocated joints which come together) enabled somehow to fall 'into place' or 'make sense'. This leads to the creation of meaning and the bringing together (fusion) of different parts of the self (*Gestalt*). Note how, as with Whiteley's account of the transformation process (things have to get worse before they get better), a breakdown is a necessary prerequisite before the breakthrough can occur. This is in keeping with the experience of crisis theorists such as Caplan (1970) and with Jones's observations on creativity, growth and systems theory (Jones, 1982).

Almond (1974) argues that therapeutic communities are a sub-set of communities in general and suggests that they are a form of healing community. These communities are distinct from non-healing communities in that they have a number of important, distinguishing features. He suggests that they have the following four features which are important to the healing effort.

- They have an internal sense of the 'specialness' of the individual and of relationships to one another; to the group and the community as a whole.

- There is a translation of this 'specialness' into charismatic roles and into behavioural norms which reflect the cohesiveness for the community and its strong espousal of a set of beliefs and practices.
- There is much devotion of time to healing activities and to the cultivation of a sense of individual and collective achievement derived from the positive results of healing efforts.
- There is a varied pattern of relationships between a healing community and its culture. This is characterised universally by a boundary between members and non-members.

Almond's perspective on the therapeutic community verges on the spiritual and inspirational and indeed, Fromm (1976), in an attempt to clarify the concept of 'religion'and place it on a wider philsophical–social plane, suggested that it has less to do with a concept of god, with idols or a system of religious belief, but to 'any group-shared system of thought and action that offers the individual a frame of orientation and an object of devotion'.

Finally, we must turn to the work of Jerome Frank in order to obtain a macro-perspective on the issue of treatment and healing settings. Frank (1989) has conducted an extensive review of non-specific aspects of treatments used in psychiatry. He was interested in those aspects of treatment methods which are not directly observable or measurable. Dominated as they are by a medical ideology, psychiatric treatment modalities tend to be 'highly visible' (Brown and Fowler, 1966) in that they are procedurally orientated, readily observed, often use technical equipment, are relatively easy to evaluate, are highly valued in hospital settings and attract social and professional acclaim, e.g. ECT, medication, etc. By contrast 'low visibility' treatment forms are non-technological, involve personal interactions at a high level of intimacy, tend to be poorly conceptualised, difficult to evaluate, are not highly valued in hospitals, are often taken for granted and attract little social acclaim, e.g. conversational approaches (counselling) or interactive approaches (social skills training).

Frank's work arose out of a concern with the placebo phenomenon and the idea of meta-treatment (Abroms, 1969). This has arisen out of a recognition that alongside the dominant treatment forms something else, less visible, less easy to define exists. This provides a context which may enhance the dominant treatment modality. Frank suggests that all legitimate treatment approaches (apart from whatever other outcomes they are assumed to effect) have to combat personal demoralisation. He argues that illness demoralises the individual and that treatments which are helpful are those which (among other things) help to combat this demoralisation process. He states that if a treatment approach does this it will often have the following characteristics:

- It provides an emotionally charged, confiding relationship with either a helpful person, group or community.
- It provides a healing setting, e.g. a clinic, hospital, day centre or community with a clear identity.
- It provides a rationale, conceptual scheme or myth which provides a plausible explanation for how or why it works or will be effective.
- It provides a ritual or a series of rituals in which the individuals may engage and participate.
- It provides hope, raises expectations and increases motivation.
- It helps the individual develop a sense of wholeness and to achieve a sense of mastery, increased competence and control over their lives.

To conclude, we should perhaps acknowledge and affirm the 'charismatic' and in many respects 'magical' dynamic which underlies therapeutic endeavours in general and therapeutic community practice in particular. This is best illustrated by quoting Maxwell Jones's observations on the lack of conceptual clarity with regard to models of the therapeutic community which has irritated so many reviewers seeking the definitive definition of the term.

> The fact is of course that we have no single model of the therapeutic community. All that we can hope to do is to mobilise the interest, skills and enthusiasm of staff and patients and give them sufficient freedom of action to create their own optimal social organisation (Jones, 1968).

PROSPECTS FOR THE FUTURE

We must conclude this chapter by briefly considering the future prospects for the therapeutic community as an approach to treatment in psychiatry. As Traur (1984) points out, the demise of the therapeutic community is more apparent than real and indeed has been 'rediscovered' in many settings outside of mainstream hospital psychiatry. With the emphasis on community care and the advent of the split between health and social care (Griffiths, 1988) it would seem reasonable to predict that the therapeutic community model would have an important role to play within social care settings (Millard, 1989; Brown and Clough, 1989). If the community care movement is to avoid trans-institutionalisation, whereby the location and size of the unit changes but custodial practices from the institution are simply transferred to the new setting, then an antidote to institutional practice such as the therapeutic community is necessary. Indeed, as the Wagner report (1988) pointed out, except in relation to the therapeutic community and the principles of normalisation, there is very little theoretical basis to much residential care provision. Kennard (1979) has pointed out that the therapeutic community model is most effective for individuals who are likely to stay around for a long period of time. It is reasonable to assume, therefore, that it is best suited to the needs of the elderly (Burton, 1989), the long-term mentally ill (Traur, 1984; Hull and Pullen, 1989), individuals with learning difficulties (Atkinson, 1989) and offenders in the probation and penal systems (Ball and Sowa, 1989; Sapsed, 1989).

The role of the psychiatric nurse (and the residential social worker) in day or residential settings is crucial not only to the maintenance of a safe supportive environment but to the establishment, development and maintenance of a therapeutically viable environment in tandem with other members of the multidisciplinary team. This requires skill in the mobilisation and management of therapeutic factors. The nurse's role is central to the therapeutic effort because his/her role is often (like the relative's) closer to the socioemotional experience of the patient (Jansen, 1983) than some of the other professionals. By utilising these insights and by responding empathetically and honestly within an atmosphere of positive regard, the nurse can make a key contribution to the establishment, development and maintenance of the therapeutic 'milieu'.

Finally, I will conclude by asserting that it would appear that the therapeutic community impulse (Kennard, 1989), in many different shapes and forms, is very much alive and well!

REFERENCES

Abroms G M (1969) Defining milieu therapy. *Archives of General Psychiatry,* **21,** 553–560.

Alexander F and French T M (1946) *Psychoanalytic Therapy: principles and application.* New York: Ronald Press.

Almond R H (1974) *The Healing Community.* Northvale, NJ: Jason Aaronson.

Atkinson D (1989) Group homes for people with mental handicap: key issues for everyday living: In: *Groups and Groupings,* eds Brown A and Clough R. London: Tavistock/Routledge.

Ball L and Sowa T (1989) Groupwork in intermediate treatment. In: *Groups and Groupings,* eds Brown A and Clough R. London: Tavistock/Routledge.

Bandura A and Walters R H (1963) *Social Learning and Personality Development.* New York: Holt, Rinehart and Winston.

Baron C (1987) *Asylum to Anarchy.* London: Free Association Books.

Barton R (1959) *Institutional Neurosis.* Bristol: Wright.

Beardshaw V (1981) *Conscientious Objectors at Work: Mental Hospital Nurses – a case study.* London: *Social Audit.*

Bion W R (1955) Group dynamics: a review. In: *New Directions in Psychoanalysis*, eds Klein M, Heimann P and Money-Kyrle R E. London: Tavistock.

Bion W (1961) *Experiences in Groups*. London: Tavistock.

Bloch S and Crouch E (1985) *Therapeutic Factors in Group Psychotherapy.* Oxford: Oxford University Press.

Bloor M, Kegany N and Fomkert N (1988) *One Foot in Eden: A sociological study of the range of therapeutic community practice*. London: Routledge and Kegan Paul.

Bridger H (1946) The Northfield experiment. *Bullet of the Menninger Clinic*, **10**(3): 71–76.

Brown A and Clough R (1989) Life in day and residential settings. In: *Groups and Groupings*, eds Brown A and Clough R. London: Tavistock/Routledge.

Brown M and Fowler G R (1971) *Psycho-Dynamic Nursing*. Philadelphia: W B Saunders.

Burton J (1989) Institutional change and group action: The significance and influence of groups in developing new residential sources for older people. In: *Groups and Groupings*, eds Brown A and Clough R. London: Tavistock/Routledge.

Cain T M and Smail D J (1969) *The Treatment of Mental Illness*. London: University of London Press.

Caplan G (1970) *The Theory and Practice of Mental Health Consultation*. London: Tavistock.

Caudill W (1958) *The Psychiatric Hospital as a Small Society.* Cambridge, Mass: Harvard University Press.

Chinoy E (1967) *Society: an Introduction to Sociology.* New York: Random House Inc.

Clark D H (1965) The therapeutic community: concept, practice and future. *British Journal of Psychiatry*, **3**(479): 947–954.

Crockett R (1966) Authority and permissiveness in the psychotherapeutic community: theoretical perspectives. *American Journal of Psychotherapy*, **XX**(4): 669–676.

De Board R (1978) *The Psycho-analysis of Organisations: a psychoanalytical approach to behaviour in groups and organisations*. London: Tavistock Publications.

Dill D (1981) The management of academic culture: notes on the management of meaning and social integration. *Higher Education*, **11**(3): 303–320.

Edelson M (1964) *Ego-psychology, Group Dynamics and the Therapeutic Community.* New York: Grune and Stratton.

Edelson M (1970) *Sociotherapy and Psychotherapy.* Chicago: University of Chicago Press.

Foulks S H (1975) *Group Analytic Psychotherapy: method and principles.* London: Gordon and Breach.

Frank J D (1989) The view of a psychotherapist. In: *Non-specific Aspects of Treatment*, eds Shepherd M and Sartarious N. Bern: Huber.

Fromm E (1976) *To Have or To Be?* London: Abacus.

Goffman I (1968) *Asylums: Essays on the social situations of mental patients and other inmates.* Harmondsworth: Penguin Books.

Griffiths R (1988) *Community Care: Agenda for Action.* London: HMSO.

Hawkins P (1989) The social learning approach to residential and day care. In: *Groups and Groupings*, eds Brown A and Clough R. London: Tavistock/Routledge.

Hillery G A Jr (1955) Definitions of community: areas of agreement. *Rural Sociology,* 2(2): 111–123.

Hinselwood R (1979) The Community as analyst. In: Hinselwood R and Manning N (eds) *Therapeutic Communities: Reflections and Progress.* London: Routledge and Kegan Paul.

Hinselwood R D (1987) *What Happens in Groups.* London: Free-Association Books.

Hobson R F (1979) The Messianic community. In: *Therapeutic Communities: Reflections and progress*, eds Hinselwood R D and Manning N. London: Routledge and Kegan Paul.

Hughes L (1990) Assessing organisational culture: strategies for the external consultant. *Nursing Forum,* 25(1): 15–19.

Hull H and Pullen G (1988) The Eric Burden community: madness and community. *The International Journal of Therapeutic Communities,* 9(2): 109–114.

Jacques E (1953) On the dynamics of social structure. *Human Relations,* 6: 3–24.

Janson E (Deputy Chair) 1983 *Mental Health and the Community.* London: Richmond Fellowship Press.

Jones M (1952) *Social Psychiatry.* London: Tavistock.

Jones M (1956) The concept of the therapeutic community. *American Journal of Psychiatry,* 112(8): 647–650.

Jones M (1968) *Social Psychiatry in Practice.* Harmondsworth: Penguin.

Jones M (1982) *The Process of Change.* London: Routledge and Kegan Paul.

Karterud H (1989) *Group Processes in Therapeutic Communities.* London: Artesian Books.

Kennard D (1979) Limiting factors: the setting, the staff, the patients. In: *Therapeutic Communities: Reflections and progress*, eds Hinselwood R D and Manning N. London: Routledge and Kegan Paul.

Kennard D (1989) The Therapeutic Community impulse – what makes it grow? *International Journal of Therapeutic Communities,* 10(3): 155–163.

Kennedy R (1987) The work of the day: aspects of work with families at the Cassel hospital. In *The Family as Inpatient: Families and Adolescents at the Cassel Hospital*, eds Kennedy R, Heyman H and Tischler L. London: Free Association Books.

Lear T (1987) The rhyme and reason of healing in the group. *Group Analysis,* 20: 351–365.

Letemendia F J J, Harris A and Willems J A (1967) The clinical effects on a population of chronic schizophrenic patients of administrative changes in a hospital. *British Journal of Psychiatry,* **113**: 959–971.

Levy M J (1952) *Structure of Society.* Princeton University Press.

Louis M (1980) Surprise and sense making: what newcomers experience in entering unfamiliar organisational settings. *Administrative Science Quarterly,* **25**(2): 226–250.

Main T (1946) The hospital as a therapeutic institution. *Bulletin of the Meninger Clinic,* **10**: 66–70.

Main T (1957) The ailment. *British Journal of Medical Psychology,* **30**: 129–145.

Main T (1977) The concept of the therapeutic community: variations and vicissitudes. *Group Analysis,* **X**(2): 129–145.

Manning N (1975) Factors affecting referrals to therapeutic communities. *Association of Therapeutic Communities Bulletin,* **17**: 7–10.

Manning N (1989) *The Therapeutic Community Movement: Charisma and Routinisation.* London: Routledge and Kegan Paul.

Menzies-Leith I E P (1988) *Containing Anxiety in Institutions.* Free Association Press.

Miles A (1972) The development of interpersonal relations among long-stay patients in two hospital workshops, *British Journal of Medical Psychlogy,* **45**: 105–114.

Millard D W and Kirk J D (1979) Personal growth in the residential community. In: *Therapeutic Communities: Reflections and progress,* eds Hinselwood R D and Manning N. London: Routledge and Kegan Paul.

Myers K and Clark D H (1972) Results in a therapeutic community. *British Journal of Psychiatry,* **120**, 51–58.

Neil A S (1968) *Summerhill.* Harmondsworth: Pelican Books.

Rapaport R (1956) Oscillations and sociotherapy. *Human Relations,* **9**(3): 357–374.

Rapaport R (1960) *Community as Doctor.* London: Tavistock.

Roberts J (1980) Destructive processes in a therapeutic community. *International Journal of Therapeutic Communities,* **1**(3): 159–170.

Rose M (1986) The design of atmosphere: ego-nurture and psychic change in residential treatment. *Journal of Adolescence,* **9**: 49–62.

Sapsed C (1989) Groups and groupings in a probation hostel. In: *Groups and Groupings,* eds Brown A and Clough R. London: Tavistock/Routledge.

Savalle H and Wagenborg H (1980) Oscillations in a therapeutic community. *A T C Bulletin,* **27**: 6–14.

Sharp V (1975) *Social Control in the Therapeutic Community.* Aldershot: Saxon House.

Stanton A H and Schwartz M S (1954) *The Mental Hospital.* New York: Basic Books.

Shenker B (1988) *International Communities.* London: Routledge and Kegan Paul.

Tierney W (1988) Organisational culture in higher education: defining the essentials. *Journal of Higher Education*, **59**(1): 2–21.

Toennies F (1957) *Community and Society*, ed. Loomis C P. East Lansing, Michigan: Michigan State University Press.

Tosquelles F (1964) In: *Encyclopédie Française de Psychiatrie*, eds Rappard P H, Ayme J and Torrulia H. Thérapeutique Institutionelle, 37930 G 10.

Traur T (1984) The current status of the therapeutic community. *British Journal of Medical Psychology*, **57**: 71–79.

Wagner G (1988) *Residential Care: a positive choice*. London: HMSO.

Weber M (1947) *The Theory of Social and Economic Organisation*. New York: Oxford University Press.

White N F (1972) Re-appraising the in-patient 'milieu': Obit 'Milieu'. *Canadian Psychiatric Association Journal*, **17**, 51–57.

Whiteley J S, Briggs D and Turner M (1972) *Dealing with Deviants*. London: Hogarth Press.

Whiteley J S and Gordon J (1979) *Group Approaches in Psychiatry*. London: Routledge and Kegan Paul.

Whiteley J S and Collis M (1987) The therapeutic factors in group psychotherapy applied to the therapeutic community. *International Journal of Therapeutic Communities*, **8**(1): 21–32.

Wilson S (1979) Ways of seeing the therapeutic community. In: *Therapeutic Communities: Reflections and progress*, eds Hinselwood R D and Manning N. London: Routledge and Kegan Paul.

Winnicott D W (1965) *The Maturational Process and the Facilitating Environment*. London: Hogarth Press.

Winnicot D (1974) *Playing and Reality*. Harmondsworth: Penguin.

Yalom I (1979) *The Theory and Practice of Group Psychotherapy*. New York: Basic Books.

FURTHER READING

Ackoff R L (1976) Towards a system of systems concepts. In: *Systems Behaviour*, eds. Beishon J and Peters J. London: Open University Press, Harper and Row.

Bion W (1961) *Experiences in Groups*. London: Tavistock.

Clark D (1981) *Social Therapy in Psychiatry*. Edinburgh: Churchill Livingstone.

Hinselwood R D (1987) *What Happens in Groups? Psycho-analysis, the individual and the community*. London: Free Association Books.

Hinselwood R D and Manning N (eds) (1979) *Therapeutic Communities: Reflections and Progress*. London: Routledge and Kegan Paul.

Kennard D and Roberts J (1983) *Introduction to the Therapeutic Community*. London: Routledge and Kegan Paul.

Manning N (1989) *The Therapeutic Community Movement: Charisma and routinisation*. London: Routledge and Kegan Paul.

Whiteley J S and Gordon J (1979) *Group Approaches in Psychiatry.* London: Routledge and Kegan Paul.
Wright H (1989) *Groupwork: Perspectives and Practice.* London: Scutari Press.
Brown A and Clough R (1989) *Groups and Groupings: Life and work in day and residential centres.* London: Tavistock/Routledge.

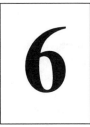

Forensic Psychiatry

Liam Clarke and Lynn Hamilton

INTRODUCTION

This chapter is set out in three sections. The first section traces the development of secure units as part of a growing concern with forensic clients. It looks at the particular way in which these units took form in one Regional Health Authority and briefly sketches the ideas which lay behind the changes. Section two concentrates on the manner by which some of these units developed their treatment philosophies. In particular, it examines attempts to implement a therapeutic community approach and the kinds of problems to which this gave rise. The concept of dangerousness is also discussed and the section ends by considering the narrow dividing line between 'prisoner' and 'client'.

Section three is a compendium of different but related issues in forensic care. It addresses the issue of violence and how nurses try to deal with it. Underlying feelings which may accompany the nursing of sex offenders is briefly introduced; this is an area, among others, where little is known. The role of research in secure units is therefore emphasised and the chapter ends with some modest suggestions for the future.

Section One

OPEN DOOR BEGINNINGS

Despite the general tendency towards an 'Open Door' policy in psychiatric hospitals during the 1950s and 1960s most hospitals retained at least one locked ward (Rees, 1957; Glancy, 1974). These wards provided a temporary locked facility for acutely disturbed patients as well as giving accommodation to long stay, 'difficult' or 'truculent' patients whose behaviour, while not overtly violent or dangerous, was nevertheless a challenge to their adequate management.

There are many practising nurses who may still remember these so-called refractory wards. As psychiatric nursing progressed through the 1970s, concern developed about the detrimental effects of custodial care (Goffman, 1960; Barton, 1959) and a growing awareness of the inadequacy of much of what passed for nursing care. As a consequence, the growing reluctance to 'lock people up', together with the progressive closure of hospitals led to a group of clients becoming increasingly difficult to deal with and there emerged a fairly clear picture of a defined client group who simply did not fit 'the system' any longer.

THE CASE OF ANTHONY LEDGER

On 5 June 1976 Malcome Dean wrote in the *Guardian* newspaper of a:

. . . disorder in a welfare machine that has battered a sick man between prison and the wrong kind of mental hospital. Anyone who believes there are not many holes in the British welfare net should meet the relatives of Anthony Ledger, who stepped before Littlehampton magistrates this week to plead guilty to assaulting three policemen and who now awaits sentence by the local Crown Court. [He was imprisoned for 18 months.] It is now two and a half years since his cousin first visited him in Wandsworth prison and noted his mentally disordered state.

Since then Mr Ledger has been in and out of prisons and mental hospitals, as his offences have become more serious, but has yet to be found a secure hospital place where his paranoid schizophrenia, which has been diagnosed by successive psychiatrists, could be treated. Instead he has only been fed into places with revolving doors – prisons which have to release their inmates at set times, or ordinary mental hospitals from which he has been able to discharge himself.

The result has been that for a few days after release he has survived on his own, living roughly in abandoned cars or buildings, but then has been picked up again. Three years ago he was arrested for stealing a toy. Last year his petty offences included stealing a bag of coal, taking a free ride on the railways, and booking in at a boarding house without any money. This year he has made two separate and unprovoked attacks on the police. 'What does he have to do before authorities will provide him with a secure hospital place?' asks his probation officer, Mr R L Brown. 'His behaviour suggests he is asking to be treated and contained. He finds it almost impossible to survive outside institutions, let alone manage the treatment programme for his mental sickness. Every doctor who sees him agrees that he is ill but no doctor will accept responsibility for him'.

In November last year, and on 19 May this year, separate psychiatrists from Broadmoor examined Mr Ledger and diagnosed paranoid schizophrenia. They both agreed that he was in need of long-term care and treatment but not a maximum security hospital.

Unfortunately for Mr Ledger, he falls between two stools. He has still not committed sufficiently violent offences to qualify for a place in one of the four special hospitals, but he is too disruptive for any ordinary mental hospital, particularly since they introduced their new open door philosophy.

Hundreds of pounds must have already been spent on Mr Ledger, compiling reports, conducting case conferences, and organising meetings between magistrates and the probation service, the probation service and the DHSS, the DHSS and doctors, and the doctors and regional health administrators. Would it not be cheaper to build a few secure places?

© *The Guardian*

This article found its mark with those in the psychiatric services where such 'high profile' cases became useful ammunition in the demand for innovation, increased resources and change generally. While the article contained unproven assumptions about the nature of 'mental illness', particularly its amelioration by the provision of institutional care, its basic humanitarianism was patent. Clearly, something needed to be done.

THE POWELL INITIATIVE

By 1959, Enoch Powell had set up a working party to examine issues of secure provision in mental hospitals and it was within this forum that the idea of medium-secure units took shape. However, the idea took an exceedingly long time to germinate. Snow (1991) believed that the reason for this was concerns over the financial outlay to implement it. More probably, the (political) perception, that local units for offenders were extremely unpopular with the general public, was the main prohibitive factor.

THE BUTLER REPORT: TREATMENT AND SECURITY

The Butler Committee (Butler, 1975) was set up on 21 July 1972 with the following terms of reference:

1. To consider the extent and on what criteria the law should recognise mental disorder or abnormality in a person accused of a criminal offence as a factor affecting his liability to be tried or convicted, and his disposal;

2. To consider what, if any, changes are necessary in the powers, procedure and facilities relating to the provision of appropriate treatment, in prison, hospital or the community, for offenders suffering from mental disorder or abnormality, and to their discharge and after-care; and to make recommendations.

On 20 April 1974 the Committee published an Interim Report recommending the provision, 'as a matter of urgency', of secure units within *each* Regional Health Authority. The following reasons were given: the units were required for those mentally disturbed persons, offenders and non-offenders alike, who did not require the degree of security provided by the Special State hospitals (which, they noted, are overcrowded anyway) but who are not suitable for treatment in the open conditions available within local psychiatric hospitals. In addition the Committee believed that:

> . . . custodial requirements cannot be reconciled with the 'open door' therapeutic policy now practised (Butler, 1974, p.31).

Because of these custodial requirements many consultants were reluctant to accept offender patients and Bluglass (1978) had indeed identified a general resistance among psychiatrists. At the same time, many agencies had come to recognise their own shortcomings in dealing with 'the mentally abnormal offender and the behaviourally disturbed individual' (Glancy, 1974; Fuller, 1985).

Although the provision of secure units had been recommended to Regional Hospital Boards by the Ministry of Health as far back as 1961 not a single unit had been built. Consequently, the Courts often had little option but to imprison offenders who were in need of treatment but, for their own and the public's safety, could not be contained in an ordinary hospital.

GOVERNMENT BACKING

On 18 July 1974, Barbara Castle stated, in Parliament, the Government's acceptance of the recommendations of the Interim Report of the Butler Committee and circular HSC(IS)61 (July 1974) was issued to Regional and Area Health Authorities urging that action be taken to treat patients in conditions of security (that is, interim units) pending the construction of new units. (At this stage the Government undertook to provide only the *capital* cost of the units.)

Little progress was made in establishing the new units as the departmental circular had urged. By 1978, six or seven units were in the planning stage but building had not yet started. Indeed, in some parts of the country there was an unwillingness even to formulate plans or give the proposals the attention the Butler Committee thought they deserved. While consultations proceeded, clear 'affirmation of intent' was lacking.

By 1983 only 20 of the planned 717 beds were open (Pilgrim and Eisenberg, 1985) and the development (of buildings, not ideas) was painfully slow. This is despite the fact that, by now, agreement had been reached that central Government would fund the running costs as well as the capital outlay of the units. Indeed, the Government did: Snow (1991) records that of £44 285 000 allocated to Regional Health Authorities from 1976 to 1982, 7 per cent was spent in 1976, rising to 40 per cent in 1982.

During this period £26 000 000 of directly allocated funds was not spent, being used instead upon general health care provision. This suggests a marked lack of enthusiasm for the project as a whole, albeit with regional variations: the particular needs of such clients were perhaps judged as having too low a priority (and public appreciation).

THE DEVELOPMENT OF THE UNITS

However, by 1985 the setting up of interim units, usually in converted wards of existing mental hospitals – some of these remain – and Regional (purpose-built) units, was gathering considerable momentum. Building and commissioning was well under way with approximately 14 interim and five Regional units established and with many more in the pipeline. By late 1984, it was hoped that 200 fully staffed beds would be up and running (Snowden, 1983).

SECURE BUT NOT SECURED

We would now like to describe the response by the South East Thames Regional Health Authority, whose units have formed the basis of the forensic experience of us both. Initially, this Authority convened a special advisory group (composed of medical doctors) and they set to work designing a clinical philosophy as a framework for detailed planning of the new service. A parallel nursing advisory group considered the philosophy of supervision, staffing arrangements and an educational programme.

The scheme proposed was that of a 'special assessment and supervisory service' (SASS). This terminology avoided the term 'security', so as to play down the unfortunate connotations which the term can suggest: it was believed that 'supervision' reflected the character and purpose of the proposed scheme. In addition, references to 'secure units' might convey misleading assumptions about the uniformity of treatment milieus being developed across the country (Fuller, 1985). In this respect, it is notable that schemes and arrangements differed throughout the United Kingdom and that this particular scheme was regarded as unique. Snowden's (1983) survey described wide variations across the country in the priorities given to the nature of the units established (for example, taking account of perceived local needs and pressures).

Fuller (1985) similarly noted wide variation, in terms of size, staffing complement, architectural layout and security arrangements but such 'ecological factors' were, he observed, uniform for the five units of this Region. At the same time, 'common denominator' factors, for example Home Office rules and Court Orders, would impinge upon every unit in the country, thus affecting whatever local policies or practices were in place.

This raises the interesting question of how the term 'medium security' would be interpreted in the absence of an overriding definition, as well as how different interpretations would be embodied in operational policies and in what way would they reflect concern over 'public safety' as well as care for the clients.

AN EARLY STUDY

Using a Correctional Institutions Environment Scale, Fuller (1985) summarised two batches of beliefs, outlined below, which he had obtained from the unit's staff.

Items with Good Inter-staff Agreement

1. Positive encouragement of patients.
2. Development of therapeutic personal relationships between staff and patients.
3. Positive involvement of staff in therapy.
4. Need for a friendly informal atmosphere.
5. Willingness of staff to give and receive criticism.

Items with Poor Staff Agreement

1. The degree of frank and free expression within the unit.
2. Clarity of rules and use of sanctions.
3. Degree of patient involvement in decision-making.
4. Specific emphases in therapeutic activities.
5. Flexibility and clarity of routine.
6. Expectations about standards of neatness in the unit.

These conclusions compare positively with findings obtained by Clarke (1991) in his study of relationships in forensic units. For example, those items with good staff agreement were the same for both studies while items 2 and 5 in Fuller's second category became terrifyingly difficult for almost everyone in the Clarke study.

THE SERVICE STRUCTURE FOR THIS REGION

In summary, an integrated Regional service was envisaged involving four tiers of care and supervision.

Tier 1.   The special maximum security hospitals
Tier 2.   A purpose-built central clinic for the region: 30 beds
Tier 3.   Five peripheral area clinics at large mental illness hospitals serving the patient's home district: 15 beds each
Tier 4.   Out-patient and community services

In retrospect, this was the most complex structure devised in the country. For example, the central clinic did not have a catchment area of its own (Snowden, 1983) although this was subsequently altered to a dual role whereby it continued to function as a central unit while acting as a defined catchment area (Delmont, 1987).

A circular, or fail-safe, system was intended to provide essential 'cover' for clients throughout the various potential progressions of their 'illness' (see Figure 6.1). Clients would move along one or all of these tiers, absorbing different levels of security and treatment orientations until judged fit to return to society. Instead of establishing one large unit (as many other Regions had) a local concept was implemented in which the severely troubled or troublesome patient could be managed near his own home.

LOCAL SCHEME

Bluglass (1978) thought that the decision to opt for this 'local scheme' stemmed from a conviction that the nature and extent of the 'forensic' problem was not known and so could not be solved simply by the provision of a mere building: such units, he thought, must relate to their potential turnover of clients as well as respond to local support agencies and surrounding National Health Service hospitals. Such a service would also provide further social links via the provision of a comprehensive community forensic psychiatric service.

However, the main emphasis was to try to avoid a 'mini-Broadmoor' arrangement (with attendant custodial mentality). To this end, a key element was a plentiful provision of staff of all disciplines. For example,

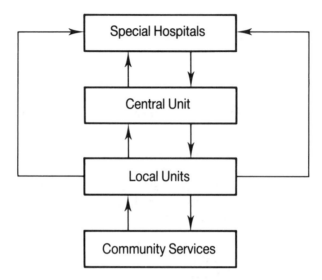

Figure 6.1   Diagram showing the possible movements of patients within the regional system following admission.

there were to be almost 40 nurses for 15 clients (not including allocated students). It was anticipated that this would also aid the security of the building – in addition to being able to 'lock it up' a sense of confidence in the security would be enhanced for both staff and clients alike by the sheer numbers of nurses.

For and Against the New System

The proponents of local medium-secure systems were clearly enthusiastic about their viability as a treatment strategy and they saw them as filling the 'yawning gap' in psychiatric provision to which the Butler Report had referred. They were particularly keen to stress that these units would definitely *not* cater for patients who were a danger to the general public, rather treating people who were seriously disturbed or a *threat to the people caring for them*. Therefore, it became important to ensure that these carers would be specially trained.

Special Training

The issue of 'special training' became a notable feature in these units especially in relation to differing views about the potential violence of clients. For many of the nurses these differences became an irresolute difficulty. There had always been a lack of precision about the exact types of clients who would be catered for and it was this uncertainty which produced much of the anxiety and bitterness about the appropriateness of various approaches to care. Although definitions had been proffered by the Butler and Glancy Reports (1974), differing interpretations of these continued and, on the part of some, careering into:

> Fantasies of murderers and rapists on the rampage in local housing estates . . . not always. . . . relieved. . . by good public relations and education (Bluglass, 1978, p.491).

Getting It Together

Project teams were established (by June 1979) for each of the five local units in the South East Regional scheme and, with Government backing, commissioning proceeded. The specialist teams provided further information designed to communicate the purposes of the system and they also published information about the new departure in a series of widely distributed pamphlets. All five units were expected to be in business by 1984 (Snowden, 1983).

The unit in which both present authors worked was named Ashen Hill. A 15-bedded unit and entirely self-contained, from the outset it proclaimed its intention to work as a therapeutic community reflecting the themes of permissiveness (relative to behavioural norms); confrontation (relating to limit setting for clients' behaviours); democratisation (relating to authority and decision-making) and communalism (relating to shared living accommodation). It hardly needs stressing that to weave such a philosophy into the workings of a secure setting is no mean task and somewhat controversial. The unit at Rainhill, which had been open since the late 1970s, also claimed to work in this way; clearly, the influence here was Grendon Underwood, a psychiatric prison which had been, generally, running since 1962 along the lines laid down by Maxwell Jones.

Section Two

THERAPEUTIC COMMUNITIES AND THE BUTLER COMMITTEE

Sharp (1975) notes the therapeutic community influence on prison reform and the rehabilitation of offenders. Gray (1973) provided an overview of therapeutic community practice in Grendon Underwood Prison and an evaluation of results. He related positive outcomes (after follow-up) with:

> . . . increased ability to understand and communicate feelings (Gray, 1973, p.23)

The Butler Committee referred to the Henderson (Belmont Unit), Grendon Underwood Prison and Garth Angharad Hospital as examples of therapeutic communities. While acknowledging the success claims of these communities in rehabilitating some of their inmates, the Report considered that 'these methods' would not be suitable for the more aggressive offenders or for those who decline treatment: such people, the Report stated, 'require secure containment' (p.91)

The characteristics noted by the committee as indicative of the therapeutic community (at Grendon) were the following:

1. Good staff–patient relationships.
2. Inmate participation.
3. Frequent meetings of:
   (a) small counselling groups;
   (b) work groups; and
   (c) psychotherapeutic groups of staff and patients.
4. Inmate committees for various activities, such as communications to staff on administration matters.

The therapeutic community was, they stated, particularly successful in managing disturbed clients by lowering opposition to authority and increasing self-esteem. However, immature clients or those of low intelligence would require more structure than afforded by a therapeutic community. They noted that clients who were violent or uncooperative were often transferred out of the community. For such violent clients or for those reluctant to accept treatment a training regime was advocated, aimed at developing appropriate patterns of social behaviour. There should be a 'realistic' provision of equal periods of work and social activity, albeit adjusted to individual needs:

> Work and activity have always been the cornerstones of eduation and rehabilitation and it is difficult to see what effective alternative regime could be offered to an offender suffering froma psychopathic disorder to enable him to find his place in the community on release (Butler, 1975, p.96).

The committee clearly reflected the philosophy of 'the devil makes work for idle hands'; so too they demonstrated an uncomplicated acceptance of the concept of 'psychopath'. These sentiments clearly echo a view of caring for forensic clients which is basically rehabilitative: the problems of these clients (especially if 'psychopathic') are recognised as social in nature and thus amenable to training and educational programmes. An affirmation of a 'common-sense' or 'down to earth' approach to clients is also reflected in the Report's pragmatic assertions and a thorough scepticim of the more radical elements of therapeutic communities prevailed.

CONTROLLERS

In some forensic units the pragmatism of the Butler Report was carried over in the attitudes of a 'controller' group of nurses, who were especially angered by the therapeutic community approach, referring to its practitioners as the nurses with 'flowers in their mouths': these flowers were the verbal representation of what the controllers perceived as the too-soft approach to serious offenders. Puzzled by the inability of the 'therapist nurses' to see the inherent dangerousness of the clients, the 'controllers' were adamant that these units could never be therapeutic communities.

DANGEROUSNESS

A particular recommendation of the Butler Report concerned the implementation of multidisciplinary systems for the processing of clinical assessments related to admissions. The importance of team assessment to evaluate suitability for admission was stressed: two principal factors were asserted to govern the admission process:

1. Does the client have a mental disorder which requires hospital admission to a secure unit?
2. Does the unit have the resources and skills to offer safe and appropriate help?

Referrals could come from a variety of sources and these are displayed in Figure 6.2.

A certain idealism understandably surrounded the descriptions which the proponents of the units provided and, to a certain extent, these may be seen as propagandist exercises. In fact, relationships between staff became, over time, less than ideal, particularly over the question of suitability of clients for admission. Arguments also occurred among nurses on the issue of whether so-called 'psychopathic' or 'sociopathic' clients were actually 'ill' or merely malingerers/criminals. The Butler committee had accepted that a concept of dangerousness could be 'valid' although it had some difficulty in trying to define it. Having entertained various (submitted) definitions they arrived at their own, as follows:

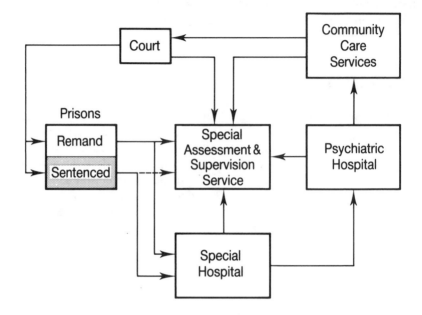

Figure 6.2   Diagram showing referrals to SASS by a number of different routes.

. . . a propensity to cause serious physical injury or lasting psychological harm (Butler, 1975, p.59)

They noted the general public's probable overriding concern with 'physical dangerousness'.

Although aware of the problems of predicting dangerousness they believed that choosing procedural safeguards would depend on 'the danger to be guarded against'. This matter was left open with room to extend the concept if necessary. However, reference was made to '. . . the impossibility of certain predictions. . .' (p.59) and that

> A balance has to be struck between the need to protect society and the right of the individual to return to the community when his detention is no longer strictly justified (Butler, 1975, p.74).

On the basis of systematic observations, Clarke (1991) concluded that nurses appeared to be guided by their 'common sense' personal judgements as to which clients constituted a danger and to what extent. Inevitably, differences emerged reflecting differing approaches to the question of security overall. A charge-nurse expressed the position thus:

There is no scientific way of demonstrating a level of dangerousness in an individual, no formula . . . most decisions are based on feelings. If someone is making a parole decision there is no graduated process of evaluation. It is a question of feeling, but the public should be satisfied (Clarke, 1991).

However, the question remains as to how best to gauge the public's criteria for satisfaction. Should one be as certain as one can be that a client is fit for parole before giving it, or should clients be given an opportunity to demonstrate their fitness outside the unit as part of the process of giving it? On the whole, those advocating a therapeutic community stance would opt for the latter, arguing that the former is both custodial and unrealistic.

THE THERAPEUTIC COMMUNITY

Before discussing the application of therapeutic community principles to forensic settings the reader is referred to Chapter 5, which describes the basic premises of these communities. In the context of forensic units, therapeutic community advocates assert that the social environment of the unit can liberate the individual inasmuch as his social interactions on the unit can prepare him for living responsibly on the outside. This notion, of course, assumes that social factors are a determining factor in precipitating mental illness, a conclusion likely to lead to debate rather than agreement. Traditional hospitals (from where secure unit nurses were recruited) had generally tended to over-stress their custodial functions; therapeutic commuities, on the other hand, were known to make their surroundings as democratic as possible. Another irritant is the likelihood of authoritarian nurses gravitating towards those areas of their hospital deemed to be most custodial (Gilbert and Levinson, 1956; Rice *et al* 1966). Whether or not this indeed happened hardly detracted from the fact that, in secure units, staff would in any case be seen by many clients as custodial; after all, most of these clients had not willingly chosen to enter the unit but were detained under various provisions of the Mental Health Act (1983). Another potentially difficult problem is that free movement into the community is obviously restricted by legalities as well as locked doors. As such, a concept most precious to therapeutic community practitioners, namely the lack of boundary between institution and community, is obliterated. What can then happen is a kind of a compensation drive by the staff to formulate therapeutic *attitudes* of an essentially non-punishing kind. However, this can conflict with the need to establish the limits to behaviour which the unit as a whole is prepared to tolerate. Some of the nurses will set about this task quickly and insist that each community member is familiarised with the various rules. The result of all of this can be a polarisation between those advocating an interpersonal, warm and socialising approach within a secure setting and those who advocate a security primacy with added-on rehabilitation elements. Disagreements on these issues may become acute, at times amounting to open hostility.

Advantages

Having noted some of the difficulties, it must also be said that the therapeutic community approach does encourage nursing staff to play a considerable part in the decision-making of their units: they have a large say in clients' therapies and there is an expectation that they will organise and facilitate groupwork as well as formulating plans, in conjunction with their clients, aimed at resocialisation along a wide variety of fronts.

This kind of sharing is one way in which nurses forego authority and enhance the control of their clients. Of course, much of this has to take place as best it can in an arena with definite boundaries in terms of key-holding, security generally and the granting of parole. Notwithstanding this, the reality of the clients' everyday lives, including the crimes which have brought them into the unit, *can* be reflected back to them and slowly integrated into a changing perspective of who they are and where they are going. In effect, everyday living problems are brought *into* the unit, specifically into the groupwork, which then becomes the focus of the client's reality-orientated therapy. A particular feature of therapeutic community practice is the regular occurrence of community meetings wherein issues of unit management and administration can be introduced and dealt with democratically. Both clients and staff participate although, again, not everyone shares the same enthusiasm for a mechanism which, potentially, can undermine professional intentions.

Professional Anxiety

Elements of high anxiety and stress accompany this kind of nursing and the business of being in close contact for long periods with people, some of whom have committed grave offences, can be brittle and tense. Staff attitudes, expectations and reactions can have a considerable effect upon the way in which the overall situation is managed. In fact, it has not been possible for these units to bypass the traditional dependence upon drugs, although some reduction has been achieved with the introduction of 'Control and Restraint': a Home Office (prison-developed) system of physical restraint and containment. Medication, however, continues to hold its place with most residents prescribed some form of the 'major tranquillisers'; and indeed, even those subscribing to the therapeutic community approach agree that some forms of medication are at times appropriate and necessary. Actually, the preponderance of so much serious mental illness among the forensic client population has led some to deprecate the very idea of therapeutic community practice as a viable option. After all, it is said, secure units were designed and resourced to manage the unmanageable: some of the residents are former or prospective Special Hospital clients or they might be prisoners who have lapsed into mental illness or, indeed, have come to a secure unit for assessment with or without treatment; in any event, it is said that the therapeutic community approach is too 'softly, softly' and that society has a right to the primacy of security.

Prisoners or Clients

One sentenced prisoner in five has some form of mental illness (Gunn, 1991). The conventional wisdom is that hundreds of such prisoners either languish unnecessarily in conditions of excessive security or are channelled inappropriately into the criminal justice system, when in fact they need psychiatric help. Having said this, most clients in secure units *have* committed serious and sometimes violent offences, including homicide. In addition, these crimes are more often associated with drinking, drug dependency and 'psychopathy' than with schizophrenia, manic depression, organic brain pathology or the neuroses (Guze *et al*, 1969). Higgins (1981) gave lists of referrals and diagnoses to his unit at Rainhill which fairly characterises the kinds of clients with which these units have to work: they are reproduced in this chapter in modified form here (see Tables 6.1 and 6.2).

Higgins's (1981) sample is interesting in that 34 of his referrals were refused admission to the forensic unit as not being disturbed enough or for having problems which had been somewhat exaggerated: forensic nurses are aware of the desire to pass on to them clients possessed of a high 'nuisance' value and part of their assessment strategy is to try to fill their places with genuinely 'disturbed' individuals for whom they can organise a workable rehabilitation package. Also notable is Higgins's statement that:

> No patient categorised as psychopathic disorder alone has been admitted as the medical and nursing have reservations about psychopathy as a diagnostic entity, its response to medical treatment, and the wisdom of attempting long-term treatment in a small closed unit lacking many social and occupational facilities (Higgins, 1981, pp.892–893).

There is a lengthy tradition in psychiatric nursing, generally, of scepticism and anger at this particular client group and a peculiar lack of tolerance shown towards them. May and Kelly (1982) identify this response as an outcome of nurses' perceptions of the psychopathic client as one who refuses to legitimise the nurse's therapeutic functions; possessing neither readily identifiable technical skills nor unambiguous authority, nurses

Table 6.1   Reasons for referral as possible admissions to secure unit

	Behaviour	Men	Women
Hospital	Violence and violent threats	14	6
	Arson	1	3
	Aggressive sexual acts	1	0
	Persistent absconding with possible		
	risk to others	5	0
	For rehabilitation	1	0
Remand Centre	Violence and violent threats	9	6
	Property offences/previous violence in		
	hospital	3	0
	Theft and absconding	0	1
	Arson	1	0
Prison	Obvious mental illness	4	1
Special hospital	No longer needing maximum security		
	for rehabilitation	12	2
Out-patient	Violence and violent threats	4	3
	theft and absconding	0	1
Total		55	23

From Higgins (1981), reproduced with permission.

Table 6.2   Diagnoses (excluding 11 re-referrals) or referrals in Table 6.1 for possible admission to secure unit

Diagnosis	Men	Women
Schizophrenia	24	9
Personality disorder	8	8
Personality disorder/schizophrenia	6	1
Affective psychosis	4	2
Brain damage/personality disorder	2	0
Epilepsy/personality disorder	2	1
Total	46	21

From Higgins (1981), reproduced with permission.

look to their interactions with clients as a means of sustaining some sort of professional identity; when their therapeutic advances are rejected – especially in the absence of 'mental illness' – then their reactions can be fierce.

Section Three

VIOLENT INCIDENTS

Secure units constitute a focus for the investigation of violence as an aspect of mental illness. While findings are still tentative there appear to be several stable features accompanying most violent outbreaks (Fottrell, 1980; Dooley, 1986; Rix, 1988). Initial violence tends to occur between clients with nurses constituting the other main group of victims; most incidences are minor (the majority of clients being non-violent) and the perpetrator tends to have a history of violence: the majority of incidences occur during the morning. Of course, comparisons between studies is made difficult by variations in perceptions of what constitutes an aggressive or violent outburst. Violence also seems to be situation-specific. In other words, a conviction for a violent crime such as rape hardly predicts a client's reactions in a secure setting.

While the actual structure of secure units is a controlling factor in itself, in line with the potential violence of some clients nurses may have to employ limit-setting techniques so as to ensure the safety and well-being of themselves and others: there is a need to identify quickly residents who possess hostile elements and to develop a capacity of becoming aware of predictable patterns which might signal impending aggressive behaviour. Early detection systems enable the nurses to initiate alternative approaches aimed at warding off overt aggression. Added to this are recreational diversions such as structured activities and counselling approaches aimed at reducing client's anxieties and promoting their sense of self-control.

Aggressive attacks do occur, however, and forensic nurses have become skilled in containing them physically when they do. Occasionally, it becomes necessary to seclude clients, a manoeuvre which, again, some find more acceptable than others. The practice is described in the Mental Health Act (1983) code of practice as: 'the supervised confinement of a patient alone in a room which may be locked for the protection of others from significant harm'. Supporters assert that the goal of seclusion is to assist clients to gain control of their aggressive impulses by reducing sensory stimulation, removing social interactions which can be frustrating and providing a safe, controlled environment. Seclusion also helps to maintain a balance between the needs of the individual and those of the larger client group within a potentially volatile atmosphere. In general, it ought to be kept to a minimum and used as a last resort; it should be used for short periods only and reviewed regularly. In a recent review, McMillan (1993) recognised that variations in its use still abound, especially within secure settings, but that the confidence being gained in using alternative approaches to violence and aggression could make a phasing-out of seclusion a realistic option.

The alternative approach to containing disturbed behaviour is by prolonged physical restraint and/or high doses of medication: however, where there is provision for an 'intensive care area', that is, a lockable, self-contained and closely supervised living space (within the unit) where disturbed individuals can be cared for away from the general area, it has been found that aggressive or violent behaviour is dramatically reduced (Kinsella *et al*, 1993). Needless to say, in the general run of events on these units, an obvious requirement is to be able to interpret and respond appropriately to bizarre ideas and challenging behaviour. This places additional demand upon the communication skills of the nurses both with other professionals and with clients themselves.

THE BELIEFS AND ATTITUDES OF THE NURSE

Feelings can sometimes run high, even among professionals; nurses possess skills but they also have feelings. All secure units have their share of sex offenders and when the victim has been defenceless and/or weak it becomes understandable if a diagnosis of mental illness fails to abolish the natural anger which most of us have in the face of such outrages. Of course, for those who see all moral problems as relative then the entire question becomes a redundant issue and, indeed, it would seem today that there are professionals who would be prepared to offer counselling to Hitler.

However, for most of us it can be difficult to face these issues or to work for people who have perpetrated heinous crimes. With this in mind, many secure units have attempted some form of staff training or therapy group where these, and other such issues, can be worked on and to some extent dealt with. To a degree, these groups have proved more attractive to the therapeutic community people than to those who are more security-minded; they have been of benefit, nevertheless.

RESEARCH

The Butler Committee had noted (pp.10–11) a marked lack of research in forensic care, a particularly strong factor in their not being able to obtain straight answers to some of the basic questions which they were asking. They recommended that the new units should contain built-in sub-systems of evaluation. The South East Thames Region was particularly well endowed for this since their central unit contained an experienced research capacity. Indeed, a fair amount of research has taken place, albeit precious little of the kind which seeks to enquire from nurses and clients how they actually feel and believe about their situation overall and the future of forensic care.

A particular development in response to assessed need has been the Court Direction Scheme. This scheme directs mentally disordered offenders from the Courts into health care settings, thus avoiding potentially harmful stays on remand. It identifies people with a mental illness as soon as possible after their arrest, offering advice to the Crown Prosecution Service, probation service and police. It also arranges for these offenders to be assessed with a view to admission for treatment to an ordinary psychiatric facility and it provides a necessary liaison service between all of the agencies involved with clients.

Hillis (1993) reports that the West Midlands Diversion Scheme has identified clear areas for future investigation; people with mental disorders who offend can, she says, be successfully diverted away from the criminal justice system with a pivotal role being played by the community forensic psychiatric nurse. The question of what constitutes mental disorder and the extent to which it should mitigate criminal activity are, of course, important issues; Hillis (1993) states that the kinds of mental disorder which might divert the client away from prosecution are psychosis, depression, potential self-harm and substance/drug abuse and always, of course, only in connection with non-serious offences. If the offence is serious (for instance, involving violence) then placement in a secure unit is considered with an informed decision being made by the Crown Prosecution Service about prosecution later on.

THE FUTURE

Twenty years ago the Butler Committee recomended 2000 medium-secure places, yet today there are but 600. The Reed Committee (Reed, 1992) suggests that the number of places offered by medium-secure units should increase substantially with an accompanying increase in the numbers of forensic psychiatric nurses describing forensic nursing as an 'under-developed speciality'. Employing authorities in conjunction with institutes of nursing should consider these implications, they argue, particularly in relation to staffing issues. Also, there needs to be a greater examination of the interface between the joint planning of health providers and the Prison Service so as to facilitate both the specialised needs of prisoners and forensic offenders. The Reed Committee similarly raised concerns about the dramatic drop in the number of places in lockable wards in psychiatric and learning disabilities hospitals. This, of course, has implications for Community Psychiatric Nurses who may have to incorporate elements of forensic nursing into their training programmes as well as provide clinical placements accordingly. Finally, there is the thorny question of the ideology of secure units, especially if they declare themselves to be therapeutic communities. Some units have seemingly dealt with this issue by ignoring it. For those who have chosen to propound a therapeutic community philosophy, the result has been a degree of confusion with not a little anger expressed by its opponents. However, in the attempt lies great merit: in trying to fashion a safe, professional approach which is yet humane and therapeutic there lies only credit.

REFERENCES

Barton R (1959) *Institutional Neurosis.* Bristol: John Wright and Sons.
Bluglass R (1978) Regional secure units and interim security for psychiatric patients. *British Medical Journal,* **1**: 489–493.
Butler R A (1974) *Interim Report of the Committee on Mentally Abnormal Offenders.* Home Office and DHSS, Cmnd. 5698. London: HMSO.
Butler R A (1975) *Report of the Committee on Mentally Abnormal Offenders.* Home Office and DHSS, Cmnd. 6244. London: HMSO.
Clarke L (1991) Therapeutic Community Principles and Practice within a Secure Environment. University of Brighton: Unpublished thesis.
Dean M (1976) The case of Anthony Ledger. *Guardian,* 5 June.
Delmont P (1987) Special Assessment and Supervisory Service: A Descriptive Study. Falmer, Brighton: Sussex and Kent Institute, Unpublished dissertation.
Dooley E (1986) Aggressive incidents in a secure hospital. *Medicine, Science and the Law,* **26**(2): 125–130.
Fottrell E (1980) A study of violent behaviour among patients in psychiatric hospitals. *British Journal of Psychiatry,* **136**: 216–221.
Fuller J R (1985) Treatment environments in secure psychiatric settings: a case study. *International Journal of Offender Therapy and Comparative Criminology,* **29**(1): 63–78.
Gilbert D and Levinson D (1956) Ideology, personality and institutional policy in the mental hospital. *Journal of Abnormal and Social Psychology,* **53**: 263–271.
Glancy J E (1974) *Revised Report of the DHSS Working Party on Security in NHS Psychiatric Hospitals.* London: DHSS.
Goffman E (1960) *Asylum.* Harmondsworth: Penguin.
Gray W J (1973) The therapeutic community and evaluation of results. *International Journal of Criminology and Penology,* **1**: 327–334.
Gunn J (1991) *Mentally Disordered Patients.* London: Home Office.
Guze S *et al* (1969) Criminality and psychiatric disorder. *Archives of General Psychiatry,* **20**: 583–591.
Higgins J (1981) Four years' experience of an interim secure unit. *British Medical Journal,* **282**: 889–893.
Hillis G (1993) Diverting tactics. *Nursing Times,* **89**(1): 24–27.
Kinsella C, Chaloner C and Brosnan C (1993) An alternative to seclusion? *Nursing Times,* **89**(18): 62–64.
May D and Kelly M P (1982) Chancers, pests and poor wee souls: problems of legitimation in psychiatric nursing. *Sociology of Health and Illness,* **4**(3): 279–299.

Mental Health Act (1983) London: HMSO.

McMillan I (1993) Special solutions. *Nursing Times,* **89**(18): 67.

Pilgrim D and Eisenberg N (1985) Should special hospitals be phased out? *Bulletin of the British Psychological Society,* **38**: 281–284.

Reed J (1992) *Review of Health and Social Services for Mentally Disordered Offenders and Others Requiring Similar Services: Final Summary Report.* London: HMSO.

Rees T P (1957) Back to moral treatment and community care. *Journal of Mental Science,* **103**: 303–313.

Rice C E *et al* (1966) Measuring psychiatric hospital opinion about patient care. *Archives of General Psychiatry,* **14**: 428–434.

Rix G (1988) Violent incidents on a regional secure unit. *Journal of Advanced Nursing,* **13**: 746–751.

Sharp V (1975) *Social Control in the Therapeutic Community.* Lexington House, Mass: Saxon Books.

Snow K (1991) Ashen Hill: from historical beginnings to therapeutic community. Falmer, Brighton: Sussex and Kent Institute, Unpublished paper.

Snowden P R (1983) The regional secure unit programme: a personal appraisal: the present state of play and future plans. *Bulletin of the Royal College of Psychiatrists,* **7**: 138–140.

7 Complementary Therapies in Psychiatry
Lynne Phair

INTRODUCTION

Complementary therapies are now being discussed and written about in all the media avenues. Nurses are becoming aware of them, if not understanding their application and use; many treat them with scorn, suggesting that they are trendy fads which can never replace conventional medicine.

It is worth explaining the use of the terms 'alternative' and 'complementary', both of which are frequently interchanged with no regard to their appropriate use. Some individuals feel that there is a fundamental gulf between the way that *orthodox* medicine views, treats and prevents disease and the way that *alternative* medicine treats disorders and the person. Others argue that both systems are working towards the same end, namely assisting the body to heal itself, using whatever method is appropriate, thus using *complementary* therapies (Holmes, 1984).

This chapter describes a number of complementary therapies, giving a brief description of their function and uses which they may have. Psychiatry is itself an evolving science. Changes occur in the treatment of clients, faster possibly in psychiatry than in any other field of medicine. Treatments which were used only 15 years ago, such as deep insulin therapy, are now only found in the history books. The theory of psychiatry is turning more and more to approaching the client in a holistic way; taking physical, psychological and social histories; using multidisciplinary teams to draw up care plans with the client which will address their mental health needs. Clients may receive counselling, occupational therapy, music or art therapy, enabling them to explore their innermost thoughts and beliefs; and, with support, work to deal with issues that may be causing them distress.

Yet, are they being helped 'holistically', are they being encouraged to take responsibility for themselves and their lives, while being supported and enabled to heal themselves? Some may argue that this does not always happen, and this is when the use of complementary therapies can work alongside the orthodox treatments agreed with the client. To illustrate this opinion, let us look for a moment at the subject of stress management, together with the cognitive approaches to the client's eventual identification of the stressor, how the stressor is dealt with and their subsequent recovery.

Teaching relaxation techniques can be a problem. Clients do not always have the capacity to identify their level of stress (unless presenting as an anxiety attack) or if they do, may not be able to concentrate on the instructions being given when learning techniques because of their own preoccupations. By using aromatherapy or reflexology a level of relaxation can be achieved, thus enabling the client to identify the aim of the cognitive methods which he is being taught. The client may also need dietary advice, or discussion about how to continue working with stress after the therapist has completed her work. An introduction to yoga, relaxation by music, or visualisation may assist the client in taking responsibility for themselves with the therapist's assistance.

Many complementary therapies work in areas which are still not understood or accepted by traditional medicine. Shiatsu, reflexology, colour therapy or iridology are examples of these. Homœopathy and aromatherapy are regarded by many to work purely by a placebo effect; yet some, namely acupuncture, hypnotherapy and chiropractic (Booth, 1993), are becoming accepted and are used in Health Service establishments.

The physical, spiritual and mental components of a human being are more complex than any one person can begin to understand. Looking after the whole person, using all of their senses, and all of the therapies, can only enhance the client's potential or ability to deal, themselves, with themselves.

Some Examples of Complementary Therapies

Many therapies can offer active help and support to people suffering from mental health problems. It is impossible to describe them all. The six therapies described here are, therefore, simply a glimpse at a world not yet fully understood or integrated into the NHS. It should be emphasised that for most therapies appropriate training and qualification should be obtained before embarking on their use with clients (Trevelyan, 1993). A few can be used with great benefit to both nurse and client, for example skilful touch, by having a little knowledge and a good understanding of the skills needed to implement them.

REFLEXOLOGY

Reflexology or Reflex Zone Therapy has been known to man since Egyptian times; hieroglyphics on pyramids depict foot massage, and in Ancient Greece, Russia, China and India the powers of foot massage were used to heal many ailments.

Reflexology is a simple yet practical and effective way of treating people of all ages in any environment. It works not by simply massaging the feet, but by a combination of massage and palpation of all areas of the foot, generating positive energies which act upon the natural energy pathways of the body. In reflexology the whole of the body and its systems are reflected in the feet and are mirrored exactly. The big toe reflects the head; the side of the small toe replicates the shoulders; and the whole of the spine is reflected along the medial aspect of both feet.

The foot is also divided into 10 vertical zones, as postulated by Dr William Fitzgerald (Marquardt, 1983). There are hypotheses that these vertical fields depict meridians which run from head to toe, commencing in the centre of the body and working outwards. The feet reflect these meridians with 10 zones, five on each foot, commencing at the head and spanning outwards.

How Has Reflexology Become Part of Today's Life?

Although there is evidence to support theories that reflexology has been practised for at least 5000 years, it has only recently become re-established as a therapy, acting by creating a homeostasis of the whole body.

At the beginning of the century Dr William Fitzgerald, an ear, nose and throat specialist, found that by massaging certain parts of the foot he could affect another part of the body. Together with a colleague, he used a dramatic demonstration to convince others of his theory's validity by sticking pins into a volunteer's face without pain, if he first applied pressure to the relevant point on the person's foot or hand (Norman, 1988). This work was continued in the 1930s by Eunice Ingham, a physiotherapist, who concluded that there were specific areas of the foot for each part of the body and mapped them accordingly. This early work has now been developed, and many foot maps now exist.

How Does Reflexology Help People?

The reflexologist has no magical powers: the therapist is there to facilitate the body to balance itself by clearing the natural energy pathways of the body, thus enabling the body to create its own homeostasis. By looking at the foot, as well as by feeling, the therapist can gain knowledge about the health status of a client. With experience it can be noticed where blemishes, callouses and corns are; the structure, tissue tones or oedema may reflect ailments which may be occurring in the body (Lett, 1983). Eczema over the oesophageal sphincter on the foot may indicate a problem of heartburn, or gastric irritation when the person is under stress; hard skin on the heel may point the therapist towards the person's lower back for investigation. This has to be taken in relation to the person, however: a blister on the big toe may not indicate migraine, but simply ill-fitting shoes! None the less, the ill-fitting shoes might cause headaches due to adverse pressure on these points.

Reflexologists are not medical people, and cannot and will not diagnose ailments or offer specific treatments. This is quite clearly the domain of the medical practitioner; but by treating the person as a whole through the foot, the practitioner can encourage changes throughout the body's energy pathways which benefit every aspect of a person's life.

The therapy has nine main functions (Norman, 1988). The most active of those is the effect on the person's stress levels and the treatment's ability to induce deep relaxation. Everyone's life-style today has an element of stress attached to it; and no one person should judge whether another person's life is or should be causing them to experience raised stress levels. So often today the fast pace of life refuses to allow the effect of everyday pressure to be dealt with (Norman, 1988). This has a knock-on effect, causing a person's 'base line stress level' to be raised. To feel the body's true level of relaxation usually requires deep commitment from the person, provided that they recognise they have a high stress level. Often an ailment which is actually stress-related precipitates in a physical form, e.g. irritable bowel syndrome, migraine, insomnia; these are the manifestations which the person wishes to treat.

By inducing a level of relaxation which is nearer to the person's base line stress level the body becomes able to commence, using its own complicated mechanisms, to heal itself (Lett, 1983). With this fundamental activity achieved the reflexology treatment can then continue to facilitate other positive benefits, as follows.

- It improves circulation. Due to relaxation of the cardiovascular system blood flow, even to the capillaries, improves.
- It cleanses the body of toxins. The lymphatic drainage system also experiences dilation with effective relaxation, thus enabling effective drainage from cells to the body's elimination systems.
- It creates homeostasis. By working with the whole of the body through the foot the person, not just an organ, receives care and attention.
- It revitalises energy. By clearing the energy pathways of the body through a series of treatments the physical and emotional energy balance will be returned.

- It acts as a prophylactic treatment. With a regular holistic relaxation technique such as reflexology the body responds proactively in its defence against infection. If the person is feeling well as a whole the immune system appears to be more efficient.
- It facilitates mental stimulation. This also, as a direct result of deep relaxation, enables the person to be more alert, less exhausted and experience enhanced concentration levels.
- It helps to formulate relationships. Particularly when caring for people with mental health problems, gaining the trust and confidence of a client is the basis for any constructive work, regardless of the nature of the illness. Gaining intimate knowledge can, for some clients, be almost impossible to divulge. The acts of reflexology for the practitioner enables a trusting bond to develop through touch. The level of care which is transmitted through the type and time spent on the client enables the practitioner to give undivided attention to their client demonstating an interest in the whole person rather than just the problem. The bond which develops is very rapid and is of a quality not easily accomplished with more orthodox techniques.
- It is rewarding for the practitioner. It is a pleasant treatment to administer to any client but the returned benefits are felt by the practitioner, if they are able to concentrate their minds on the activity which is happening within that room. The relaxation and positive energy flow returns to the practitioner, recharging themselves with every session.

Reflexology in Practice

The use of reflexology with clients suffering from physical illness is becoming more widely accepted in many areas of general medicine. To find such treatments being used in NHS establishments is still, however, rather unusual. There are conditions which should not be treated with reflexology. These include acute infections, deep vein thrombosis, unstable pregnancies and some malignancies (Evans, 1990). Areas such as postnatal care (Evans, 1990) and palliative cancer treatment and anxiety management (Thomas, 1989) are, however, being treated successfully with this technique.

Its direct use in psychiatry has, to date, been documented only in a limited way. When deciding the projected effectiveness of the treatment the client's mental state must be considered carefully. Fragile ego boundaries may make touch difficult or inadvisable; however, for a defensive withdrawn client touch in a safe area such as the feet may encourage a relationship. Elderly confused people who wander or clients who are agitated may find the stationary nature of the treatment difficult. However, the average length of a treatment time of 40 minutes may be altered to suit the individual needs and abilities of the client. Alternatively, the practitioner may begin the treatment programme by working on the hands (as the reflex zones are also mirrored here) (Norman, 1988), and once the client feels comfortable with the practitioner the therapy can be transferred to the feet. The average course of treatment is between six and 12 sessions, depending on the severity of the ailment and how long the person has been suffering. They may feel no benefit until after the third or fourth treatment, when a variety of effects may occur. As the body begins to excrete the toxins and the energy begins to flow the person may feel tired, lethargic or energetic; experience diarrhoea, polyuria or rhinitis. Whatever the individual experiences, however, is unique to them and is the body's way of dealing with unwanted waste. If warning is given to the client of these effects, anxiety can be allayed.

Most psychiatric conditions would respond favourably to reflexology but objective evaluation of the cause of improvement, as with most psychiatric nursing interventions, would be difficult to conclude. Thomas (1989), however, demonstrated the benefits of reflexology in anxiety management, compared with more traditional techniques, proving that it was not simply physical contact which promoted a positive response in clients.

Snapshot Histories

A 59-year-old man with long-standing emotional problems due to the break-up of his marriage, lacked confidence, was indecisive and had a very poor sleep pattern. He received six reflexology treatments, and complained to the therapist after five that he had missed his alarm call by oversleeping. His counsellor reported that he was more confident and decisive about his life situation. The man agreed with this, and felt more able to deal with unresolved issues.

An 83-year-old woman had an aggressive dementing husband; she was restless, agitated, not wanting to go out, unable to climb the stairs to her daughter's flat, and ruminating about the situation. She could not identify in herself any tension and described herself as the same as she had always been; she refused a relaxation tape, having tried it once before and had not been able to follow the instructions. After eight treatments she slept all night, was able to walk up the stairs and was also able to identify the feeling of relaxation. She was reintroduced to the relaxation tape with which she now felt comfortable; and was also pleased to join a women's support group.

A 44-year-old professional woman, divorced but with a boyfriend, had been consuming eight aspirins a day, she thought, for 20 years as she always felt 'rotten'. She was unable to identify specific features except lethargy, melancholia, poor sleep pattern and weight gain. Her GP had found nothing abnormal. On examination tender areas were found on the thyroid reflex and the stomach reflex; however, the client was treated holistically and after three treatments reported weight loss and improved sleep pattern. Her aspirin intake had dropped to four per day. After nine treatments there had been a cessation of her aspirin intake and she felt energetic enough to take her son on a 5-mile walk.

AROMATHERAPY

Aromatherapy means 'a therapeutic effect brought about through smell'. Smell is an underestimated sense in today's world, yet how often do we find our gastric juices flowing as we pass a bakery, or visualise a summer's day as we savour the sweet smell of a fuchsia? (Wise, 1989).

Alongside many complementary therapies, there is evidence that using essential oils was part of the life-style of the ancient Egyptians. In the tomb of Tutankhamen, opened in 1922, a number of ornate pots and stone jars were discovered containing essential oils. Hieroglyphics from the Ebas papyrus dating from the eighteenth dynasty showed recipes to cure inflammation (Tisserand, 1990). The Bible makes reference to the use of oils, including 'cinnamon, myrrh and holy anointing oil' (Exodus 30: 22–25). In seventeenth century England pomanders of oranges and cloves were worn to ward off the Black Death. During the nineteenth and twentieth centuries, however, with the development of chemistry and synthetic drugs, the use of natural essential oils became unfashionable and more traditional remedies were overshadowed (Westwood, 1991).

Interest in the use of oils was rekindled in 1937 when a French chemist, René Maurice Gattefosse coined the word 'Aromatherapy'. He rediscovered the power of oils when he burned his hand. He plunged it into the nearest bowl of liquid which happened to be lavender oil; his hand healed with exceptional speed, and recognising the antiseptic qualities of this oil he researched the properties of other oils. From this time, the use of essential oils has been developed until it is now a well-practised science.

The Properties of Essential Oils

The term 'essential oil' can be defined as referring to an odorous, volatile product obtained by a physical process from a natural source (Williams, 1989). Different oils come from various parts of the plant or tree:

Sandalwood: wood of the tree trunk
Bergamot: outer rind of the fruit
Geranium: leaf
Ginger: root
Ylang-ylang: flowers

To obtain these oils, a number of methods of extraction need to be used. The most common method is steam distillation, where the essential oil is separated from cooled condensed water. Another method used for fragile flowers is that of solvent extraction. The flowers are placed in layers of wax and solvent which is changed daily; these are then centrifuged and distilled, the process taking up to 20 days; consequently these oils are expensive. Citrus oils are obtained by expression. This method involves crushing the fruit, or machine abrasion of the outer rind, depending on the locality of the oil.

Because of the specific location of the oils, vast quantities of the source plant may be needed to obtain therapeutic doses. Two thousand grammes of basil is required to obtain 1 g of essential oil; 70 g of rosemary is required to obtain 1 g of oil, and 100 g of dried *Anthemis nobilis* is required to obtain 1 g of Roman Chamomile (Williams, 1989).

It is a widely held misconception that essential oils are no more than pleasant-smelling perfumes and their effect is purely placebo in nature. Closer examination of the oil however, reveals that their chemical construction contains active chemical compounds. The process of smelling is also more than simply a pleasant addition to the sensory system. The sense of smell in humans is not used as actively today as in past years. Smelling one's enemy or detecting food sources are skills lost in modern times (Tisserand, 1990). The physiology of smell has not yet been explained well. Olfactory nerves are in direct contact with the air and it is thought that the messages are translated into sensation or coded impulses. The fibres of the olfactory nerve are in direct communication with the limbic system of the brain, wherein rests the centre of feelings and emotions (Williams, 1989), thus having a direct effect on the mood and emotions of the person.

The oils have a complex mixture of chemical compounds; all the constituents are organic and fall into two main classes, hydrocarbons and oxygenated constituents. Within these classes, there are main groups of chemicals: terpenes, alcohol, phenol, aldehyde, ester and ketones. Different oils have varying combinations of these main components, thus giving oils their specific and wide-ranging properties (Williams, 1989).

Practical Uses of Aromatherapy

Aromatherapy enables essential oils to be used in a variety of ways, all of which are therapeutic, yet a different method of adminstration can be suggested depending on the nature of the ailment and the character of the person in receipt of the treatment.

Massage

The most traditional and most well-known use of essential oils is massage. The recommended oil is added to a base oil at a ratio of between 1–3 per cent depending on the client, and is massaged into the body using techniques which work on the sympathetic nervous system and on the lymphatic drainage system. Massage, therefore, has three effects. It is a powerful relaxing agent and the use of lavender has been identified to reduce heart rate, respiratory rate, blood pressure and pain in patients in an intensive care unit (Hewitt, 1992). It activates the release of toxins from the body cells, and it enables essential oils to be absorbed through the skin and have a therapeutic effect. A successful massage may often induce a mass excretion of toxins from the body about 8–12 hours after the treatment, usually in the form of a charge of energy, bowel evacuation or polyuria.

Bathing

Bathing can be used as a support to massage treatment or as an independent treatment. For someone suffering from insomnia a 5 ml blend of camomile in a bathful of warm water will aid relaxation and induce sleep. Soaking for about 10–15 minutes enables the oil to be absorbed adequately. Bathing can be suggested daily. By this means, if the person is suffering from depression or an anxiety state, this treatment encourages them to take more responsibility for themselves.

Inhalation

This is a useful technique for relieving congestion and catarrh. Placing two drops of a decongestant oil such as eucalyptus into two pints of boiling water and placing the head over the bowl covered by a towel effectively relieves cold and 'flu symptoms.

Compresses

These are useful in first aid. Placing a compress of water and oil on a bruise or damaged part of the body can bring immediate relief.

Vaporiser

By using an essential oil burner the small reservoir of water with the oil of choice is heated and vaporises. The room is then scented and the effects of the oil are absorbed by the olfactory sytem. Oils which have an antiseptic property, for example teatree and lavender, are able to act as an antibacterial agent inhibiting airborne transmission of disease. In hospital settings a pleasant aroma can, in itself, assist in alleviating new clients' anxieties about their unusual surroundings (*Journal of Aromatherapy*, 1988).

Foot Bath

If a client is unwilling or unable to have a full bath, soaking the feet can enable the absorption of oils to be just as beneficial. The soles of the feet are considered to have a high absorbency rate and oils can be massaged here, too, rather than all over the body to obtain a therapeutic effect.

Using Aromatherapy in Psychiatry

By offering the client time and personal attention the psychological benefits of aromatherapy are unquestionable. When used by competent qualified practitioners, blends of oils can offer relief to many clients with mental health problems.

Snapshot Histories

An 87-year-old man who suffered with Alzheimer's disease was constantly shouting out and trying to get up from his chair although he did not have the strength to do so. A blend of marjoram, geranium and neroli used regularly in the bath and as a foot massage enabled the man to be more at ease.

A 34-year-old woman whose son was born profoundly deaf was informed, when he was five-and-a-half years old, that he had Ushers Syndrome, a genetic disorder that had a degenerative process that would cause him to be blind by his teenage years. She was very distressed and experiencing morbid thoughts about herself and her son. She was receiving counselling but was emotionally and physically exhausted, due to insomnia and ruminating thought patterns. A body massage and baths three times a week with a blend of melissa, geranium and frankincense enabled her to sleep, relax and regain control of her thought processes and to work through her fears about the future.

The use of Aromatherapy in psychiatry will be seen in the future as a normal part of the holistic approach, which is needed to ensure that people can find treatments to suit their own needs. This treatment should not be used unless an experienced aromatherapist is monitoring closely the treatment and progress of a client.

A Selection of Essential Oils Beneficial to Clients with Mental Health Problems	
Oil	*Psychological uses*
Lavender *(Lavandula officinalis)*	Hyperactivity; insomnia; mood swings; worry about the future; suspicion; anxiety attacks
Basil *(Ocimum basilicum)*	Poor memory; poor concentration; mental stimulation
Bergamot *(Citrus bergamia)*	Anxiety; depression; obsessions; lack of confidence; stress
Clary sage *(Salvia sclarea)*	Compulsiveness; insomnia; restlessness; stress; relaxation; negative thoughts
Frankincense *(Boswellia thurifera)*	Bereavement; fear; insecurity; perseverance; worry; irritability
Geranium *(Pelargonium odorantissium)*	Mood stabiliser; body balancer
Marjoram *(Origanum marjorana)*	Hyperactivity; overwork; agitation
Melissa *(Melissa officinalis)*	Humility; anxiety about the future
Camomile *(Anthemis nobilis)*	Restlessness; anxiety; worry; insomnia; low mood
Ylang-ylang *(Cananga odorata)*	Anger; impatience; low self-esteem; suspiciousness; anxiety; guilt; feeling of unworthiness

For more information, see, for example, Westwood (1991) and Tisserand (1990).

MASSAGE

Of all the complementary therapies massage is probably the one therapy which will cause people to raise their eyebrows and snigger. The term has been linked to immoral activities, and so the therapeutic value of the treatment has been undervalued. The action of massage, confusing sensuality with sexuality, causes people from a British social culture to at least deprive each other and themselves of the relaxing activity of touch. Adults take opportunities to substitute the lack of touch in their lives by stroking animals or cuddling children and babies. In some cultures touch is quite acceptable and so, in turn, is massage.

Massage is a systematic manipulation of body tissues which has a therapeutic effect on the nervous and muscular systems of the body. The body has the ability to automatically redistribute body fluids; the calf muscle, for example, acts as a pump within the legs which during contractions favours the return of blood flow towards the heart from the feet. Massage is therefore a manual substitute for normal body activity.

Along with other therapies, massage has a history which is recorded in the scriptures of ancient times. Hippocrates recorded the use of massage in treating sprains and dislocations of joints and muscles. Ancient Greek and Roman literature advocates the use of massage before and after sport, during convalescence and after bathing to treat melancholia, asthma and digestive problems (Maxwell Hudson, 1988). In India massage has always been greatly valued, and the art of massage is used by mothers on their babies, and in turn by the children on their parents. Massage is mentioned throughout historical literature; for example, both Sir George Simpson's *Voyage Around the World* and Captain Cook's accounts in 1779 describe treatments of massage for sciatica and general physical ailments.

It was a Swede, Per Henrik Ling (1776–1839) who developed a systematic approach to massage which formed the basis of the therapeutic massage known today, by identifying five basic movements and simple sequences. The various levels of muscle tissue can be reached and massaged in a therapeutic fashion. The nature of his work is still recognised and 'Swedish Massage' is the correct term to use to describe the types of movements undertaken. However, because of other associations that have been attached to this term, 'Therapeutic Massage' may be more commonly used.

Enabling the client to become relaxed by using physical and personal techniques began to lose attraction after the First World War, when mechanical and chemical relaxants were developed. Slowly, today, the personal skill of therapeutic massage is once again being discovered, as side-effects of chemical treatments are becoming more well-known.

The Function of Therapeutic Massage

Per Ling identified five types of movement which together formed a therapeutic massage technique.

1. *Effleurage*: a stroking movement laying one or both hands flat on the part being treated, placing firm pressure in the direction of the venous flow; moving in a rhythmical fashion enables an increase in venous circulation; improvement in the arterial circulation by removing congestion in the veins; improves lymphatic circulation; improves both desquamation and relaxation.

2. *Pétrissage*: all pressure movements which enable picking up and moving the muscle away from the bone in a firm, controlled manner. The muscle tissue may also be moved along the line of the muscle and reversed to promote an even distribution of pressure. This movement

causes compression and relaxation of the muscle, ensuring filling and emptying of veins and the lymphatic system; this in turn eliminates fatigue, assists the breakdown of adipose tissue, relaxes hard muscle, and momentary contraction by this movement strengthens them. Kneading of the alimentary tract affects the involuntary muscle and stimulates the action of peristalsis.

3. *Friction*: the skin is moved by the fingertips and pressure is put on the fibre by pressing on the underlying bony surfaces. This movement enables a breakdown of adipose tissue and fibrous thickening, assists in the dispersal of oedema and stimulates the circulation.

4. *Tapotement*: all movements are percussion, which includes the popular image of massage movements such as hacking and cupping; all are performed on the larger muscles of the body. These movements strengthen the muscle, cause dilation and contraction of the superficial vessels, stimulate the nervous system, increase tissue activity and break up fatty deposits.

5. *Vibrations*: this movement applies to the stimulation and relaxation of the nerve endings by the fingertips. The effect of this movement stimulates the nerves, relieves pain and loosens both scar tissue and adhesions.

Psychological Benefits of the Physiological Action of Massage

It is quite clear that the action of massage has obvious physical effects on the body. These physical effects in turn assist in creating positive psychological energies which benefit the client by improving the circulation, releasing muscular tension and toxins, and creating a calm rhythmical action; the client benefits by: feeling more relaxed; trusting the practitioner and allowing their body to find its own level of rest; this in turn ensures that the breathing slows and deepens, the heart rate slows, blood pressure lowers and the parasympathetic nervous system is enabled to take a balanced control of the body systems (Ashton, 1984).

The action of the massage enables the practitioner and client to form a trusting relationship; sometimes the client is not confident enough to express themselves verbally or is unable to recognise the tension being held within them. By using massage it enables doors to open and a closer relationship to develop between the two people (Passant, 1990). It also prevents the client and therapist from playing psychological and non-verbal games which can develop in traditional counselling techniques. Barriers have to be broken down due to the intimacy of the treatment, and trust will develop (Byass, 1988).

The benefits for the practitioner must not be underestimated. The practitioner, by ensuring a focus of attention on the client, can control their breathing and muscular tension, as successful treatment cannot be given if the practitioner cannot control their own level of tension; it also enables the practitioner to have permission to communicate non-verbally to the client, a skill which is particularly beneficial if the clients are unable to communicate verbally or to understand verbal support. It is also a beneficial therapy in areas when physical care, by the nature of the client group, takes priority over psychological care, and staff wish to take time to encourage relationships with their clients. Using massage ensures the same relaxing quality for both the giver and receiver (Maxwell-Hudson, 1988).

Snapshot Histories

A 45-year-old man suffering from manic-depressive psychosis was experiencing a hypomanic phase in his illness. The man, more than 6' tall and weighing 16 stone, had been administered phenothiazine medication, but was still experiencing over-activity and flights of ideas. He was becoming physically exhausted and distressed. He was given a back and neck massage in a quiet darkened room. After 30 minutes he settled and fell asleep while the massage was occurring. He slept for 8 hours.

An 87-year-old woman had been admitted to hospital for respite care. She had no clinical diagnosis of psychiatric disorder but was unkempt, antisocial and refused help for her arthritis. She had painful rheumatism in her hands and found moving them difficult, and feeding herself impossible. A hand massage was administered every day for 1 week, when she was able to use her hands more easily and was able to feed herself again.

A 74-year-old man suffering from multi-infarct dementia was becoming distressed as he could not open his bowels. He was continually looking for the toilet, although he found it difficult to articulate his needs. He refused medication. An abdominal massage was performed and within 12 hours he opened his bowels and became quite settled in the ward.

BACH FLOWER REMEDIES

Bach Flower Remedies, by the nature of their name, are sometimes confused with aromatherapy as both are prepared from plants. The fundamental difference, however, is that the remedies and essential oils are prepared in completely different ways. Essential oils are highly concentrated and prepared usually by complicated means, whereas remedies are produced from whole flowers or plants and the remedy is extracted by relatively simple means.

What Are Bach Remedies?

The 38 remedies discovered by Dr Edward Bach in the 1930s are all elements of plants and flowers, which Dr Bach intuitively felt could assist people in their fight against disease. The remedies work on the principle that people are affected mentally or emotionally by both physical and psychological disease, and by healing the mind the body would also be healed.

Dr Bach trained at the turn of the century in orthodox medicine and practised these methods; however, he later turned to homœopathy as a way to treat the whole person. It became unacceptable to him that only people's physical symptoms were treated, and in the 1930s he left London. After wandering the countryside, often sleeping under the stars, he found that he was developing a sensitivity towards plants and their energy (Davis, 1991). He became so sensitive to plants and their curative abilities that he would develop symptoms of that condition the closer he became to the source of the cure.

Working completely with the emotional aspects of physical and psychological disorders, Dr Bach emphasised that these remedies were not miracle cures, and the length of time the disease had been evident will reflect on how long it would take for the person to benefit from the remedies. It may also become apparent that as one set of emotions are dealt with, another different picture will present itself. It is felt that this may be due to a blockage in the energy flow of vitality and until this is remedied there will not be a positive response and harmony will take longer to achieve (Evans, 1991).

The Theory of How Bach Remedies Work

Proponents of Bach Remedies follow the beliefs of Dr Bach that life is a oneness of the higher self, of mind and body, and in obtaining an equilibrium the body would be able to heal itself properly (Ramsell, 1991). It is accepted that some people may not have the intellectual ability to identify what emotional effects a disease may be having on them, and it is at this time that a skilled practitioner may be able to assist in identifying the best remedy, or combination of remedies, to assist the spiritual body to heal the physical body.

It is advocated that remedies cannot necessarily heal disease, but if a person's emotional state is stable and the person is in a position of equilibrium, fears of the future, of the course of the disease or the impending knowledge of death can be dealt with confidently.

The Production and Use of Bach Remedies

Dr Bach advocated clearly defined methods of collection of the flowers and plants; and methods of preparing the 'mother tincture'. This included the time of year that the flower should be picked and how it should be prepared, particularly using unpolluted water and harvesting the flowers on a bright sunny day (Weeks *et al*, 1990). The tincture, after being preserved in brandy, sometimes indefinitely, is decanted into stock bottles and then in turn, diluted with mineral water, and put into a treatment bottle. The dose, ultimately resembling a homœopathic remedy, thus results in the tinctures working on a very subtle level (Davis, 1991).

The 38 remedies cover every negative state of mind known to man and Dr Bach requested that his discoveries should never be added to; his key word was 'simplicity', feeling that nature itself would hold the answer to man's ability to deal with diseases, whether fear of AIDS today or diphtheria in the 1930s (Ramsell, 1991).

It is propounded by the Edward Bach Centre that the remedies are not addictive and have no side effects (Ramsell, 1991). It is therefore appropriate for people to read the literature for themselves and select remedies to relieve their emotional trauma. Alternatively, an experienced practitioner may be able to select remedies more specifically depending on the character and emotional disposition of the client.

Probably the best-known remedy in general terms is the Rescue Remedy. It can be used in every kind of emergency, both physical and emotional (Davis, 1991). Rescue Remedy is a combination of Cherry, Plum, Clematis, Impatiens, Rock Rose and Star of Bethlehem. It is advocated to assist with every eventuality from a sudden emergency, examination nerves and visits to the dentist to helping a person in the terminal stages of their illness, dealing with inevitable eventualities with serenity (Evans, 1991).

Snapshot Histories

A 2-year-old boy, while playing at home, fell and sustained a 5 cm cut over his eyebrow. He was understandably distressed, and despite his mother applying direct pressure to the wound and comforting him, his screaming caused increased vasodilation and bleeding would not stop. Four drops of Rescue Remedy was administered sublingually and within 45 seconds the child was calm and the bleeding stopped. The mother was able to transport the child unescorted to hospital for sutures.

An elderly woman was suffering from rheumatoid arthritis. She was depressed due to the nature of her illness, her rigidity and pain, fear of the future and the course her disease might take. A remedy combination of Rock Water, Mustard and Mimulus was administered. The pain decreased, her mobility improved and her outlook became less rigid and severe (Evans, 1991).

TOUCH

The subject of Touch as a complementary therapy needs to be considered in two separate ways of using the same medium. Therapeutic Touch, called by other names 'psychic healing' or 'faith healing', is a specific therapy requiring the development of certain skills, which can be used to the benefit of people suffering specific diseases. The other form of touch therapy is less formalised, and yet it is documented as being valuable to all people when used skilfully by the carer: Skilful Touch.

Therapeutic Touch

Under a variety of names healing has been practised over centuries both in industrial and non-industrial societies. It is defined as a transfer of energy to support an individual's coping abilities by the laying-on of hands (Turton, 1986). In the USA it has now become an accepted technique to learn and is taught in at least 33 United States teaching departments as a formal course for the profession to utilise (Turton, 1984).

It is felt by many to be a gift; a direct act of God or spiritual intervention. However, the theory that the practice of the laying-on of hands does not have to be initiated in connection with any religious belief or divine intervention is receiving increasing support. Work by Dolores Krieger has identified specific theories and hypotheses surrounding the therapy. It is her theory that human beings are open systems, receptive to all energy fields, inorganic, organic, psychic and conceptual, which make humans receptive to all energies. The healer has to be an individual whose health gives them an over-abundance of energy. Known as 'Prana' and combined with a strong sense of commitment, this enables the healer to project this energy for the well-being of another. The healer therefore channels this energy-flow over the ill person to re-establish the impaired energy-flows of the ill person (Turton, 1986).

Krieger identifies four components to the process of therapeutic touch. The nurse or healer must:

1. be in a quiet and relaxed state;
2. be able to assess the energy field of the patient for clues to differences in the quality of energy flow using their hands;
3. mobilise by stroking or unruffling motions the areas of the body perceived as being energy-blocked; and
4. consciously direct her excess body energy to the client.

In one study where therapeutic touch was investigated, Krieger, together with Estebany, examined the effect of laying-on of hands on haemoglobin levels. The results showed that the group 'treated' by touch showed a rise in the level, whereas the control group showed no significant change. The same experiment was repeated using nurses trained in the skills. The results were the same, identifying the potential for this therapy within the health care profession (Turton, 1986).

Work with cancer sufferers also shows that therapeutic touch can benefit the client in a palliative way. Through these techniques a 50-year-old man suffering terminal illness felt that touch, combined with oils and massage, assisted him by communicating care, reducing his physical pain, reducing his sense of isolation, enhancing his will to deal positively with life despite his prognosis, and enabled him to return love and affection to his wife (Turton, 1989).

Skilful Touch

Touching people does not always happen in Western cultures as a matter of habit. Yet the need for touch is accepted in children and babies and in intimate relationships. The custom of touch is referred to metaphorically in the English language, implying its importance: 'keep in touch', 'handle with care' and 'rubbing someone up the wrong way', these figurative terms creating an unconscious reference to touch. During childhood, touch is a means of learning and discovering, and deprivation of early tactile experience may compromise a child's learning as well as his capacity for more tactile communication; as adults, touch becomes less evident in everyday life (Le May, 1986). However, touch is important in adult life, in intimate relationships or establishing relationships, expressing care and concern, or showing emotional support and understanding, and professionals in helping roles such as nurses, teachers or social workers should have a heightened awareness of these gestures (Hargie *et al*, 1983). The knowledge of touch and its interpretation is also invaluable to professional people. So many messages can be given; for example, establishing a relationship or destroying it by the professional's knowledge of personal space, obtaining permission to enter the client's personal space or the type of handshake offered and the messages it carries (Pease, 1985).

Touch in the nursing profession should be used as consciously as any other form of supportive technique. Watson identified two categories, Instrumental Touch, which is a deliberate physical contact needed to perform a specific task, and Expressive Touch, which is a relatively spontaneous contact offering psychological support (Le May, 1986). There are groups of people who are deprived of expressive touch, particularly the elderly (Hollinger, 1980). Despite the nurse's unsubstantiated belief that touch is used regularly, it is not used consciously to assist people in expressing themselves. Studies have suggested that touch helps people to compensate for bereavement, dependency and altered body image; it also helps to increase reality orientation in sensory deprivation (Le May, 1986).

The elderly are often exposed to long episodes of non-touch care, unless it is to perform a physical, often embarrassing, task. Prolonged episodes of bedrest have been found to cause behavioural changes including anxiety, hostility, dependency and discomfort (Hollinger, 1980). As a part of a client's psychological care, touch used in a skilful way can help to formulate relationships built on trust. If the nurse uses touch in a smothering way, it can be considered patronising and can destroy a relationship.

A small structured study carried out by Langland and Pannicucci (1982) indicated that touch is important in relational aspects of communication with elderly confused clients. Increased touch enhances communication and prevents sensory deprivation, and it is important that the skill is used effectively with clients of all ages – particularly those who are elderly and confused.

Snapshot Histories

A 47-year-old woman was experiencing some sleep disturbance and depressive feelings, which she claimed she had no reason for. She avoided eye contact, sat on the edge of her chair and played with her wedding ring. At a time felt appropriate by the therapist she placed her hand on the woman's forearm, and allowed a conscious silence. The lady began to cry and slowly began to talk about her fear that her husband was committing adultery.

An 87-year-old man suffering from Alzheimer's disease was wandering aimlessly around the ward. He was becoming breathless and his ankles were oedematous, and was in obvious need of rest. The nurse took him by the hand and sat him down, continuing to hold his hands in a comforting fashion, and began to talk about his family and late wife. He slowly became less anxious and talked about his life with the nurse.

REFERENCES

Ashton J (1984) In your hands. *Nursing Times*, 9 May: 54.
Booth B (1993) Chiropractic. *Nursing Times*, **89**(22): 52–54.
Byass R (1988) Soothing Body and Soul. *Nursing Times*, **84**(24): 39–41.
Davis P (1991) *Aromatherapy An A–Z*. Saffron Walden: C W Daniel.
Evans M (1990) Reflex zone therapy for mothers. *Nursing Times*, **86**(4): 29–31.
Evans J (1991) *Introduction to the Benefits of the Bach Flower Remedies*. Saffron Walden: C W Daniel.

Hargie O, Saunders C and Dickson D (1983) *Social Skills in Interpersonal Communication.* London: Croom Helm.

Hewitt D (1992) Massage with lavender oil lowered tension. *Nursing Times,* **88**(25): 8.

Hollinger L (1980) Perception of touch in the elderly. *Journal of Gerontological Nursing,* **6**(12): 741–746.

Holmes P (1984) Holistic nursing. *Nursing Times,* 18 April: 28–29.

Journal of Aromatherapy (1988) Aromatherapy on the Wards. *Journal of Aromatherapy,* **1**(2): 8.

Krieger D (1979) *The Therapeutic Touch.* Hemel Hempstead: Prentice Hall.

Langland R and Paniccucci C (1982) Effects of touch on communication with elderly confused clients. *Journal of Gerontological Nursing,* **8**(3): 152–155.

Le May A (1986) The human connection. *Nursing Times,* 19 Nov: 28–30.

Lett A (1983) Putting their best feet forward. *Nursing Times,* **79**(33): 49–51.

Marquardt H. (1983) Reflex zone therapy of the feet. In: *A Text Book For Therapists.* Wellingborough: Thorsons.

Maxwell Hudson (1988) *The Complete Book of Massage.* London: Dorling Kindersley.

Norman L (1988) *The Reflexology Handbook. A Complete Guide.* Bath: Piatkus.

Passant H (1990) A holistic approach in the ward. *Nursing Times,* **86**(4): 26–28.

Pease A (1985) *Body Language.* London: Sheldon Press.

Ramsell J (1991) *Questions and Answers Clarifying the Basic Principles and Standards of the Bach Flower Remedies.* Oxfordshire: Albey Printing Co.

Thomas M (1989) Fancy footwork. *Nursing Times,* **41**: 42–44.

Tisserand R (1990) *The Art of Aromatherapy,* 11th edn. Saffron Walden: C W Daniel.

Trevelyan J (1993) Aromatherapy. *Nursing Times,* **89**(25): 38–40.

Turton P (1984) The laying on of hands. *Nursing Times,* 2 May: 47–48.

Turton P (1986) Joining forces. *Nursing Times,* **19**: 31–32.

Turton P (1989) Touch me, feel me, heal me. *Nursing Times,* **85**(19): 42–44.

Weeks N, Weeks I and Bullen V (1990) *The Bach Flower Remedies Illustrations and Preparations.* Saffron Walden: C W Daniel.

Westwood C (1991) *Aromatherapy. A Guide for Home Use.* Christchurch: Kerbina Ltd.

Williams D (1989) *Lecture Notes on Essential Oils.* Sudbury, Suffolk: Bush Boake Allen Ltd.

Wise R (1989) Flower power. *Nursing Times,* **85**(22): 45–47.

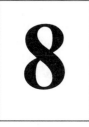

8 Nurses and Psychology
Liam Clarke

INTRODUCTION

Two central problems confront anyone setting out to describe psychology within a psychiatric nursing context. The first is to state what is meant by modern-day psychology. The second is to place this description into a psychiatric nursing context which will make sense to the average practising nurse. These are both formidable tasks: the second, in particular, is often neglected since few psychologists show much interest in the problems or interests of present-day nurses. In the first instance, therefore, it seems logical to describe what is meant by psychology before attempting to link it to the concerns or interests of nursing practice.

AN OVERVIEW OF PSYCHOLOGY

Let us state at the outset that potential students often misunderstand exactly what psychology is. Quite often they are attracted to a subject which they imagine focuses attention on the more dynamic aspects of human existence; a fascinating world of unconscious processes perhaps, ready to reveal its secrets to (their) inquiring minds. It must certainly come as a shock to discover that nowadays a pre-condition to the study of psychology is a working ability with mathematics. It must also come as a let-down to discover that most psychologists are hardly interested in people at all (that is in the sense of persons living out their lives in social situations) but concerned instead to tackle problems which typically involve *specific elements* of human or animal performance. For example, a substantial part of my education as a psychologist involved complicated experiments with Siamese fighting fish: many hours were spent on experiments designed to show that these fish displayed certain behavioural characteristics when exposed to a circular rather than to a triangular or square-shaped object when this was lowered into the water in which they swam! Now, I have little doubt that part of the rationale for this was to encourage my use of 'the scientific method' and to a certain extent this worked; however, since it had always been my intention to work with people I sometimes wondered if my psychology course could not have been better organised with this in mind. Certainly I was awarded my Degree without ever having to confront either my own or anyone else's values, attitudes or feelings about even the simplest aspects of human life.

In that not only can the subject-matter of psychology surprise us, so the sheer complexity of the issues with which it tries to deal can, to some extent, defy a neat description. Before proceeding to examine several of these issues in some detail, especially in the context of mental nursing, we should first try to define what psychology is as well as some of the terms it uses which, if poorly understood, can lead to considerable problems in the practice area.

DEFINITION OF PSYCHOLOGY

Psychology is the scientific study of human and animal behaviour. Ponder this definition carefully and note some of its terms. Immediately it will be seen how – just as in the case of sociology in Chapter 9 – it becomes necessary to continue to define terms within this original definition, in order to keep clear what it is we meant in the first place. As Burns (1991) points out, the term *behaviour* contains no moral implications and psychologists are hardly concerned about what the layman might regard as 'good' or 'bad' behaviour. Instead, they use the word to designate the totality of responses of which humans and animals are capable. Clearly, such behaviour functions at different levels and while some psychologists may be interested in, for example, human memory, others may be working out pathways and connections in the nervous systems of monkeys. One needs also to look at the words 'scientific study': this suggests that the methods used to examine behaviour are at least *similar* to those used in the physical sciences, namely the identification of an hypothesis about some aspects of behaviour and its manipulation within controlled conditions to see whether or not it behaves according to the hypothesis. The latter approach to the study of psychology has necessarily meant psychologists examining minute *aspects* of behaviour which, because minute, can be rigorously controlled.

Looking at this problem in a slightly different way leads us to try to define what a psychologist *is*.

Psychologist
Someone who has followed a university course (usually of degree standard) and obtained a degree in psychology.

Discussion

While it would be permissible for someone to describe themselves as a psychologist on the bare essentials of the above definition, this would only be in the sense of someone with an English degree calling themselves a writer. A more accurate occupational use of the term psychologist would be: someone who has attained the above requirement but has supplemented it with further specialised education or training in a particular aspect of psychology (see p.167). The following discussion summarises the work of some practising psychologists. It will become apparent that the groups which are of most relevance to our discussion are those psychologists who opt for clinical work as a career.

Clinical Psychologist

Someone who, having attained the educational standard of a psychologist, as defined above, has taken a further qualification in clinical work. This qualification implies supervised experience working with children or adults needing psychological help in a variety of situations. Although this experience is often in behaviour therapy, there are a growing number who offer a wide range of interventions under the guise of eclecticism.

Discussion

In other words, having taken a first psychology degree such people have chosen to work with people who have psychological or mental difficulties. In order to do this, however, they have had to undergo a training lasting 2 or 3 years in ward or community mental health settings and under the supervision of senior clinical psychology practitioners.

It is extremely difficult to obtain placements on recognised courses offering this training. This is because British universities churn out psychology graduates in large numbers every year and the 'clinical psychology option' is an extremely popular specialty among new graduates. Competition is desperate and many are disappointed. An interesting aspect of the selection of new graduates for this training is that training centres sometimes require that the graduate has spent some time (perhaps a year or more) working closely with psychiatric clients as a nursing assistant. One final point concerns the nature of the clinical training which the average British trainee undergoes. Almost invariably, this will be behaviourist in orientation: at the same time there exists a strong eclectic element in much British work so that the behaviourist theme has not unduly affected good working relationships within clinical teams of doctors, nurses and psychologists.

Psychiatrist

Someone who has graduated from a university with a medical degree and thus has become eligible to practise medicine. He/she has chosen that field of medicine which purports to deal with mental illnesses. Some may become even more specialised, working with the old or with adolescents. The psychiatrist is generally regarded as having overall responsibility for patient care and assessment. (This is a bone of contention among radical therapists from a variety of professions.) While not necessarily hospital based, psychiatrists invariably work from the standpoint of a 'medical ethic' and their strong propensity for physical treatments usually means that psychological treatments must take a back seat.

Discussion

It might seem, on reading the above definition, that the differences between the psychologist and the psychiatrist are more apparent than real. The essential difference between them is that the psychiatrist has had a medical training leading to qualification as a medical practitioner. In other words, he or she could have proceeded to undertake postgraduate training in general practice, paediatrics or dermatology; instead they chose to specialise in mental illnesses. In making this choice, they would have had to undertake postgraduate training (lasting approximately 3 years) in order to obtain the specialist qualification enabling them to practise psychiatry (and become eligible for a consultancy appointment after a reasonable amount of experience). Psychiatrists are the group with whom psychiatric nurses work most closely and, historically, doctors and nurses have usually been very closely linked in the management of patient care. (A small point here is that it is customary to refer to psychiatrists, as indeed all medical practitioners, as doctor; psychologists are not normally addressed as doctor.)

TRAINING

An interesting feature of the training of both these groups, psychiatrists and psychologists, is that the content of their training is almost entirely knowledge-based in the sense of being made up of a series of factual propositions which are said to be grounded in clinical observations and empirical evidence. Although there has been a modest move away from the biological elements, the budding psychiatrist is still rigorously examined on the 'facts' of illnesses, their diagnoses and pharmacological treatment. There are very few, if any, 'experiential' elements in their training: instead, the student psychiatrist is prepared in the mould of 'expert', educated in the traditions of diagnosis and prescription. There is a dramatic absence of emphasis on the 'person-to-person' aspects of psychotherapeutic relationships.

British psychiatric nursing, on the other hand, is almost exclusively experiential in terms of its training programmes; the knowledge-base is almost non-existent in some places and traditional examinations have been largely abandoned (something which medical schools would never do). Yet, extraordinarily, these two groups have continued to work hand-in-hand in the care of psychiatric patients.

How to Explain This

It would surely come as a great surprise to an outsider were he to look at the respective ways in which the different disciplines prepare their students, especially the astonishing divergences between the nurses and doctors. I would suggest that the explanation for these divergences has to do with power. Outside the clinical areas, for example in journals, conferences, seminars, and particularly in schools of nursing, nurses proclaim an interpersonal and counselling approach which even questions the traditional assumptions of medical practice. For example, they might ask if depression in women is partly due to social circumstances and marital pressures and not, strictly speaking, an 'illness' at all (see discussion on depression in Chapter 9). Most psychiatric nurses are nowadays familiar with such anti-'medical model' discussions. When these issues emerge in clinical settings, on the other hand, the medical profession simply act to obliterate this 'person-to-person' approach and insist upon their prescriptive right to diagnose and treat the patient. One result of this is that outside specialist centres such as the Cassell Hospital, it becomes difficult to find nurses practising in a non-medical and non-hierarchical manner. One outcome of all of this is that British nurses are not doing what, for so long now, they have *told us* that they are doing.

Notable exceptions to this are those small groups of behaviourist nurse therapists whose training has been so markedly influenced by developments in psychology. Behaviourism evolved within psychology, of course, and not psychiatry and it has remained the province of psychologists, although lately some nurses have become highly skilled in the use of its principles. The successful uptake of behaviourism by these nurses raises interesting questions of professional divisions within multidisciplinary teams. The nurse therapist is recognised as an autonomous practitioner in many respects and empirical studies (Marks *et al*, 1977) have shown that they are as efficient in their work as their clinical psychology colleagues.

Of course, the nurse therapist has achieved this without recourse to a psychology degree, rather undergoing a training in behaviourism sensationally more economical than psychology degree courses.

Examining the Complexities

Having thus looked at some of the roles of those involved in the practice of psychology it becomes necessary to return to an examination of the complexities of the subject itself. These complications operate at two levels, or categories. First, the term 'psychology' can be used in a rather loose sense to describe different aspects of personal relationships (and this is the commonest use of the term). Alternatively, it can refer to defined areas of human performance which are subject to disciplined inquiry by psychology academics designed to enlarge man's knowledge of human behaviour. We can examine both of these categories in turn by reproducing the kinds of 'psychological' statements which humans produce every day. Some examples are: 'Hey! You've got a bad attitude!' or: 'He's got a very nice personality,' or, even more precariously, 'Of course that's what you meant subconsciously'. Many people particularly resent the latter kind of 'psychologising', especially when it is directed at them! However, we should not become unduly worried about these examples of 'loose psychologising' since they can usually be demolished quite easily. For instance, 'attitudes' and 'personalities' cannot be good or bad, nice or ugly, big or small. They are words which represent what psychologists call 'hypothetical constructs'; that is, they are terms used to sum up or define aspects of thought and emotion which are *believed* to govern or affect human behaviour. They have no basis in brain physiology that we know of. We will never examine or touch someone's memory. Indeed, words like 'memory' and 'attitude' are simply a means of communication; 'word constructions' used to describe or define elements which are beyond direct observation – psychologists are (of necessity) quite good at inventing words to describe their work, although not nearly as good as sociologists! Put another way, if the word 'attitude' did not exist we would have to invent it to describe what we mean by 'attitude'. The following case study illustrates the point.

Case Study 1: The Trouble with Frank

Frank, a student nurse, was asked to attend a disciplinary interview with his senior nurse tutor. At one stage during the interview Frank was critically informed that he had a 'bad attitude' towards nursing and the nursing profession in general. Somewhat astonished, he asked for the evidence to support this: as far as he was concerned this was an amazing judgment on his character and behaviour. The senior tutor proceeded to tell Frank that, on more than one occasion, he had arrived late for his shifts, that he had long hair and that he occasionally looked dishevelled. The latter allegations being somewhat obvious left Frank feeling momentarily dumbfounded. Quickly, however, he recovered and made his reply:

> If I was always early and if I got a haircut; if I bought a two-piece suit and a shirt and tie are you saying that that would mean I had a *good* attitude?

Perhaps you would like to reflect on Frank's response, asking yourself when it *would* be possible to accuse *anyone* of having a bad attitude and the kinds of evidence you would need. Certainly, few of us would agree that short hair and accurate time-keeping constitute a 'good attitude' towards nursing. On the contrary, such simple, if highly visible, 'good' behaviours might indeed camouflage an otherwise poor nursing performance. Perhaps if the senior tutor had simply tried to deal directly with the late time-keeping and the long hair without recourse to psychological concepts he would have had more success. This is precisely the advice which contemporary psychologists would give in this situation: namely, deal with the behaviours since there is little to be gained by theorising.

On the other hand, there are occasions when a student might not be as obliging as Frank in providing such obvious attitude-indicators as long hair and poor time-keeping. Indeed, a student's behaviour might be subtle enough to require some degree of interpretation. For instance, a student might continually interact with clients in a manner which suggests a patronising or condescending approach: this may be based on the fact that the student uses a particular tone of voice, sullen looks and so on. In such situations as this it might indeed make sense to introduce a construct such as attitude so as to try to make sense of what the person is doing or why they are doing it.

In their professional lives nurses make such inferences all the time: for example, when they respond to client's talk by defining it as an indication of some underlying construct such as anxiety, sadness, guilt or denial. In fact, it could be said that it is the task of the nurse to make sense of the statements of her clients by forming hypotheses about what might lie behind the statements. We shall examine this aspect more fully when we come to deal with counselling psychology.

'A Clash of Personalities'

One often hears such a phrase as this from students who are attempting to explain why their ward supervisor gave them a poor report. It is yet another example of the kind of 'loose psychology' which people commonly employ so as to describe relationships. 'He has lots of personality!' is a frequent variation, as is 'She is a bundle of personality!' Of course, a person *cannot* have lots of personality: his personality is what it is and may actually vary in relation to different situations and circumstances: the latter point is something which holds true for all psychological characteristics to a greater or lesser extent. However, while people are rarely constant in this world there do appear to be some aspects of the self which are relatively enduring and stable across a wide variety of social situations and for these enduring and stable characteristics we use the word 'personality'.

Personality Problems

When we use the word 'personality' we are inclined to consider only those characteristics which we see as 'attractive' or 'exciting' and to quantify them in the person by saying that they have 'bags of personality' or whatever. When these attractive qualities are absent then we tend to say that the person has no personality (rather than that they are boring, or vague, for example). Similarly, when people refer to others as having a 'bad attitude' or a 'good attitude' what they often mean is that they are either repelled or attracted to these people in terms of how they see them, as either pleasant or unpleasant.

However, the formation and expression of attitudes and beliefs about other people are rarely objective processes. This is because our perceptions are largely an outcome of what we *want* or *need* to see in a particular situation or circumstances. As Immanuel Kant put it: 'We see things not as they are but as we are' or in the perhaps more telling words of the old saying: 'Beauty is in the eye of the beholder'. This last remark helps us to connect with the third and final aspect of loose psychology, namely the idea of the subconscious mind.

The Hidden Depths of the Mind: Fact or Fantasy?

In the case of the 'subconscious' remark (above) it must be reckoned that its fairly common usage does reflect a general, if vague, acquaintance with the notion of 'things not being what they seem'. Certainly, Freud's theory of unconscious life came to permeate almost every aspect of human existence and endeavour so that it comes as no surprise to find his terminology bandied about. I wonder, however, to what degree people realise the extent to which modern psychology holds much of what Freud wrote in mild contempt?

We may ask why has Freudian and/or psychodynamic theorising diminished: what went wrong with the Freudian dream? However, before attempting to examine the present-day place of psychodynamic psychology we had better define what we mean by these terms.

Psychoanalysis

Psychoanalysis is both a theory and a method. Originally devised by Sigmund Freud (although not entirely from original elements) as a theory it holds that all human behaviour and thought is determined by unconscious forces. It is also a method of therapy whereby an attempt is made to realise the nature of these unconscious forces. Both the theory and the practice of psychoanalysis have undergone considerable change and development since its inception. However, its practice is grounded in the fundamental principle of 'the transference': this lies at the heart of psychoanalytic therapy. The terms 'psychodynamic' or 'dynamic' and 'psychoanalytic' or 'analytic' may be taken as synonymous.

Before defining the role of psychoanalysts let us look more closely at the concept of transference which many psychiatric students find vague and elusive.

Transference

The transference represents the manner in which feelings produced by the patient (psychoanalysts continue to use the word 'patient') and directed towards the analyst are said to 'properly belong elsewhere'. For example, it might be said that the love or hate which the patient feels for the therapist is simply an expression of love and/or hate which lies unresolved from earlier relationships, with parents for instance. In other words, the therapist becomes a kind of receptacle for 'used' feelings. The following case study may help to flesh this out.

Case Study 2: The Hidden Meaning

Jim Ryan has been in psychoanalysis for almost a year: over the last few weeks Jim has started to argue with his therapist who, he feels, is not providing him with sufficient guidance and Jim links this with the cost of the therapy. A lot of anger is expressed by Jim towards the therapist.

This is a common enough event in therapy/counselling and there are a growing number of people who think that Jim may have a valid point of view: what, they might ask, is he getting for his money? However, particularly in psychoanalysis, there exists a tradition whereby such matters are presumed to contain a 'truer meaning' and that it is the job of the therapist to discover this meaning by interpreting or getting beneath the (apparent) 'mundane' statements of the patient. In this instance Jim's anger is interpreted as not being merely about money and the nature of the help he is getting, but rather represents a deeper anger against a father who was rarely present when Jim needed him; indeed, a father who demanded emotional payment of some kind if ever he *did* give attention to Jim. In other words, the arguments about money are an echo of unresolved feelings from the past which continue to rankle in the present. The feelings of anger (about payments) reflect deeper hatred of an unsatisfying father and a longing for love.

Transference Boosting

Analysts use certain techniques to enhance the transference. For example, the frequency of sessions (usually three to five sessions a week) increases both its occurrence and intensity: the darkened room with the patient facing away from the analyst encourages the transference on the rather sensible grounds that the more 'blank' the therapist is the more he can be used as a 'blank screen' to 'write' feelings upon. In order to remain as blank as possible the analyst will talk much less than other therapists/ counsellors, reserving his thoughts for infrequent interpretations similar to the one given to explain Jim's anger. The use of a couch where the patient lies down (if he wishes) is also said to enhance the transference. Additionally, the retention of the term 'patient' helps to define a passive partner in a relationship where the acceptance of the interpretations of a powerful therapist is encouraged.

> *Psychoanalyst*
> A therapist who practises psychoanalysis. He/she will have undergone a lengthy training involving a 3–5-year period in which they themselves have had psychoanalytic sessions at least three times weekly. They need not possess any academic or medical credentials (in Britain). The emphasis is upon their having undergone the lengthy novitiate of personal analysis. In America they *must* possess a medical degree.

Shifting Sands

Why did this once dominant brand of psychology reach such a low ebb in Great Britain? Well, the 'psychology of the unconscious' diminished in stature, as did all 'loose talk' about personalities, precisely because these concepts did not easily lend themselves to quantifiable measurement. Psychotherapies are essentially semantic in nature and contain few elements which are capable of being measured or tested scientifically: this is because the scientific method is all about numbers. In brief, modern psychology wanted to be a science and with the coming of behaviourist practice, which did emphasise observable (and thus measurable) phenomena, this seemed at least vaguely possible. Dynamic psychology, on the other hand, rested upon the theoretical *assumptions* of its founders and their acolytes and regardless of how brilliant or earthshaking (in the case of Freud) these assumptions might be, they were suspiciously incapable of verification. Let us examine this point.

Obsessional states

Freud stated that obsessional neurosis was an outcome of unresolved conflict occurring at about the time when children were being toilet-trained: he believed that a preoccupation with order and cleanliness revolved around initial encounters with faecal matter at a time when we are unable to make sense of the parental demand to disown it or let it go. Basic observations tell us that babies are by no means averse to their faecal matter. Equally, basic observations suggest that attempts to persuade growing infants to comply with social requirements can lead to extreme fractiousness. In some cases where the baby is uncooperative one suspects that considerable anxiety may be infecting everyone involved. However, the question is: how can one *prove* that a failure to overcome this conflict – between social demand and primitive (blissful) ignorance – leads to a later preoccupation with cleanliness and order? It is an attractive and fanciful idea but how do you test it?

Testing Assumptions

In trying to solve this problem, Paul Kline (1984) performed a longitudinal study in which the toileting behaviours of a range of babies were measured and compared with their performances later in life. Kline (1984) found no evidence to support the Freudian hypothesis: in other words, there was little or no connection between variations in potty training and adult mental health. Kline's evidence is enough for many and his work forms part of the successful assault upon Freudian and other 'speculative' psychologies which became fashionable in the 1950s and which have lasted (Eysenck, 1957; Gellner, 1985). However, not all of Kline's findings went against Freudianism (see Kline, 1984) and one wonders if there is not yet a great deal in Freudian psychology which simply does not lend itself to measurement but is life-enhancing nevertheless, or 'true' but from a non-measurable perspective. One is reminded here of D H Lawrence's dictum that water was two molecules of hydrogen and one of oxygen 'and something else': presumably the something else which makes it feel wet. One would not set out to measure poetry, for example, or put the latest novel to the scientific test, yet many find truth in the novel or poem; the fact is, there will always be those who find the Freudian kind of theorising about human nature irresistible and it is perhaps unsurprising that Freud's work was to prove a power stimulus to much of modern art, both literary and visual.

Look at the words of this old music hall song:

I want a girl just like the girl that married dear old dad.

Reflect on these words for a few seconds and try to imagine what they might mean. Next, let us see if we can find a meaning for them by considering one of the central tenets of psychodynamic psychology.

The Oedipus Complex

Taken from Greek antiquity it tells of Oedipus, who killed his father to gain possession of his mother: obviously an idea which is anathema to our contemporary beliefs and attitudes about families and relationships. Now, of course, dynamic psychologists do not believe that we go about our daily business with incest playing on our minds but they might suggest that, at some level of awareness, the idea persists as a repressed aspect of our overall sexuality. This question is of direct significance to us today, given our greater willingness to acknowledge incest and child abuse as a social reality. (Whether this greater degree of openness implies some degree of acceptance – a lessening of the anathema – is a vexed question yet to be discussed.)

We know from his case studies that Freud was presented with such material by some of his female patients: he eventually defined these 'stories'as fantasies inasmuch as the young women who told them to him were, in his view, giving expression to repressed elements of their sexuality. In fact, Freud believed that these fantasies of child abuse formed the core of the neurosis of those who held them.

The world has moved on and we are now prepared to recognise incestuous behaviour much more so today. As such, some are of the view that Freud got it wrong: these women *had* been abused but Freud, because of *his* unconscious complexes (resulting from his social upbringing in a different age), could not himself face the traumas of these, his patients. His solution was to cloak reality with a self-serving theory.

So – returning to the words of our song – *do* boys want a girl just like the girl that married dear old dad? Goodness knows, it's often said that men want their wives to be their mothers and intuitively we (men) certainly seem to shy away from thinking of our mothers in a sexual way. Shakespeare recognised this (centuries before Freud) in his portrait of Hamlet, who displays an obvious inability to come to terms with his mother's marriage to his uncle; but is it only the unseemly spectacle of a quick marriage which upsets Hamlet, or is it rather the impropriety of his uncle's usurpation of his father's place? And what is that place if it is not the bedchamber? Well, perhaps and perhaps not. You certainly cannot prove it and for those who find mystery distasteful, those who seek 'proof', such intellectualising about what lies underneath people's beliefs and actions may all seem a little preposterous. But is it?

MAKING USE OF PSYCHOLOGY

In fact, it is not my intention to suggest that such loose usage of psychological terms – 'psychologese' – is of no consequence: quite the contrary. There are many important areas of living in which our implicit theories of life (what we tend to refer to as our 'hunches') play an important part; for instance, whether or not you are given the next job you apply for will depend in large part upon the impressions your interviewers form of you, since few candidates assist their interviewers by *behaving* inappropriately. Most candidates have good references (we always supply 'safe' names); most candidates dress appropriately and they tend to supply the kind of information they hope their prospective employer wants. Indeed, my own experiences of interviewing potential student nurses are of my acceptance or rejection being based upon the kind of hypothesising which we discussed in the attitudes section earlier; it is simply often a question of 'hunch'. One takes a gamble because one cannot *know*: it simply is not possible to predict human behaviour, so one guesses (hopefully intelligently). Try to imagine a world in which it was possible to predict behaviour!

The Need for Certainty

We wonder endlessly about Hamlet's dilemmas and misfortunes, not knowing why he acts as he does yet feeling we might do the same; however, is it not this which fascinates us? Do we want the 'answer' to Hamlet? Psychologists such as Paul Kline might be tempted to say that we do, or the behaviourists might seek to ascertain the stimuli which condition poor Hamlet to respond as he does. Either way, they are looking for certainty. So many of us today believe that there is a psychological 'reality' – a kind of higher plane of psychological 'truth' which takes precedence over the actual lives we lead and the ordinary language we use when trying to lead it. For example, many of us are not averse to beginning sentences with: 'Psychologically speaking, of course . . .'

Perhaps this is the major fault of psychology in the modern age, particularly counselling psychology; namely, that it suggests that there *is* a psychological answer to all of our problems (if we would just listen to the counsellor).

When the American sociologist Garfinkel (1967) instructed counsellors to respond to clients with stock answers chosen *at random* he found that the clients were satisfied with their counsellor's responses *even when told of the nature of the responses they had been given.* Not for nothing have counsellors been called 'the secular priests' (North 1972) and Garfinkel's experiment is ample proof of the esteem in which many people hold counsellors: nor is the counselling role a difficult position to maintain with demoralised clients receptive to practically anything that may be thrown at them. Of course, experienced and/or better prepared therapists/ counsellors recall Freud's remark about 'taking away the neurosis so that people can get on with the ordinary miseries of life' and cut their therapy-cloth accordingly. The danger today with so much of what passes as counselling is that even the ordinary miseries are subjected to analysis and cure leading to a situation which can only be described as the psychologisation of everything. The problem we face with many of the new counsellors is that while the theories and languages they use are 'loose' and weak (sometimes obviously so), the ideology of counselling is ferociously strong: woe betide he who criticises the counselling classes!

The point at issue here is not to deny that the loose usage of psychological terms is without meaning: but we need to ask how this loose psychologising differs from psychology 'proper'; indeed, what do we mean by 'proper psychology'? Perhaps we should examine this now.

But I Could Have Told You That!

Perhaps the best way to do this is to consider yet another common saying, this time often produced by lay people in response to their being told the findings of some psychological experiment. Most teachers of psychology are familiar with the response, 'But I could have told you that!' or 'I already knew that!'.

Common sense and basic intuition do indeed suggest many 'truths' to us: they are called home truths when someone else has to bring them to our attention! However, much will depend upon the meaning of the phrase 'to know'.

Contemporary psychology seeks answers to questions which can, broadly speaking, be communicated in such a manner that if the experiment which produced the answers was performed again the same answers would be obtained. A brief reflection on this will suggest the following.

1. The experiment and its findings will need to be expressed in as mathematical a fashion as possible so as to facilitate repeating it.
2. The problems it seeks to solve will need to be very closely identified and labelled.

These two requirements help to explain the Siamese fighting fish experiment which I introduced at the beginning. The problem with this mathematical approach is that while it enables us to give answers that are concise, factual and repeatable, the content of the answer is of little use to human affairs. Does it really matter if Siamese fighting fish respond to a circle rather than to a triangle? Yes, it is interesting when psychologists demonstrate, via exhaustive tests, that humans can typically recall seven snippets of information within a defined period of time but, apart from the interest, what does it tell us about Hamlet, love, hate, jealousy (or any of the other great strands of life)?

THE CONCEPT OF PSYCHOLOGY

Broadly speaking, academic or 'proper' psychology fits within a paradigm of science best defined as quantitative. By this is meant that the subject matter with which psychology deals must be capable of being measured in a mathematical way; in a way which can be communicated either by numbers or, at least, in a manner which can be easily replicated. What this invariably leads to is a severe restriction on the investigation of those areas of human life which many people might *think* are the province of psychology, so that it comes as a surprise to learn that psychologists have little patience with ideas or assertions which cannot be quantifiably verified, favouring instead issues such as depth perception in water-deprived rats or object perception in Siamese fighting fish. Even in the field of human social psychology, there is an emphasis on accurate measurement where a typical experiment might be designed to ascertain the effects of short (as opposed to long) rest periods on typing speeds, or factual recall of number sequences. Indeed, having surveyed the current interests of psychologists, a leading (if unorthodox) psychologist summarised the current picture as 'Man buried under the debris of a million investigations' (Shotter, 1975). In fairness, it must be added that most of this refers to research or 'academic' psychology. However, even in the field of applied psychology the picture is remarkably similar, a situation which has come about with the advent of Behaviourism.

Behaviourism
This school is now fairly dominant within British psychology. Essentially, it states that psychology should restrict itself to those aspects of human performance which can be observed, measured and thus more easily predicted or altered. In this instance the connection with other sciences becomes obvious. Further, its practitioners take the view that behaviour is *learned*, so that so-called mental illnesses are actually examples of poor or maladaptive learning.

This view has given rise to an approach to therapy which is much favoured by British clinical psychologists, and not a few nurses (Barker, 1985): the similarities with academic psychology are clear. To begin with, behaviourists treat those syndromes (very effectively) which have distinct parameters and which by their nature can yield the sort of improvements which are clearly measurable and communicated: phobic states and compulsive disorders are good examples. The theoretical background is diametrically opposed to the psychodynamic theories of Freud which we discussed earlier and, hence, the therapeutic approach differs too. Recall Freud's theories on obsessional behaviour, especially the presumed link with the unresolved difficulties surrounding the parent–child relationship during potty training. In dynamic therapy the method is to find the unresolved complexes which lie deep in the patient's unconscious and which are making him obsessional. In a sense, obsessional behaviour is the client's forlorn attempt to 'undo' the guilt which surrounds the anxieties about what may or may not have happened during the early period. Behaviour therapy, on the other hand, is *dramatically* different. For a start, it takes little account of so-called unconscious motives, although nowadays it *does* attend closely to the conscious thoughts of the client (in which case the behaviour therapist may call himself a cognitive–behaviour therapist or other synonym). However, the overwhelming emphasis is upon the here and now. The following case study highlights these differences.

Case Study 3: The Housebound Prisoner

Mrs Jones has remained inside her house for almost 4 years, frightened even to open her front door. In addition to the many problems which this poses for her it also poses many difficulties for her family. It is hard to imagine Mrs Jones's position and that of others like her as anything other than a living torment.

Behaviourists take the view that Mrs Jones has *learned* to behave this way. Perhaps one day while shopping in a supermarket she became giddy and frightened. She discovered that it paid to withdraw from the supermarket since such avoidance brought relief from the sense of fear. This process (of avoidance) continued all the way from the supermarket, down the main street, through side streets, up the garden path and finally into her house. In other words, because each of these stages had made her anxious in turn, she was quick to avoid each in turn, thus reinforcing her feelings of relief but unfortunately ending up as a prisoner in her own home.

Discovering the Antecedents

It is important for behaviourists to discover the antecedents which led up to Mrs Jones's panic in the supermarket: these can and will be written down. Next, the feelings which surround these antecedents must be carefully notated and Mrs Jones can write these down herself. Better still, she can attach a number of them in terms of how she perceives their severity. In this way she is invited to construct a hierarchy of her anxieties ranging from mildly threatening to utter panic. The therapist (nurse) can then begin to expose Mrs Jones to her demons gradually, slowly sensitising her to the realisation of how groundless her fears about them really are. She is *literally* shown that walking down the high street is safe and that her notions of panic are misguided.

Opponents of behaviour therapy often fail to recognise its tremendous value in getting people back into circulation again. Usually the client will be back in the supermarket in about 6 to 18 weeks. As such, behaviour therapy is 'effective'; it produces 'results' which are capable of being observed and measured and it is economical of therapeutic time. Not surprisingly, it is the counselling approach most favoured by cost-effective-minded managers. Indeed, on occasions the behaviour therapist may deputise a member of the family (for example, a husband) to implement and support the ongoing therapy. Again, this is very viable in economic terms but it also raises interesting therapeutic issues, as the following anecdote suggests.

Case Study 4: The Reluctant Wife

Many years ago I worked as a staff nurse on a ward where electric treatment was given in a cavalier fashion. A depressed woman had been admitted and was shortly afterwards prescribed electric treatment. However, she retained sufficient self-control and determination to be able to refuse persistently to have it. Having failed to persuade her, we hit upon the idea of enlisting her husband's support: accordingly, he was drafted in to persuade her to give consent and he succeeded in this over a period of time. Justifiably proud of our ingenuity we soldiered on, oblivious to the possibility that her husband might very well have contributed to her depression. For all we knew or cared he might well have been the reason for her mental problems.

This is not simply a question of ethics: transactional analysis is a psychological concept (Berne, 1964) which holds that people's 'problems' are a function of interrelationships and other social processes. Most of us could probably agree with this to some extent. Behaviourists, however, imbued as they are with the notion that human behaviour is at the mercy of (apparently) random environmental stimuli, seem incapable of reckoning with the more subtle complexes which comprise human affairs. I suspect that because they deal with people whose problems are manifest, the 'ordinary subtleties' of living take a back seat and people are grateful for getting some release from their more gross compulsions and obsessions. Ironically, it turns out to be the behaviourists who fulfil Freud's dictum: it is they who remove the neurosis so that people can get on with the 'ordinary miseries of life'.

Nurses and the Practice of Psychology

Behaviourism, in fact, is an area of psychological practice which has taken strong root in nursing in recent years. This followed the findings (Marks *et al*, 1977) that psychiatric nurses (following appropriate training) were as effective in its implementation as clinical psychologists. This has led, in Great Britain, to the provision by the English National Board of a statutory (1 year, full-time) training for the qualification of Nurse Behaviour Therapist.

This is not without its problems, however. Many Community Psychiatric Nurses, for reasons which relate to ethical problems of control and power, are wary of behaviourism as a therapeutic tool. Their criticisms stem from the same framework as those who criticise behaviourism generally: namely that it smacks too much of control of client's lives, as well as being superficial and incapable of getting close to the deeper emotional problems of clients. Yet it is intriguing that the complementary English National Board course leading to a similar qualification in psychodynamic therapy is rarely available, and with an uptake (or demand) which is extremely limited. Why should this be so?

One answer is that behaviour therapy may be seen by cost-effective managers as more measurable in outcome terms. As stated, behaviour therapists tend to deal with clients whose problems are such that any improvement, however temporary, will be clearly seen and so easily chalked up as a positive result; for example, diminution in external rituals, lessening of phobic anxiety and so on. Managers *like* such observable improvements which they in turn can demonstrate as an effective use of resources. Unsurprisingly, perhaps, behaviour therapy courses are the ones which they are most likely to support.

So Is Psychology Relevant to Nurses?

At this point we are much better placed to answer our initial question concerning the extent to which psychology is or is not relevant to psychiatric nursing. We are in a better position because we can now see the need to narrow the focus: many of the problems of therapeutic research arise from the fact that questions are formulated in very general terms; for example, 'Is psychotherapy effective?', and so on. We need to be more specific than that. Therefore, we can now see that *some* psychology, behaviour therapy, is relevant to some nurses but by no means to all. Most other psychology *could* be relevant if only there was not the extraordinary distance between the findings produced by increasingly artificial and complex studies (by university-based psychologists) and the vicissitudes of daily living. If we take an example from psychiatry we can see that the exact connection between the neurotransmitter substances (for instance, dopamine) and a 'schizophrenic' person shouting obscenities in public is fraught with exactly this problem. Between his dopamine and his behaviour, so much intervenes in the adult life of a schizophrenic person. Contemporary psychology deals with this problem by a process of scientific bypass: it simply refuses to regard life events as scientifically valid since they are not measurable – with the exception of behaviourism and so-called cognitive interventions. In this instance, nurses have also learned that it is 'acceptable' to approach a client's problems in a pragmatic manner, as the following example shows.

Case Study 5: The Organisation Woman

Jane Slocumbe has been referred to her local Mental Health Centre where she is allocated (under supervision) to a student psychiatric nurse. Miss Slocumbe finds it difficult to carry out daily living tasks and complains of feeling morose. Friendless, she becomes apprehensive at the thought of meeting people in much the same way as she becomes anxious at the thought of having to do household or other chores. Behind in her work for the same reasons, she says that she is rarely happy but is moderately content when not faced with the impending drudgery of having to do something.

Having listened to Jane, student nurse Baily advises that a task-orientated schedule be implemented. Jane, she feels, has a problem with her time management and might be better motivated if given a printed schedule. This schedule could specify a variety of tasks to be completed within a predefined time span. A separate column could be used for Jane to record her feelings and thoughts when carrying out these tasks so that they can be examined later: student nurse Baily opines that Jane's position is, overall, illogical, based as it is upon Jane's contention that being active increases her feelings of anxiety. Hopefully, says student nurse Baily, when the illogicality of her position becomes clearer, Jane should improve. The student quickly passes over Jane's comment on her father's death one year earlier as 'probably irrelevant' and of little use in the practical application of her therapy.

Pragmatism and the Nurse

Of course, British nurses have often been characterised as pragmatic, realistic and 'can do' people; certainly, the general public admire their angelic commitment to a kind of work which most would find disturbing or unacceptable. Who, other than nurses, would wish to immerse themselves in the intimate daily lives of other people? Only nurses, it seems, are moulded to take care of life's messes, be they physical or emotional. Should we, therefore, expect them to let go of their pragmatism when engaged in the business of trying to disentangle client's psychological problems? What I am saying here is that even when the British psychiatric nurse adopts the mantle of 'counsellor' it is still a pragmatic undertaking; the 'counselling' becomes a new tool, a 'talking tablet'; a treatment protocol to be applied to a client which in this instance becomes 'a patient by any other name'. This may even be true in the way nurses handle the 'softer psychotherapies'. One is reminded, here, of Menzies' (1960) contention that nurses surrounded themselves with tasks and rituals as a defence against anxieties induced by coming 'too close' to their patients. Perhaps the more recent uptake of 'the counselling approach' is but a more subtle barrier against intimacy: the feigned intimacies of the counselling relationship being a facade which *suggests* that we are helping clients but which is really a re-expression of an age-old control as well as a desire to be *seen* as a helping profession in tandem with others.

Other Problems

Having said this, however, it must be recognised that the greatest barrier to the practice of psychological therapy by nurses is the 'hit and miss' nature of its delivery. This is because nurses, unlike all other psychological disciplines, do not work in a discretionary manner: they are mandated to manage wards or caseloads *not of their choosing* and with a time frame (the shift) which is radically different to other professional frames.

Nurse–client relationships are always a function of the settings in which care is delivered. In typical psychiatric wards it becomes difficult to implement even the most basic tenets of the counselling relationship. For example, in the contracting phase of the counselling relationship it is considered desirable to:

1. initiate matters by agreeing to the number of meetings to take place;
2. outline the length of the counselling sessions; and
3. regard as crucially significant the concept of confidentiality.

Let us briefly examine these points in turn. First, it is difficult to agree on a number of meetings when the nurse may be called away, for example to another ward. Secondly, the length of the counselling sessions cannot be agreed with confidence. What, for instance, if another client becomes disturbed: can the nurse–therapist continue to function with *her* client if this happens? Lastly, in the context of confidentiality, what assurances can be given to a client that conversations will remain as private utterances between the client and the nurse–therapist? Very few, since tradition demands that almost all nursing material becomes part of the multidisciplinary team's discussions.

Professional Identities

These are the problems of a discipline which has yet to find its professional identity. I would define contemporary nursing as possessing an incoherent identity and this makes it all the more difficult to answer questions about the relevancy of psychology – or, indeed, anything else – to its practice. We have stated that psychology, in the form of behaviourism, is clearly relevant. On the other hand, we know that many nurses dislike behaviourism and attempts to identify mental nursing practice with behaviourism (Barker, 1982) have foundered. Other psychological therapies have had a major influence on psychiatric nursing practice: for example, the humanist approach to therapy popularised by Carl Rogers (1965) has had considerable influence upon British psychiatric nurses. Over and above this, however, is the manner by which the managerial/household responsibilities of nurses, handed on through generations of institutional care, militates against a discretionary application of such therapies. Indeed, this has sometimes resulted in psychiatric nursing being conceptualised as a mechanical undertaking forever aligned with (psychiatric) medical treatments. For instance, how many nurses today would claim to work *psychologically* with their clients as opposed to implementing psychiatric (usually physical) treatments? A conventional and very popular response to this question has been: 'Why not both? Surely it is possible to apply a psychological treatment, for example counselling, while giving a physical treatment?' I well recall such responses to my apprenticeship enquiries about the issue of talking to patients while bathing them. 'But what', I would ask 'if I want to talk to them *rather* than bath them? What if I just want to talk to them?' To such questions I was invariably given a muttered, resentful and non-committal response.

A Psychological Practitioner?

This is the central issue which surrounds the idea of whether the nurse can or can not be a psychological practitioner: the issue of *being required* to administer physical treatments (whether agreeing with them or not). This will always work against the nurse implementing the therapy of his or her choice. Having said this, there is certainly scope for nurses to acquire psychology skills and knowledge, of the applied rather than academic kind. This will mean a nurse better equipped to deal more effectively with both clients and fellow professionals. Becoming more 'psychological' will thus enhance the standing of nurses. Time will tell whether or not it encourages greater autonomy of practice: in plain speaking, whether we will see the delivery of therapeutic programmes to clients that are based upon sensible psychological and social principles.

REFERENCES

Barker P (1985) *Patient Assessment in Psychiatric Nursing.* London: Croom Helm.

Berne E (1964) *Games People Play.* New York: Grove Press.

Burns R B (1991) *Essential Psychology,* 2nd edn. London: Kluwer Academic Press.

Eysenck H (1957) *Sense and Nonsense in Psychology.* Harmondsworth: Penguin.

Garfinkel H (1967) *Studies in Ethnomethodology.* Englewood Cliffs: Prentice-Hall Inc.

Gellner E (1985) *The Psychoanalytic Movement.* London: Paladin.

Kline P (1984) *Psychology and Freudian Theory: An Introduction.* London: Methuen.

Marks I, Hallam R S, Connolly J and Philpott R (1977) *Nursing in Behavioural Psychotherapy.* London: Royal College of Nursing Publications.

Menzies I (1960) A case study in the functioning of social systems as a defence against anxiety. *Human Relations,* **13**: 95–121.

North M (1972) *The Secular Priests.* London: George Allen & Unwin Ltd.

Rogers C (1965) *Client Centred Therapy.* London: Constable.

Shotter J (1975) *Images of Man in Psychological Research, Essential Psychology Series,* ed. Herriot P. London: Methuen.

9 | Sociology and Mental Nursing
Liam Clarke

INTRODUCTION

Most 'sociology for nurses' textbooks follow a path whereby the student is provided with a definition of sociology, given an overview of its development as a discipline, followed by a static presentation of its main topics in an ordered sequence. We may surmise that practising psychiatric nurses would want to go a little deeper than this, however: they would want to know the *relevance* of sociology to their job; they would enquire how different sociological categories 'fit in with' or at least accompany the practice of nursing. 'What', they might ask, 'has sociology to do with nursing? Can there be such a thing as sociological nursing?' Or, putting the question more modestly, 'Is it possible for nurses to work in a sociological manner?' Dingwall and McIntosh (1978) argue that nurses *ought* to know more about sociology so as to achieve a better understanding of their own situation as well as that of their patients. Similarly, Briggs (1984) states that a systematic study of the social role of nurses is:

> natural as well as necessary for the committed nurse who wishes to understand more about herself, about her patients and about her relations with other people with whom she works (Briggs, 1983, p.xv).

Nursing is of natural interest to sociologists since it is the major caring profession (Cox, 1979). Additionally, sociologists, including nurses, desire to examine the different dimensions of caring (Morse *et al*, 1991) and especially the various models of health care which currently lie at the heart of most nursing discussions. Psychiatric nurses have absorbed much from their counselling colleagues in recent years, particularly following the implementation of the 1982 English National Board Mental Nursing Syllabus. The language of caring, for instance, merges imperceptibly with that of psychotherapy. Indeed, the counselling relationship described by Rogers (1967) lies at the heart of psychiatric nursing, which aspires towards a caring rather than a curing model.

THERAPY IS ABOUT RELATIONSHIPS

Therapy is frequently said to be about relationships: relationships lie at the heart of therapy (Egan 1986) and the preparation of today's psychiatric nurses largely derives from this premise. Placing this directly in a nursing context Briggs (1983) states that,

> The whole concept of care and of nursing as a caring profession can be grasped only if relationships are considered as well as tasks. Nor is it possible to isolate the problems and processes of nursing from the social context . . . within which we all live (Briggs, 1983, p.xv).

So if sociology is essentially concerned with relationships and groups it follows that anything which assists the nurse in building positive relationships with clients will aid the client's well-being. Of first importance here is the ability of nurses to evaluate the social context of care delivery; specifically, the conditions in which they are expected to work.

This is not an idle issue, since nurses work 'at the coal face' for many hours at a time and not always in salubrious conditions: they are entitled to inquire about the real-life applications of theories and models which are usually developed outside the workplace. Indeed, even when practising nurses are included in the process of, for example, curriculum development many practitioners still question the 'real-life viability' of the programmes which may result.

Nursing is, by definition, a social activity: indeed, I would suggest that nursing is an occupation partly characterised by the determined hustle and bustle of its workplace encounters. This intensity may be largely true of many forms of nursing; however, the mental nurse regularly encounters the peculiar intensity generated by people who may actively despise relationship formation at all: I refer of course to the mentally ill.

However, it is impossible to imagine any kind of nursing which does not involve forms of social encounter: this is a statement which needs examining.

THE NATURE OF SOCIAL ENCOUNTERS

It might be said that some activities are essentially 'private' in the sense of belonging to the individual alone: for example, planning and preparation are two nursing activities which can be carried out alone and do not seem to require any social contact. However, even when planning nursing interventions alone there is a social element at play. Whether it is preparing the environment for an incoming patient or preparing mentally in anticipation of a trying or stressful day, all such 'activities' are about preparing for interactions; they are a rehearsal in the sense of anticipating the meaning of encounters and how they may be improved if one is adequately prepared for them. It is sometimes said that the good teacher is the prepared teacher. Indeed, if there is one thing which separates psychiatric nursing today from the past it is precisely this principle of intentionality, of trying to avoid hit or miss interactions with clients and instead engaging with them in the knowing way which comes from anticipation and preparation. This kind of purposeful interacting is enhanced greatly when infused with theory; indeed, the very notions underpinning readiness come from reflecting about the nature of what one is doing: nurses currently make sense of their interactions with clients by referring to a model or theory of practice. Although these models cannot take account of the myriad of elements of social encounters, they provide a framework whereby psychiatric nurses can begin to discuss issues with each other with a view to developing some sort of coherent philosophy of practice. In other words, models allow nurses to effect a necessary transition from

(a) preparation of self to
(b) theoretical reasons for such preparation to
(c) exchange of theorising so as to
(d) arrive at an ever more coherent of substantive theory of nursing care.

DEFINITION

The function of this chapter will be to examine some of the well-trodden paths of sociology but within the context of their relevance to mental nursing practice. However, while keeping to the general approach of sociology texts, I intend to provide a definition of the subject which leaves aside the history of the topic. I will then introduce and discuss a small number of sociological topics of direct relevance to nurses. Let us begin with the notion of a definition.

Cox (1983) refreshingly admits that a concise definition is elusive. If such conciseness is proposed, for instance: 'The Science of Society, its Laws and Nature', it will instantly be seen that this is so wide as to be pretty meaningless. At the same time, such tight definitions do suggest certain relevant aspects. Clearly, for example, we are interested in *society* and not the *individual* and we can straight away make a distinction between the study of psychology (see Chapter 8), which is essentially about individuals and sociology, which concentrates on groups and social movements. We can state that sociology does this in two ways.

1. *Macrosociological Studies.* This approach takes a broad view of society and its movements and is therefore the term used to describe the effects of societies and their organisation upon people. Such a study

might examine properties of change in the overall provision of health care and its effects upon patients.

2. *Microsociological Studies.* This approach, being more focused, attempts to examine the manner by which subunits within a society work and the way in which they also affect people. A microsociological study might, for instance, examine the effects of different staff groups (shifts) within a ward and how they are perceived by the patients, or a study might demonstrate how patients perceive the role of student nurses in comparison with their charge nurses (Shanley, 1984).

THE SOCIAL WORLD AND THE INDIVIDUAL

A distinction needs to be made here: sociology is essentially a study of group processes; it is about *society* either in whole (the provision of medical care to all) or in part (the role of midwifery in a defined social group). It is not, however, about *individuals* as such. The science which examines individuals within groups (indeed any aspect of the individual within society) is called social psychology. We can distinguish between sociology and social psychology by looking at an emotionally charged football crowd which begins to sway and chant as the match progresses. A sociologist will develop an interest in the crowd as an entity, in the sense of it 'having taken on a life of its own'. In other words, he will take as his starting point the maxim, 'The whole is different from the sum of its parts'. A social psychologist, however, will wish to enquire about how different individuals or groups of individuals (subgroups) will contribute, as constituent elements of the crowd, to the overall behaviours of the crowd. In the long run the distinction is one of emphasis, albeit an important one. At the same time, it serves us well to remember that these are somewhat artificial divisions and that concepts derived from one area may be enhanced if taken up and developed by another.

THE BIOLOGICAL AND THE SOCIAL

Narrowing the area of definition further, and putting it into a health context, clearly we are interested in how people are affected by social processes rather than, for example, internal biology. Having said this, we are then faced with the vexed complication that many biological effects are socially mediated. Few would disagree that malnutrition leads to rickets, anaemia or confusion, for instance. Similarly, few would deny that there is an intimate relationship between poor diet and social class, occupation and economic background. More pertinent, from the point of view of psychiatric practice, is the occurrence of voluntary starvation and the role of social processes such as family relationships in its development. The 'condition' of anorexia nervosa properly belongs in a psychiatric textbook and will not be examined here; but it is important to recognise its younger sister (brother?) 'dieting', and the connection with gender, upbringing and the kinds of social persuasions exerted by peer pressure and the media; more precisely the advertising dog which wags the media's tail.

FEMINIST THERAPIES

Feminist perspectives have provided an impetus for the study of some of these issues with a vigorous literature which often has direct bearing on psychiatric practice. For example, Orbach (1978) shows how some women therapists approach problems of obesity, anorexia and weight loss. While these methods are still being discussed they are a creative departure which help people in an area where patients/clients still die. They are also an example of how contemporary sociology throws light on and has a direct bearing on the work of therapists including nurses. This is true for a wide range of 'conditions' where factors such as race, gender, family, class and sexual mores (to name but a few) are now freely accepted as background (possibly causative) factors. Aspects of both race and gender will be discussed more fully later in this chapter.

A DESCRIPTIVE DEFINITION

At this point we must give up any pretence of producing a tight definition of sociology. The canvas is too wide and the brushstrokes are neither smooth nor precise enough. Instead, we must rest content with the kind of synoptic account which leaves us without a memorable definition. Does this matter? By their nature, definitions tend always to leave out material which is pertinent to the subject under discussion, thus tending to mislead as well as to inform. However much we may crave tight definitions we are probably better served by acknowledging the difficulties of pigeonholing a subject: we are better served in accepting its complexity.

The Table of Contents

Having produced a definition, however, most texts then set out, at various levels of difficulty, the different elements of the subject.

The following is a typical Basic Menu:

1. Methods of investigation
2. Population: trends and directions
3. Education
4. The family unit
5. Social class and structure
6. Religion in a secular world
7. The provision of health: changing concepts
8. The industrial future
9. Gender: roles and expectations
10. Housing for all
11. Government: institutions and patterns

Some books may be more esoteric and have chapters on language or architecture, perhaps, or more likely these days, sexual mores and behaviours (see, for example, Brettell, 1988).

Another area of growing interest is transcultural or multicultural descriptions and analyses of various kinds. Multicultural factors are currently an emerging feature of the way in which psychiatric care is delivered to different ethnic groups in Britain where there is, today, almost general agreement that we are a multiracial society. Indeed, this is reflected in recent psychiatric examination papers (see English National Board RMN Paper, 25 September, 1989).

RACE

The sociology of race is of particular relevance to psychiatric practice since the abuse of minority groups by practitioners is slowly coming to light. Generally, this abuse takes two forms. One is outright prejudice, discrimination and abuse of people in psychiatric institutions; this behaviour might be called bad psychiatric practice. In other words, prejudicial activities towards minority parties are perpetrated by bigots who happen to be psychiatric practitioners. The other form involves the more subtle workings of prejudice, whereby certain symptomatology or behaviours exhibited by minority groups are defined in a racial or cultural context or where, perhaps, certain expectations are set up given the racial background of a particular client or client group. Examples of this are a recent survey of in-patients compulsorily detained in a hospital in Birmingham (England) where it was found that about two-thirds of (black) West Indian patients, as opposed to one-third of the whites, were diagnosed as 'schizophrenic' (McGovern and Cope, 1987); and in Nottingham, where a study showed that the diagnosis of schizophrenia given by white psychiatrists to black people (assessed in a variety of settings) was 12 times more than would be expected for a white group (Harrison *et al*,

1988). Questions of diagnosis are intimately connected with treatment so that it comes as little surprise to find that:

> In the case of psychotherapy blacks are less likely to be offered it, and more likely to be given powerful phenothiazine drugs and electro-convulsive treatment (Crowley and Simmons, 1992, p.1079).

These topics are still sensitive enough to be given a wide berth. For example, Cox (1983) writes as if Britain was an all-white society, a not untypical approach. Another basic text, by Chapman (1987), does have material on race and culture and, indeed, avoids some of the pitfalls into which most of us fall. For example, she refrains from using the word 'immigrant' as a description of black people wherever they are born rather than to describe real immigrants such as come from (for instance) Ireland. The curious neglect of the Irish in sociological literature (for instance Crowley and Simmons, 1992) begs many questions: one way of explaining it is to say that Irish people (unlike some of the black nationalities) lack what is called 'exotic salience'. You might like to reflect on the extent to which this is simply another 'derision category', however. You might also like to look at Cochrane's (1983) summary of the Irish position as well as other minority groups. For a full *and telling* discussion of these issues see Fernando (1991) and Littlewood and Lipsedge (1989). Look also at Millett's (1991) personal account of her 'treatment' for manic depression, particularly her harrowing experiences in an Irish mental hospital.

In the main, however, the Basic Menu, as outlined above, is representative of the sort of book which is typically presented: what it involves is a résumé of essential research findings of each of the categories, including a presentation of 'facts and figures' such as regional variations; for example, in aspects of health care, together with a measured amount of informed opinion presented in a detached manner intended to avoid any suggestion of bias. Of course, the issue of objectivity applies to the style of sociological research as much as to particular books, with some scholars approaching their subject matter in a way which does little to hide their personal orientation, but with others taking a more objective stance. What this means in practical terms is that some would see little problem in working in a hospital ward for 3 months and then presenting their findings as written observations: others would take the view, perhaps, that this was subjective and in serious need of the kind of research controls which ensure reliability, validity and so on. Cox (1979) has emphasised the need for academic rigour and the dangers of 'ideology in disguise'.

The 'better' textbooks score highly on their elegant (including graphic) presentation of the 'facts and figures' and they are low on bias, although the best efforts of writers can sometimes fail to conceal their points of view. Although the latter books make for interesting reading (see, for instance, Haralambos and Holborn (1990), and Bilton *et al* (1987) and are a necessary aid for those engaged in academic courses. They tend to ignore the ongoing concerns of health workers which revolve around the practical delivery of care, whether in wards or community settings. As if to plug this gap the last 10 years or so have seen the emergence of a small number of texts written by and directed towards nurses. Writers such as Cox (1983) and Chapman (1987), for instance, adopt the usual framework (outlined above) but then proceed to construct a second framework within which the menu is applied to different aspects of nursing care, for example, *Sociological Aspects of Nursing the Mentally Ill* (Cox) or *Nursing as an Occupation* (Chapman).

Hand in hand with this kind of descriptive writing has been occasional research which examines some of these topics at greater depth; for example, Kath Melia's (1987) examination of the *Occupational Socialisation of Student Nurses*. Although this is a study of general nursing, the picture of a nursing world constrained by bureaucracy, shortage of staff, mind-bending routine, lack of time and the overriding ethos which stresses getting the work done will ring bells for nurses of all kinds.

In addition to the use of sociology *in* nursing there is 'barely beginning but beginning nevertheless', a sociology *of* nursing; that is, attempts to examine the role of nursing within society (chapter 8 of Chapman's (1987) book attempts this). Especially worth mentioning in this respect is the seminal text edited by Dingwall and McIntosh (1978), where the authors bring together a readable batch of papers on such nursing topics as:

1. Ideologies of nursing
2. The doctor–nurse game
3. Ritual and magic in the control of contagion
4. The faces of Florence Nightingale
5. The division of labour in nursing
6. Teamwork
7. Good girls – bad nurses

Another important text edited by Skevington (1984) reflected a growing interest in nurses by non-nursing academics. It, too, contained a wealth of information on a wide range of topics. See, for instance, chapter 6 on how women and men perceive each other in nursing and which has a strong emphasis on psychiatric nursing (Skevington, 1973). Another topic is the way in which different environments of nursing affect the manner of the delivery of care. Although this kind of sociology writing speedily goes 'out of date', nevertheless much in this text is useful, not least its reference sections. A more narrow focus, perhaps, but extremely fashionable, are books about policy issues, planning and management in nursing (Robinson *et al*, 1992). These concentrate on factors such as manpower planning, the requirements of managers and the supply of labour.

The Medium is the Message?

At this juncture it is worth stating that the sociological books aimed at professional nurses are devoid of the kind of neologistic writing that has made much of sociological output a laughing stock. So many readers are alienated by what they see as unnecessary jargon that it becomes interesting to speculate as to why some sociologists write in this manner. One reason may be that since sociology is a relatively new discipline its practitioners have attempted to compensate for its junior status by adopting a language which is esoteric; almost, in a sense, trying to emulate the technical discourses of the physical sciences! Another reason may be that such language systems are a defensive posture aimed at anyone who might question the 'scientific validity' of sociology. In other words, sociologists may be trying to blind us to the essential emptiness of their subject matter by the 'scientistic' languge which they used when deploying their subject.

While conceding some of this, sociologists might argue that any presentation of social events which aspires to be objective and dispassionate must avoid colloquial language styles and search instead for a technical and impersonal presentation; hence the ornate and sometimes arcane use of language. In a recent guest editorial in the *British Journal of Advanced Nursing*, Christine Chapman (1989) stated that:

> Many writers forget that the people reading their articles may not be familiar with the words that they use. Jargon is the barrier to much understanding (p.1).

Chapman proceeded to call for British article writers to submit work which would be clearly understood by the reading public, in this case, practising nurses.

STATIC PATIENTS: UPWARDLY MOBILE NURSES

It is early days, of course, but British nurses do appear to be aware of the pitfalls of too academic a literature-base devoid of the concerns of day-to-day practice. At the same time, the role and status of nurses are changing, both within the profession and in terms of how it is evaluated by others. A recent example of this is the manner by which nurses were occupationally designated into grades, each grade defined by tasks and responsibilities. At the same time other groups of nurses have gravitated towards the universities or other policy-making spheres and, of course, the *training* of all future nurses will be university-based. Nurses must examine these changes – especially the extent to which they may or may not contribute to an ever greater widening of that timeworn gap called the 'Theory–Practice Divide'.

THE REALITY GAME

It may well be that however 'academic' or upwardly mobile some modern nurses become they yet retain some sense of what it means to practise nursing; what it means to cope with multiple problems of groups of patients over lengthy (and unsocial) periods of duty: the latter militates against women who want to combine their work with motherhood, especially at a time of absent or high-cost crèche facilities.

The sociology of management tells of the dangers of career advancement in terms of the concurrent loss of clinical contact with patients. It has been argued (Cormack, 1976; Caudill *et al*, 1952) that the move from the bedside to higher management means a loss or abrogation of the nurturing functions of nursing (incidentally, functions which Benner (1984) believes to be intrinsically female). We have seen how this move can occur through academic mobility, one consequence of which has been the production of 'learned articles' of which many lack the 'rattle and hum' which is part and parcel of the working lives of nurses. In essence, what we are faced with is a general drift of nurses away from the bedside for a variety of reasons. It remains for researchers to try to work out the underlying factors which drive these changes. One issue which is already taking shape in the nursing literature is that of the relationship of male to female nurses and the manner by which each of these groups acquires different areas and levels of interests and responsibilities. For example, Pascall (1986) notes that (recent)

> developments in nursing have tended to strip female authority. The so-called Salmon reforms have replaced Matrons with a hierarchical structure in which 'management skills' replace nursing skills as criteria for promotion. NHS reform has further entrenched the management ethos. These developments have favoured male nurses. Men have not yet taken over the top places in the hierarchy, but they are working their way up. Thus, while 10 per cent of all nurses are men, the percentage of men to be found at District Nursing Officer level [is] 36 per cent. At the Regional level the percentage of male administrative nursing staff is 36 per cent (Pascall, 1986, p.190).

Drawing from a variety of sources, Pascall goes on to place these figures and the changes that they represent into a wider cultural context of class and race, as well as gender issues.

GENDER OFFENDERS

We can see how the development of a discussion about gender, and particularly the emergence of a feminist health literature, are beginning to influence thinking about health care delivery. Indeed, we have already touched on this in relation to dieting, weight loss and the manner in which such behaviours are influenced by advertising and the media. However, in nursing generally, gender issues such as male–female power relationships remains a neglected area. For example, in the aforementioned texts by Cox (1983) and Chapman (1987), Chapman barely mentions gender, and while Cox (1983) indirectly raises the issue of woman's status she does so in a manner which evaluates women's behaviours in terms of how they affect men and families. This is regrettable, since nursing plainly mirrors society's stereotypes of men and women (Webb, 1982), especially the manner in which the nurturing role is ascribed to women and the related functions which accompany it. Two papers which address these issues directly are by Pollock and West (1984, 1987) and they also contain handy reference sections.

Outside nursing a substantial library of female writing has already been produced, covering a wide range of topics such as the following.

1. Childbirth
2. Reproduction
3. Contraception
4. Infertility
5. The provision of health care
6. The role of men in the delivery of health care
7. Midwifery
8. Nursing
9. Chronic disability
10. Ageing
11. Psychiatry and women
12. Behavioural control and women

Obviously, a wealth of information is contained within each of these headings. Some have received rather more attention than others, however, and I propose to highlight this point by dealing with one of the more neglected issues – gender – in a way which is particularly relevant to psychiatric practice. Specifically, I want to refer to:

1. The tentatively emerging scandal of women being sexually abused within psychiatric therapy.
2. The general issue of managerial subservience of women to women in nursing.
3. Contexts of psychotherapy and somatic theories within which the above abuses take place.

SEXUALITY

Sexuality is an important element of many human relationships and it merits recognition in terms of how it influences relationships within nursing. Salvage (1987) observes:

> That there are many signs that sexuality is receiving greater acknowledgement within nursing. The nursing press is less wary of publishing articles concerned with sexuality or sexual health . . . and books on these subjects are multiplying (Salvage, 1987, p.1).

Salvage's (1987) book is the core text for this subject at present. A particular focus for psychiatric nurses is the manner in which sexuality may constitute an element of the exercise of power by male therapists over female patients.

Man's World, Woman's Place

In her book *Man's World, Woman's Place*, Elizabeth Janeway (1977) notes how 'traditional' qualities of womanhood can lead to woman-power but speaks of this as a private (individual) power for which public (collective) submission must take place; the sense of women's power, in this instance, coming from the mythical notion of the 'giver'; although, as Janeway observes, '. . . how can one give if one does not possess riches and substance?'. This notion of mythical care-giver defines the nursing role as an expression of maternal instincts and devoid of what might be called a 'professional' approach: indeed, in those instances where female nurses exercise professional autonomy, especially in a managerial capacity, it becomes necessary for some to identify and define their role in masculine and aggressive terms. Certainly, there remains in nursing the paradox of a caring profession seemingly failing to reward, at an administrative level, those nurturing qualities deemed to be essential to basic nursing care (Pollock and West, 1984).

The role of males in nursing is equally important, of course, but particularly in relation to the workings of a profession numerically dominated by women while being controlled administratively by the minority of men who work within it. This flags up the issue of power in nursing and the reader is referred to the works of Carpenter (1977), Salvage (1985) and Pascall (1986, chapter 6), all of whom discuss these issues as well as providing up-to-date bibliographies. Worth mentioning at this point is the curious anomaly of nursing historians producing work that appears to judge mental nursing as unworthy of discussion: some of the most famous books in nursing barely articulate the existence of mental nurses. Contemporary books on such topics as ethics or politics are similarly blinkered (see, for instance, Clay (1987) and

Melia (1989)), so that while issues such as gender and so on are being discussed in British nursing, this is usually within a general nursing context.

Male Therapists: Female Clients

For our purposes, the role of women as a minority 'at the receiving end' of psychiatric therapy is central. In his recent book, *Against Therapy*, Jeffrey Masson (1988) describes the 'emotional battering' of women by using case material and commentaries provided by women themselves. Masson writes of the psychotherapeutic alliance as a privileged relationship which can easily give rise to the kind of abuse and denigration which Dorothy Tennov (1976) calls 'psychobattery'. While both of these texts are aggressively antitherapeutic they nevertheless raise issues which conventional psychiatry seeks to avoid. Also, in pointing to the abuses which can come about through psychiatric relationships they cause havoc to traditional assertions about psychiatry being an objective activity, whereby an expert therapist ministers to a 'flawed' individual so as to cure or ameliorate her problems. Instead, Masson and Tennov define therapy as an activity within which traditional forms of sexual and power relationships can be used to demean and offend. Certainly, if there is one aspect of psychotherapy on which most of us could agree it is the current lack of supervision governing its practice.

Blowing the Whistle

A recent paper by Aileen LaTourette (1987) has blown the whistle on sexual assault by male psychotherapists. Having undergone therapy for a considerable period of time, LaTourette has come to believe that it contained the seeds of 'inflexibility and even oppressiveness'.

> It was no secret that my therapist found me sexually attractive and that the potential of sexual engagement between us was present in his mind. At one point during a session the therapist asked me to remove all of my clothes. I refused. My refusal was accepted, but I felt that although I was right, this was seen as a moment of life-refusal . . . and had I been a freer healthier person I would have done so *sans* problem (LaTourette, 1987, p.75).

While LaTourette highlights abuses which occur in private practice and while a literature pertaining to these matters in National Health Service practice has yet to emerge, at the same time it becomes necessary for all practitioners to avail themselves of the messages contained in these studies. This does not mean that solutions will emerge from a mere study of the evidence. Masson (1988), for instance, draws attention to the manner by which feminist therapists themselves ape the theories and practices of mainstream therapeutic camps; for example, Tennov is an advocate of behaviourism while other feminists espouse Freudian or other 'classic approaches' (see Penfold and Walker, 1984, chapter 10). We should note that criticisms of traditional practice of the sort typified by Masson, LaTourette and Tennov appear to be almost ignored by psychiatric practitioners.

Mad, Bad or Just Plain Sad?

On the whole, nursing is at one with other disciplines in preferring a literature which compliments rather than criticises. Perhaps we resent critical material because it robs us of our treasured assumptions that what we do with patients is an objective expression of our professional lives: that it is something into which right and wrong do not and can not enter. It may be that suspicions of sociology are precisely that it raises those social issues which question the nature of how and why people relate to each other as they do. Unlike psychiatry, it does not cloak people's actions with a veneer of diagnoses or symptoms (at least not to the same extent). As an example of how psychiatry does this, witness the following 'therapeutic evaluation' of a man who sexually assaulted his daughter: such a man did not behave

> out of conscious choice at that point in life; self-abuse and abusive behaviour was the only response he could make to discharge the chronic state of low self-worth caused by unmet needs. The father–offender (or any offender) will stop being an offender when he is taught to become aware of all his needs for self-realisation and to become personally responsible for meeting them (Masson, 1988, pp.264–265).

SOCIAL ORIGINS OF DEPRESSION

The kind of anguish associated with mothering children can drive women 'mad'. Persuasive evidence for this may be found in Brown and Harris's (1978) study *The Social Origins of Depression*. In summary, this study discovered unsuspected rates of mental illness among women. Specifically, high rates were found among 'working class' women with young children: the younger the woman's children or the greater the number of children were two factors which increased her likelihood of becoming depressed. Overall, the rates of depression were considerably higher than for groups of women in the 'middle classes'. The authors defined four conditions which might predispose women to becoming depressed. These were:

1. Lack of intimate relationships
2. Loss of their mother at an early age
3. Three or more children at home under 14 years
4. Lack of employment

Pascall (1986) notes that other studies confirmed these findings adding that:

> The concentration on stress and depression is an important counterweight to the rosy imagery [of motherhood] of the more popular media (p.99).

Nobody pretends that a social perspective such as this gives all the answers and Pascall (chapters 1 and 3) should be read for an evaluation of some of the issues raised. Further, the temptation to supplant a psychiatric perspective of women's problems with a sociological one may function as a subterfuge which avoids confronting directly the issue of male domination. For their part, psychiatric nurses have (for too long) persisted in playing 'fellow travellers' to psychiatrists who, in turn, ignore the manner in which human misery can sometimes be an outcome of social effects. Instead, they prefer a neater perspective of 'mental illness' whereby the patient's illness is defined as a biochemical abnormality for which drugs or electric treatment are invariably prescribed. Penfold and Walker (1984) have compiled impressive evidence showing how women are more likely than men to be prescribed drugs. Rarely do nurses reflect on the central question of their role as an occupational group (or profession) in the administration of these treatments either for or with psychiatrists. Indeed, the overall role of psychiatric nurses as dispensers of 'treatments', usually pharmacological, is camouflaged by élitist 'professionalisers' who promote notions of what nurses *ought* to be doing as opposed to what they *actually* do (whether it be in wards or anywhere else). Cormack (1976) elegantly distinguishes between a descriptive and prescriptive literature on nursing, whereby the latter presents a picture of therapeutic activity which is poorly matched by the former. The suggestion is that nurses do not appear to do what they say they do. More recent work (Melia, 1987) appears to support Cormack's (1976) findings. In particular Ussher (1992) has started to describe the past from a feminist perspective in the context of explaining its relevance for psychiatric practice and women.

HOW OTHERS SEE US

This leads us to speculate on how others see us as a professional group. This is difficult, however, for in recent years we have tended to ignore other disciplines in a headstrong (and misguided) drive for professional 'standing'. (It is crucial to emphasise the difference between this headlong rush to professionalism and the reluctance to argue for a clinical independence which might separate us ideologically from the psychiatrists.) Here is what Lucy Johnstone (a clinical psychologist) has to say about nurses:

> Nurses do not decide who should be admitted and why; they have to stand by the psychiatrist's decisions. It is . . . rare for nurses to mount an effective challenge to a psychiatrist's medical model decisions. . . . Nurses are left to work out their own unsatisfactory compromises on a day-to-day basis in the demoralising muddle of treatment approaches (Johnstone, 1989, p.53).

It may be that the move of psychiatric nurses into community-based care will stimulate new perspectives of role and motivation: for the time being, however, nurses continue, predominantly, to practise in medically orientated contexts irrespective of the geography of care.

HOSPITAL OR COMMUNITY?

Until recently, psychiatric nurses have worked in large, impersonal institutions. Today the predominant emphasis appears to be on community psychiatric nursing, an umbrella term covering a multitude of activities. Community psychiatric nursing may indeed indicate the delivery of care inside the client's home by a seemingly autonomous practitioner functioning within a local mental health team. Few would have difficulty in accepting this as a 'reasonable ideal', the client being helped to recovery while remaining in her natural habitat by a therapist who sees this habitat as a natural 'curative factor' in the process of recovery. But to what extent is this an accurate picture?

Hospital Closures

'Now that they're closing down the hospitals . . .' is a frequent preamble to a lot of talk these days, but quite how much has closed and how much has shifted is an unexplored issue. Even more vague is the nature of what takes place when hospital wards do 'move into the community'. Do such moves represent merely a shift of resources and personnel or does there take place a shift of attitude as well? Or, in fact, do the various changes make for more feasible conditions within which change becomes more likely? I would suggest that in many instances what we have witnessed is a shift of resources and personnel with sometimes little or no alteration in the belief systems of those involved. Indeed, where the shift took place from ancient institution into District General Hospital, we can even presume that medical approaches to care were enhanced (bearing in mind that some might see this as appropriate).

As for the satellite units which now dot the urban landscape it is an open question as to how the hospital-trained nurses who staff these units see their roles in the light of their changed surroundings; equally, one might ask if such shifts have *imposed* change upon them and induced new perspectives among them. These are areas which are rich in their potential for the development of a sociology of mental nursing practice as well as extending our knowledge base about institutional change generally. For there can be no question but that we do need institutions.

A Haven, a Place of Rest, a Home From Home?

Although institutional nursing does not now possess the awful qualities beloved of 1950s and 1960s critics (Jones, 1952; Goffman, 1968; Barton, 1959) it is still a fair bet that ward-based nursing lacks the charisma (and certainly the autonomy) of the community approach generally: by community approach we mean individual community nurses working in clients' homes. However, some doubts can be voiced about this: it is entirely possible that even in a community context the nurse may work in a manner such as to confirm in the patient's mind a sick or dependent role. The work of community psychiatric nurses is rarely observed other than by students, and often they are appointed to their posts without having had any training in social policy or therapies or 'community psychiatric nursing': indeed, appointments are sometimes made on grounds of expediency. We cannot use the term Community Psychiatric Nurse with any certainty about what it means; the nature of the nurse's interventions or their beliefs and attitudes about social institutions also remain unexplored terrain. Johnstone (1989) observes how community psychiatric nurses:

> . . . receive direct referrals from GPs and can thus build up their own case-load and style of working away from the hospital, by basing themselves in clinics and surgeries and visiting patients in their homes. Traditional nurses, some of whom still wear uniforms, stick mainly to carrying out the basic tasks of ward management, pill dispensing, or, in the community, giving slow-release injections of medication (Johnstone, 1989, p.158).

Complementing Cormack's (1976) findings about the mismatch between what nurses do and what they say they do, Pollock (1989) established that the reality of community psychiatric nursing diverted sharply from the pleasant myths which had come to surround it: she outlined a service within which community psychiatric nursing was that which the individual practitioner said it was and that this was governed less by nursing theory and more by financial (and other) shortages and constraints. What is being suggested here is that definitions of good practice which have as their starting point the geography of care are fallacious. In the early heady days of community psychiatric nursing some community staff harboured a superior attitude towards ward-based nurses. When the hospitals began to decant their patients into local units a community psychiatric nurse friend of mine remarked: 'I see that you are bringing the hospital to us'. What he meant by this was that our proximity represented a contamination of the 'values' of the community psychiatric ideal by the institutionalisation of the old hospital system.

The Challenge of the Old

Yet those patients who have remained in what is left of the Victorian asylums present psychiatric nursing with a most formidable challenge. This is the challenge of how to develop styles of living for those who remain (and will continue to remain) in institutional care. Any serious attempt at this must involve some effort by nurses to de-professionalise their activities in favour of working with people in a way that recognises that they have been socially deprived, often for many years. This means re-defining the nature of a 'ward' and what it means to live in one for a long period of time, regardless of where it is situated. Groups such as SPRING (South East Thames Psychiatric Rehabilitation Interest Group) are composed of multidisciplinary practitioners trying to find their way around these problems without being necessarily seduced by the charismatic allure of 'the community'.

Gold is Where You Find It

That mental hospitals came to be seen as detrimental to the welfare of patients was a reflection of the growing egalitarianism which followed the Second World War and crept through the 1950s and 1960s. The issue of whether hospitals were good or bad was fought on a battlefield of imagined and symbolic effects: those of us who said that hospitals were bad were as naive as we were ignorant. From a sociological standpoint we had read the wrong books! Instead of the polemical broadsheets which attacked 'the system' (most of which were American and often irrelevant) we should perhaps have heeded those cooler voices which warned of shortages of provision, oncoming financial stringency and the need for attitude change on the part of the public. Dramatic as it sounds, some mentally ill people walk the streets today partly because we failed to appreciate their vulnerability, preoccupied as we were with 'progressive' self-imagery. We had forgotten the unfashionable fact that some of the most important experiments in psychosocial nursing had taken place *in hospitals* such as Rapoport's (1960) study of the Henderson Hospital (arguably, the most influential sociological text of the 1960s in Britain). Rapoport's book provided a new vocabulary for those who were trying to follow Jones's (1952) methods. While only a minority of psychiatric nurses subscribed to the democratic approaches described by Rapoport, other texts which followed continued to describe patients in interpersonal terms. Texts by David Cooper (1970) and R D Laing (1967) can be described as sociological (especially Cooper) in as much as they stressed the relationship factors which lay at the heart of schizophrenia. Laing and Esterson's (1964) interviews with the families of patients are not without flaws, but for the first time the idea of 'madness' as a social phenomenon was made dramatically visible by these two writers. Cooper (1970) took up the Laingian concept of schizophrenia, which pointed a finger towards punitive families and developed this into a broader Marxian critique of conventional psychiatry.

Failing to Take Account

A singular failure of many of these studies was their failure (as always) to take account of the position and relative influence of nurses. Even when studies are comprehensive and critical, there is a peculiar disregard of the nurses; those who interact most frequently with patients in all settings. For example, Clare's (1976) influential book, *Psychiatry in Dissent*, addresses most of the major issues confronting the theory and practice of contemporary psychiatry while blithely disregarding nurses, the very people who arduously and intimately accompany patients on all of their journeys. Reading a book like this is like discovering an educational text which sets out to describe life in classrooms but without mentioning the teachers. Nurses themselves, of course, write few books and while this is changing rapidly there is as yet only a modest examination of their role in society or of the different elements within that role. Aspects such as power, gender, race, befriending patients in a helping and not a 'professional' manner, treatments and relationships with doctors are some of these elements. Instead, in recent years nurses have almost driven themselves crazy by an interminable fascination with their role as 'a profession' in the company of other prestigious disciplines. This would be fine if it involved a desire to examine this role with some degree of social perspicacity. On the contrary, however, it has involved us in a drive for social status with hardly a passing glance at what this means. It is this short-sightedness which has led us to compliantly accept imposed super-structures such as the Project 2000 scheme, a scheme which (in its implementation) is beginning to look more and more like someone else's fantasy: a cache of unexploded bombs whose doubtful outcomes are only now beginning to be realised.

Making a Nursing Contribution

If we are to make a *nursing* contribution, then we should appraise realistically the needs of those whom we set out to help. If before doing this we set aside those patients who are acutely ill, in other words those who primarily require a medical (psychiatric) treatment rather than a nursing intervention, it might become apparent that most so-called 'nursing needs' are either social or interpersonal in nature. Among social needs we may cite housing, adequate finance, home help services and so forth. Interpersonal or relationship needs might well include counselling, companionship, advocacy or a listening ear, to name but a few. In any event, it is likely that most clients' needs will combine factors from these two categories. (It is not denied that these kinds of responses may be given to the acutely ill; only that they are not therapeutically crucial.)

The old question: 'What is nursing?' can only be answered concisely by reference to that which motivates nurses as they try to deal with the extraordinary array of needs and responses outlined above; certainly, it cannot be answered at all in terms of what nurses actually do. This is because they do too much.

It may be that the spectacle of mental nurses standing behind medicine trolleys is quite properly a logical response to mental illness: what makes it sad is that this stance is presented as a legitimate method of dealing with *all* of those who fall short of normality or wellness.

No Mental Nurses

It may be that there is no such thing as a mental nurse. What this means is that the role and function of the mental nurse will be determined by the wall-to-wall needs of patients. Only occasionally will these be clearly seen as medical or clinical in nature. Rather, we have seen how wide-ranging clients' needs are and suggested that the incredible array of skills and talents needed to deal with them probably falls outside the capacities of any individual or defined group. In addition, it has been asserted that nurses could profit by examining their place in the organisation and delivery of care and treatments to patients *but in the context of society, its mores, traditions and expectations.* So what does this mean for nurses and how should they respond?

Responding

First, it calls for mental nurses to discuss these matters in a manner which recognises their branch of nursing as possessing its own history, recognising its right to evaluate its position in the light of the needs of those (the clients) whom it claims to represent. In particular, in carrying out this task in a way that does justice to the needs and aspirations of nurses also. I would say that the endless professionalising may be avoided if the nurses include the patients in their discussions; either literally or, at least, in principle.

Secondly, where the problems are not those of the immediately acutely ill, this may mean engaging in processes whereby patients and nurses work out living-styles together: for example, in an institutional setting this might involve nurses 'giving away' pretences of officialdom or guardianship; indeed, trying to work out programmes of actual disengagement. To do this, nurses do not need a 'role': there are far too many of these name tags whose usage has far outstripped any practical meaning they might have had. They need, instead, to find a way in which they can become valued as the people who take on to (partially) live with and work through the social problems faced by people whose difficulties have been brought about by past or present mental illness and who are not currently amenable to medical treatments.

REFERENCES

Barton R (1959) *Institutional Neurosis.* Bristol: John Wright and Sons Ltd.

Benner P (1984) *From Novice to Expert: Excellence and Power in Clinical Nursing Practice.* California: Addison-Wesley.

Bilton T *et al* (1987) *Introducing Sociology,* 2nd edn. London: Macmillan.

Brettell K M (1988) Patterns of evaluations of accents amongst Health Visitor students. *Journal of Advanced Nursing,* **13**: 33–43.

Briggs A (1984) Foreword. In: *Understanding Nurses: The Social Psychology of Nursing,* ed. Skevington S. Chichester: John Wiley and Sons Ltd.

Brown G W and Harris T (1978) *Social Origins of Depression: A Study of Psychiatric Disorder in Britain.* London: Tavistock.

Carpenter M (1977) The new managerialism and professionalism in nursing. In: *Health and the Division of Labour,* eds Stacey H, Reid M and Heath C. Beckenham: Croom Helm.

Caudill W *et al* (1952) Social structure and interaction process in a psychiatric ward. *American Journal of Orthopsychiatry,* **22**(2): 314–334.

Chapman C (1987) *Sociology for Nurses,* 3rd edn. London: Baillière Tindall.

Chapman C (1989) Guest Editorial. *Journal of Advanced Nursing,* **14**: 1–2.

Clare A (1976) *Psychiatry in Dissent.* London: Tavistock Publications.

Clay T (1987) *Nurses: Power and Politics.* London: Heinemann.

Cochrane R (1983) *The Social Creation of Mental Illness.* London: Longman.

Cooper D (1970) *Psychiatry and Anti-Psychiatry.* London: Paladin.

Cormack D (1976) *Psychiatric Nursing Observed.* London: Royal College of Nursing.

Cox C (1979) Who cares? Nursing and sociology: the development of a symbiotic relationship. *Journal of Advanced Nursing*, **4**: 237–252.

Cox C (1983) *Sociology: An Introduction for Nurses, Midwives and Health Visitors.* London: Butterworth.

Crowley J J and Simmons S (1992) Mental health, race and ethnicity: a retrospective study of the care of ethnic minorities and whites in a psychiatric unit. *Journal of Advanced Nursing*, **17**: 1078–1087.

Dingwall R and McIntosh J (eds) (1978) *Readings in the Sociology of Nursing.* London: Churchill Livingstone.

Egan G (1986) *The Skilled Helper*, 3rd edn. California: Brooks/Cole Pub. Co.

English National Board (1989) State Final paper for RMN Examination (25 September).

Fernando S (1991) *Mental Health, Race and Culture.* London: Macmillan in association with Mind Publications.

Goffman E (1968) *Asylums.* Harmondsworth: Penguin.

Haralambos M and Holborn M (1990) *Sociology: Themes and Perspectives* 3rd edn. London: Unwin Hyman.

Harrison G *et al* (1988) A prospective study of severe mental disorder in Afro-Caribbean patients. *Psychological Medicine*, **18**: 643–657.

Janeway E (1977) *Man's World, Woman's Place.* Harmondsworth: Penguin.

Johnstone L (1989) *Users and Abusers of Psychiatry: A Critical Look at Traditional Psychiatric Practice.* London: Routledge.

Jones M (1952) *Social Psychiatry.* London: Tavistock.

Laing R D (1967) *The Politics of Experience.* Harmondsworth: Penguin.

Laing R D and Esterson A (1964) *The Families of Schizophrenics.* London: Tavistock Publications.

LaTourette A (1987) The kindness of strangers. In: *The Power of Psychology*, ed. Cohen, D. Beckenham: Croom Helm.

Littlewood R and Lipsedge M (1989) *Aliens and Alienists: Ethnic Minorities and Psychiatry.* London: Unwin Hyman.

Masson J (1988) *Against Therapy.* London: Fontana/Collins.

McGovern D and Cope R (1987) The compulsory detention of males of different ethnic groups, with special reference to offender patients. *British Journal of Psychiatry*, **150**: 505–512.

Melia K (1987) *Learning and Working: The Occupational Socialisation of Nurses.* London: Tavistock.

Melia K (1989) *Everyday Nursing Ethics*, A Nursing Times – Macmillan Education Book. London: Macmillan.

Millett K (1991) *The Looney Bin Trip.* London: Virago Press.

Morse J M *et al* (1991) Comparative analysis of conceptualisations and theories of caring. *Image: Journal of Nursing Scholarship.* **23**(22): 119–126.

Orbach S (1978) *Fat is a Feminist Issue.* London: Paddington Press Ltd.

Pascall G (1986) *Social Policy: A Feminist Analysis.* London: Routledge.

Penfold P S and Walker G A (1984) *Women and the Psychiatric Paradox.* Milton

Keynes: Open University Press.

Pollock L C (1989) *Community Psychiatric Nursing: Myth and Reality*, Royal College of Nursing Research Series. London: Scutari Press.

Pollock L C and West E (1984) On being a woman and a psychiatric nurse. *Senior Nurse*, **1**(17): 10–13.

Pollock L C and West E (1987) Women and psychiatry today. *Senior Nurse*, **6**(6): 11–14.

Rapoport R N (1960) *Community As Doctor: New Perspectives on a Therapeutic Community.* London: Tavistock.

Robinson J *et al* (1992) *Policy Issues in Nursing.* Milton Keynes: Open University Press.

Rogers C R (1967) *On Becoming A Person: A Therapist's View of Psychotherapy.* London: Constable.

Salvage J (1985) *The Politics of Nursing.* London: Heinemann Nursing.

Salvage J (1987) *Nurses, Gender and Sexuality.* London: Heinemann Nursing.

Shanley E (1984) Evaluation of Mental Nurses by their Patients and Charge Nurses. Unpublished PhD Thesis, University of Edinburgh.

Skevington S (ed.) (1984) *Understanding Nurses: The Social Psychology of Nursing.* Chichester: John Wiley and Sons Ltd.

Tennov D (1976) *Psychobattery: The Hazardous Cure.* New York: Doubleday and Co.

Ussher J (1992) *Women's Madness: Mysogyny or Mental Illness.* London: Prentice-Hall.

Webb C (1982) The men wear the trousers. *Nursing Mirror*, **13**: 29–31.

10

Perspectives in Counselling
Stewart Whitehead

INTRODUCTION: WHY COUNSELLING?

. . . If I can create a relationship characterised on my part:
   by a genuineness and transparency, in which I am my real feelings;
   by a warm acceptance of and prizing of the other person as a separate
   individual;
   by a sensitive ability to see his world and himself as he sees them;
Then the other individual in the relationship:
   will experience and understand aspects of himself which previously he
   has repressed;
   will find himself becoming better integrated, more able to function
   effectively;
   will become more similar to the person he would like to be;
   will be more self-directing and self-confident;
   will become more of a person, more unique and self-expressive;
   will be more understanding, more acceptant of others;
   will be able to cope with the problems of life more adequately and more
   comfortably. . . (Carl Rogers, 1967)

In the above quotation, Carl Rogers describes the essence of client-centred or person-centred counselling. It is a particular kind of therapeutic relationship, which is characterised by the three central components of genuineness, acceptance and empathy in the counsellor, these in turn enabling the client to develop his/her own potential, and move towards becoming a fully functioning person. It is an approach which was initially developed by Rogers in the 1950s, and has been extended and used by many others in a variety of different settings since that time.

What relevance does counselling have for the mental health nurse? In this chapter I will explore the nature of counselling, and examine the particular relevance of counselling to the mental health setting. A distinction will be made between counselling as a particular kind of therapeutic intervention, and counselling skills, which may be used in a number of different ways. I will go on to look more closely at the core elements of the counselling relationship, and at the skills which may be used when working from this perspective. Some different approaches to counselling and the value of an eclectic approach will also be considered, followed by a section on the professional development of the counsellor, including supervision, personal growth and ethical issues. Finally, some examples from clinical practice will be presented.

In looking at how counselling and counselling skills might be used, I will be using the perspectives of both person-centred counselling and mental health nursing, and considering how these two can be integrated. I will also show how counselling can form part of a wider multidisciplinary approach within the mental health setting.

Three central themes will emerge:

1. To the client presenting in a mental health setting, there are many things on offer.
2. The person-centred approach says listen to the client, and trust his/her 'process'.
3. If we as counsellors listen carefully, the client will tell us what he/she is open to and what he/she can use, and when.

These themes form the basis of the chapter.

DEFINITIONS OF COUNSELLING

The British Association for Counselling in its Code of Ethics and Practice for Counsellors states that the task of counselling '. . . is to provide an opportunity for the client to work towards living in a more satisfying and resourceful way'. The code describes the term counselling as including '. . . work with individuals, pairs or groups of people . . .' and '. . . concerned with developmental issues, addressing and resolving specific problems, making decisions, coping with crisis, developing personal insight and knowledge, working through feelings of inner conflict or improving relationships with others' (British Association for Counselling, 1990).

For the purposes of this chapter, a distinction will also be made between 'counselling' and 'counselling skills'. This distinction is recognised by the British Association for Counselling, who state: 'Only when both the user and the recipient explicitly agree to enter into a counselling relationship does it become "counselling" rather than the use of "counselling skills" ' Although counselling skills are a fundamental part of the process of counselling a distinction here is useful, because counselling skills may be used in a whole range of interactions and interrelationships. For the nurse working in the mental health field, an ability to use these skills will be invaluable in all her/his interactions with patients/clients, even where a more formal counselling relationship is not possible. At the same time, counselling in the formal sense, where a counsellor contracts with a client to provide regular, time-limited sessions, may well be the intervention of choice for some clients.

APPLICABILITY OF COUNSELLING SKILLS IN MENTAL HEALTH NURSING

Mental health nurses carry out the many and varied aspects of their role in an equally varied range of settings. These include: inpatient facilities such as acute admission wards, where individuals may be highly disturbed or suffering acute distress; residential settings, such as group homes; community settings such as Day Centres or Day Hospitals, where often a range of services, including counselling, are provided; and in people's own homes, where Community Psychiatric Nurses may provide counselling interventions of various kinds. Specialist units, providing specialised services for people with particular kinds of problems (e.g. drug and alcohol abuse services), also use interventions where counselling skills may be particularly appropriate.

Within all these settings, mental health nurses develop relationships with their patients/clients through a variety of different interactions. These include, at one end of the scale, social interactions such as those which occur in the ward situation or rehabilitation setting, to very specific therapeutic interactions in individual work (including counselling), group work or family work at the other end of the scale. Patients or clients may present with any number of mental health problems. The picture is further complicated by the range of approaches or models used, which may also include quite specific nursing models. Where multidisciplinary teams are the norm several different models may be used, integrated into an eclectic approach.

The development of counselling as a profession reflects changes in society as a whole, as well as changes in the way in which professional helpers see themselves and their clients. The trends in recent years towards community care, preventative mental health work and health promotion have all meant an increasing emphasis on approaches which see the healthy individual as one who takes responsibility for him/herself, and encourage the development of the individual's own coping abilities in order to deal with problems. As Hershenson and Power (1987) have stated: '. . . mental health counselling does not seek to cure illness . . . but rather seeks to promote healthy development and coping'. Even in settings where a medical model predominates, the emphasis has increasingly been on the encouragement of self-responsibility and self-reliance among patients.

In non-mental health settings also, there has been an increasing emphasis on the use of counselling skills. For example, Tschudin (1981) describes the counselling skills needed in working with patients suffering with brain tumours, Hopper and Jesson (1991) and Jeavons (1991) have both emphasised the importance of counselling skills and specialist counselling in midwifery, particularly in relation to parents who have lost their babies, and Swaffield (1990) has highlighted the value of counselling skills in health promotion. While mental health nursing is a specialist field, mental health issues do not confine themselves only to mental health settings, and nurses in all kinds of settings are recognising the importance of a counselling approach.

It is my contention that, in keeping with these trends, a counselling approach offers a way forward in mental health work. Counselling skills can be applied in almost any interaction with clients, and enable the nurse to relate more effectively and helpfully in virtually any situation. A nurse who has developed these skills will be better equipped to deal with the wide range of often very difficult problems which she/he is expected to face. Such skills will be useful whichever approach is being used. In addition to this, nurses who through further training go on to develop the appropriate skills will be able to offer clients counselling as an approach in itself. The nature of counselling and the philosophy behind it mean that the skills are widely applicable. It is an approach which is equally relevant when working with clients, carers and relatives, and indeed other staff with whom the nurse has a professional relationship, whether within a clinical, educational or management context.

Nurses will begin developing counselling skills from the beginning of their training, and will become familiar with the theory behind a number of different philosophical approaches. However, nothing can take the place of experience, and it is only through the experience and practice of these skills, supported by the opportunity to evaluate and develop them within a supportive, well-supervised structure, that a full level of competence will be achieved.

PERSON-CENTRED COUNSELLING: CREATING A HELPING RELATIONSHIP

The Necessary and Sufficient Conditions for Counselling

Rogers outlined three central components of the counselling process, which he believed to be both necessary but also sufficient to create a truly helpful relationship: genuineness, acceptance and empathy.

Genuineness
This was also referred to by Rogers as 'congruence'. For therapy to occur, Rogers said that '. . . it seems necessary that the therapist be, in the relationship, a unified or integrated, or congruent person'. In other words, the therapist or counsellor is as he/she is, not acting through some kind of facade or pretence. This does not necessarily mean sharing everything about how he/she is, but an awareness of self by the counsellor is certainly necessary.

Acceptance
The second element, acceptance or 'unconditional positive regard', involves being caring and accepting of the client as a separate individual, with permission for him/her to have his/her own feelings, experiences and meanings. This caring acceptance applies to both positive and negative feelings. It implies also that the client is not being 'judged' by the counsellor.

Empathy
Empathy, the third element, is described by Rogers as where the counsellor is '. . . experiencing an accurate, empathic understanding of the client's world as seen from the inside'. In other words, the counsellor senses the client's feelings as if they were his/her own, but without his/her own feelings becoming caught up in these. In advanced empathy, the counsellor is able to communicate not only an understanding of what is clearly known to the client, but also patterns of meaning of which the client is scarcely aware.

If the client experiences these three elements as being present in the counsellor, then the environment for a helping relationship can be established. The client will feel heard and accepted as he/she is, and will experience the counsellor as working hard to understand what he/she is communicating, rather than trying to 'impose' an agenda. The counsellor will be experienced as genuine and open, and this will help to create an atmosphere where trust is able to grow. If the client then has a willingness to change, further progress can take place.

Rolfe (1990), in his article on the assessment of therapeutic attitudes in the psychiatric setting, has provided a useful summary of research evidence which illustrates that these three attitudes of genuineness, respect (acceptance) and empathy are beneficial to the client. He quotes several studies which correlate the three attitudes with therapeutic experience and successful outcomes in therapy. The consistent findings in these studies were that clients did best when they felt that their meanings and feelings were being understood, when they experienced a sensitivity to their attitudes from the therapist and when they felt they could trust the therapist. Truax and Mitchell (1971) have also carried out a review of the literature on these three qualities and conclude that:

> Therapists or counselors who are accurately empathic, non-possessively warm in attitude and genuine are indeed effective. Also, these findings seem to hold with a wide variety of therapists and counselors, regardless of their training or theoretic orientation, . . . with a wide variety of clients or patients, . . . in a variety of therapeutic contexts and in both individual and group psychotherapy or counseling (Truax and Mitchell, 1971).

Once a therapeutic environment has been established the process of counselling continues, with the counsellor using a repertoire of both basic and advanced skills to facilitate further development, change and growth in the client.

For the purposes of simplicity, during the following sections the term 'he' will be used to denote the client, while 'she' will be used to denote the counsellor or nurse. The use of these terms in no way implies any assumptions concerning the gender of clients or professionals involved in the counselling process.

Basic Counselling Skills

If the Rogerian concepts of genuineness, acceptance and empathy represent a 'core' approach to counselling, then in a similar way the skills which are used to convey these qualities are central to the process. These skills can be summarised as follows.

Non-verbal Messages and Physical Attending

We all send out non-verbal messages through our bodies, and it is important that what we say in words is reinforced rather than contradicted by these messages (i.e. is congruent with them). The counsellor can indicate that she is attending physically by the following behaviours, which can be summarised by the acronym SOLER:

S: facing the other person *squarely* lets him know that she is available to work with him
O: adopting an *open* posture lets him know that she is open and non-defensive
L: *leaning* towards him emphasises her listening and responding, and conveys the message of being with him
E: good *eye contact* without staring shows her interest in him
R: maintaining a *relaxed* posture conveys her competence and helps the other relax also

Verbal Skills and Techniques

The counsellor can also indicate that she is attending by a variety of verbal techniques. This process of *active listening* is promoted by the use of facilitative listening skills, which may include the following.

Para-verbals – the use of 'mmm', 'ah-ha', 'sure . . .', 'right . . .', and other para-verbals may facilitate the listening process, if used appropriately and sparingly.

Continuation remarks – words and phrases such as 'and . . .', 'then . . .', 'so . . .', 'but . . .', 'go on . . .', 'tell me more . . .', 'say a bit more . . .', 'and then . . .', 'keep going . . .' and 'stay with it . . .' may also be helpful, although once again these need to be used with delicacy and caution.

Reflecting content – particular words which the client may use are reflected back. Usually these are words which are emphasised or repeated by the client.

Other techniques which the counsellor may use to help clarify what the client is saying often involve longer responses, aimed at creating a fuller understanding of the client's experience, and in particular the feelings behind what the client is bringing. These include the following.

Identifying feelings – clients may express what they are feeling by using single words, e.g. 'I'm unhappy'; by different phrases, e.g. 'I'm down in the dumps'; by making behavioural statements, e.g. 'I feel like crying'; or by describing an experience, e.g. 'I feel like there's a black cloud over me'. The task of the counsellor is to help the client to identify the feeling expressed, e.g. 'You're feeling sad', although it should also be remembered that a client's particular word or phrase may sometimes be important.

Paraphrasing – the counsellor reflects back the content of what the client is saying using her own words. This usually applies to fairly short statements.

Summarising – longer passages of speech are reflected back, with the counsellor highlighting the main points or themes as they emerge. This technique is particularly useful when reviewing a session or with themes which may have emerged over a longer period of time.

Open questions – these may also help the client to explore further and convey more information. An open question is one which often starts with words such as 'how' or 'what', encouraging the client to speak more, rather than closed questions, which encourage 'yes', 'no', or other one-word responses. Generally, questions should be used sparingly, as too many may feel like an interrogation or may shift the emphasis away from the client and on to the counsellor.

Use of statements – these enable a more tentative approach and tend to appear less judgmental than questions. For example, 'you responded in that way because you were upset?' does not appear judgmental, whereas 'why did you respond in that way?' may appear critical and the client may become defensive.

Tone of voice – with all the above verbal skills and techniques, the tone of voice of the counsellor is vitally important in conveying interest and intention, and as with non-verbal cues should be congruent with the messages which are being given verbally.

Advanced Counselling Skills

In advanced counselling, the counsellor uses all the above skills, but may take a more 'confrontational' approach. Thus, while staying within the context and content of what is being said, the counsellor may reflect back to the client '. . . feelings and meanings that are buried, hidden, or beyond the immediate reach of the client' (Egan, 1986). In this sense confrontation may be seen as 'an invitation to be aware'. It is through being with the client very closely that the counsellor is able to develop advanced empathy, becoming aware of the half-implied clues and clues outside the client's awareness, as well as the overt expressions which the client may bring. The counsellor, while 'staying with' the client, is able to move things on by enabling him to look more deeply into his own feelings, attitudes, values, beliefs and behaviour, and develop a greater understanding of himself.

It should be emphasised here that one of the key assumptions of the person-centred approach is that human nature is essentially constructive, and that '. . . all human beings have within them the innate capacity to grow towards their own unique fulfilment' (Mearns and Thorne, 1988). This means that the counsellor should always be led by the client, and where confrontation takes place it is always carried out in a respectful way, with the counsellor consistently checking back with the client in a way that allows him to either accept or reject what the counsellor is offering. The client always remains in control, with counsellor and client working cooperatively together. Implicit in this is the acceptance that the pace of change cannot be forced, and that the client will be able to make the right decisions about when he is ready to deal with aspects of himself that are painful or difficult.

This process is illustrated by Rogers, who believed that the aim of counselling is not for the client to move from one fixed point to another, but rather to move from a state of 'fixity' to one of 'flowingness'. He described a series of seven stages which he believed occurred during this process. Thus personality change can be seen as occurring on a continuum, with individuals moving from a more rigid point to a more flexible one. This process of change '. . . involves several threads, separable at first, becoming more of a unity as the process continues', and '. . . occurs when a client experiences himself as being received, welcomed, understood as he is' (Rogers, 1967). With respect to a readiness to change, Rogers said that in one of the threads along this continuum '. . . there is a change in the individual's relationship to his problems', characterised by a gradual movement from no recognition of problems and no desire to change, to a recognition that they exist, to an increasing sense of self-responsibility for the problems and a recognition of the individual's own role in contributing to the problems.

Selection Issues and Assessment

Before embarking on a formal counselling relationship, it is necessary to ensure that the client is appropriate for counselling and able to use this kind of help. How the client is assessed will depend to some extent on the setting in which the client is seen, and for the nurse working in a mental health setting it will also be necessary to ensure that this is the appropriate setting. In general terms, the most important factors will be the client's willingness to change and his readiness to work on his problems in this particular way. It will also be necessary to ensure that there are no contraindicating factors, such as where the client is actively suicidal or psychotic. Other factors which will need to be considered will include whether the counsellor is willing to work with a particular client, and whether the client is willing to work with a particular counsellor. This may occur, for example, when a counsellor believes that a client's difficulties are outside the range of her competence, or where a client wishes only to see a counsellor of the same sex.

The importance of full and appropriate assessment cannot be overemphasised, as without it the basis on which counselling is offered may be misguided. Accurate assessment will help to ensure that the most appropriate form of help is offered, and for this reason it is important that careful thought is given to how clients are assessed, the criteria which are used and the arrangements for referring on should this be necessary.

Goal Setting and Contracting

As part of the assessment process, the counsellor and client will need to set a number of mutually agreed counselling goals. These will arise from the presenting issues brought by the client, and will take into account his strengths and weaknesses, as well as what the client hopes to achieve through counselling. Both short- and long-term goals may be set. It should be noted, however, that the assessment process, including goal setting, is an ongoing process and goals and achievements will need to be reviewed from time to time. Appropriate goal setting and review ensures that expectations are realistic and achievements can be acknowledged, or if necessary alternative options can be sought. Tschudin (1991), in her article 'Just four questions', suggests some useful questions which the nurse counsellor can use, and which may aid the goal setting process. These are: 'What is happening?', 'What is the meaning of it?', 'What is your goal?', and 'What are you doing about it?'. These questions may help both the client and the counsellor to focus on the process, and offer a useful way of thinking about goal setting.

Once counselling goals have been agreed, the counsellor and client agree a contract for counselling. This is essentially an agreement about what each party contributes to the process, and typically will include such things as the length of the sessions, the number of sessions, and other housekeeping matters such as timekeeping and arrangements for cancellation. The existence of a contract ensures that both client and counsellor understand and are in agreement about the nature of the therapeutic relationship which is to take place from the very outset.

Mental Health Counselling: An Eclectic Approach

So far several counselling skills have been described, and the person-centred approach to counselling has been outlined. This approach in its purest sense has its place in the mental health setting. In looking at mental health nursing, however, it may be helpful to take a broader view in order to consider how best the range of philosophical viewpoints and corresponding approaches can be accommodated in order to offer the best help to the client.

Other approaches to counselling may involve much more interpretation of the client's thoughts and behaviour (e.g. in psychodynamic counselling), or more directive interventions (e.g. in counselling based on behavioural principles). Burnard (1989) describes these and a number of other counselling approaches, including the cognitive, transactional analysis, personal-construct, *Gestalt*-therapy and eclectic approach. It can be argued, however, that characteristics of the person-centred approach may be used even within these differing philosophical perspectives. Furthermore, Heron (1986) has devised what he calls 'six category intervention analysis' which, he argues, describes all possible therapeutic interventions, transcending any particular theoretical perspective. This analysis can also be used when thinking about counselling interventions. Heron describes two broad categories, authoritative and facilitative, each of which can be subdivided into a further three categories, i.e. prescriptive, informative and confronting, and cathartic, catalytic and supportive, respectively. He describes each of the six interventions as follows.

Prescriptive interventions – explicitly seek to direct the behaviour of the client, suggesting a particular line of action.

Informative interventions – seek to offer new knowledge or information to the client.

Confronting interventions – challenge the client by giving direct feedback about restrictive attitudes, beliefs or behaviour.

Cathartic interventions – encourage the client to release tension by expressing painful emotions, e.g. crying, storming.

Catalytic interventions – encourage the client in a process of self-discovery and self-direction.

Supportive interventions – affirm the worth and value of the client.

If Heron's analysis can be seen as exhaustive, it may also provide a format for a consideration of counselling interventions which steps back from a particular philosophical stance, and takes into account other factors. The approach offered may depend on the philosophical standpoint of the professional offering her services, or the personality of the counsellor, but will also depend on the nature of the client's problems, and perhaps most importantly on the preference of the client and his willingness to accept the help on offer. Although a client may accept a particular kind of help, the likelihood of his responding to that approach will depend to a large extent on whether or not he is 'accessible' to it.

This idea has been developed by Ware (1983) in his article on 'personality adaptations'. Ware describes how people's 'energies' make them more accessible at different levels (feeling, thinking and behaviour) and that the approach that the counsellor/therapist chooses may usefully be determined by this. He describes what he calls 'doors to therapy', the 'open door' being the place at which the counsellor and client can make contact initially, the 'target door' being the area through which change will occur, and the 'trap door' being the area which is initially best avoided. For example, with a client whose personality adaptation is predominately 'passive–aggressive', it is helpful to start with a behavioural approach, while avoiding thinking or analysing. Later, by moving on to the feeling level, change is enabled to occur.

The idea of clients being more or less accessible to different approaches depending on their personality adaptation is a key one. A client's level of accessibility may also vary for other reasons. For example, a client may be more accessible at a particular time in his life, or his level of energy may vary and make him more ready to seek and accept help at some times than at others. An unwillingness to accept help can be seen as defensiveness or resistance. It can also be seen as a healthy protectiveness, with the client only making himself available and 'open' to help (consciously or subconsciously) when it is safe to do so.

In the mental health setting, clients usually come for help at a time of crisis or in a state of considerable disturbance. Thinking in terms of a mental health continuum, they may be seen as being at the end of the continuum where their coping abilities are at their lowest (at least in some areas of their life). At such a time, the apparently contradictory situation arises where the client may need to protect himself most at a time when he most needs to allow himself to be open to receive help. For this reason, it is particularly important that those who come into contact with the client in a helping capacity, including nurses, respond in a way that is sensitive to the client's needs at this time. The basic counselling skills will be very helpful here but in addition to this, a flexible approach becomes even more important. Obviously, any given professional can only offer what is within the scope of her experience and competence (or within the experience and competence of those in the setting in which she works or to whom she can refer), but a readiness to be as flexible as possible is essential. The response to any request for help should be determined by the needs of the client, as opposed to the 'dogma' of the helping professional. By trusting in the client and in the 'innate capacity to grow', it becomes possible to see how a particular approach may or may not be helpful at any given time.

The need for flexibility can illustrate the value of an eclectic approach, i.e. one which allows different models and approaches to come together in determining the best form of help for any one client. An argument against eclecticism is that it may lead to the 'dilution' of the models involved, with the worst of all worlds and the best of none being the result. The alternative view is that an approach is used more appropriately within the context of the client's needs, allowing the client a more realistic choice about the kind of help offered.

The argument can be taken further in that it can be seen as applying to approaches to mental health in general as well as counselling in particular. Thus it may be possible for medical, psychological, social and other models to work effectively together and side by side. A counselling relationship is not offered, for example, to a client whose problems fall into the category of 'psychotic illness' at a time when his 'symptoms' are not under control. Then a medical approach may be more helpful. This is not to say that a counselling approach only has value when working with clients who are suffering from problems of a 'neurotic' type. Rogers *et al* (1967) demonstrated research findings which showed that a high level of accurate empathy led to a reduction in schizophrenic symptomatology and, as has already been postulated, counselling skills are often helpful at times when a formal counselling relationship is inappropriate. Buchan (1991) has highlighted some of these points in a discussion of issues involved in nurse counselling in clinical areas. He notes that 'depending on the mental state and needs of the individual, a more directive approach may be needed, especially initially, but with the aim always of moving towards the "mutual participation" or "adult-to-adult" model'. Buchan argues that 'the patient may be helped in terms which are meaningful to her or him, and using a mode of intervention that is appropriate to the circumstances and setting', but which can still be seen as preserving the principles of person-centredness.

The need for flexibility and an openness to the particular needs and circumstances of the client can also be seen when counselling is offered to clients from different cultural backgrounds. Wright (1991) observes that in many non-Western cultures decisions and problems may be dealt with in collective ways, rather than in ways that emphasise individual responsibility, that understanding emotions, conflicts and difficulties in environmental rather than 'intra-psychic' terms may be the norm, and that clients may have quite different expectations of their counsellors. For example, Wright says that '. . . in some cultures, clients expect therapists to provide an assertive and protective role involving the giving of advice rather than the traditional Western non-directive approach'. He warns against a naive concentration on the core concepts of genuineness, empathy and respect, without consideration of 'legitimate concerns about the treatment of certain populations, and specific cultures within them'. His article is certainly challenging to any simplistic assumptions which may be made about these concepts, and all counsellors need to develop a clear awareness of the complex issues involved in cross-cultural counselling. In particular, the need to listen carefully and sensitively to our clients, and to trust in their own knowledge of what is helpful, becomes paramount.

Professional Development of the Counsellor

In order to work at the optimal level, an ongoing process of support and development for the counsellor is necessary. This may be seen as having three main components: supervision, training and personal development. Although these overlap to a large extent, as will be seen below, it is useful here to consider them separately. Furthermore, a full consideration of ethical issues is necessary, and these will also be briefly examined.

The Concept of Supervision

Munroe *et al* (1983) describe four different models of supervision:

1. Supervision as teaching, where skills acquisition is the primary goal.
2. Supervision as counselling, where personal growth and self-insight are the primary goals.
3. Supervision as administration, where organisational administration and case management are the primary goals.
4. Supervision as aspects of all three, but with the primary focus being the counsellor's 'survival' in an agency through the development of an understanding of influence, power and agency politics.

These models include the three components described at the beginning of this section, but supervision can be seen as having a further and even more important role in its own right. In particular, in order to do justice to the client, a regular forum where the often demanding relationship which has been developed can be 'brought' is essential. It is an opportunity to share what is happening with an 'independent' person, who has the skills and experience to be able to offer advice and support throughout the counselling relationship.

Supervision may take place in an individual setting or in a group, both having their advantages. Obviously the counsellor will receive more individual attention through individual supervision, while in a group the shared experience of a number of counsellors bringing their work together (see section on ethical issues and confidentiality) has many benefits. Many counsellors will arrange to participate in both settings for these reasons.

The British Association for Counselling (1990) emphasises the role of supervision in its Code of Ethics and Practice for Counsellors: 'Counsellors should monitor actively the limitations of their own competence through counselling supervision/consultative support, and by seeking the views of their clients and other counsellors'. Such supervision 'refers to a formal arrangement which enables counsellors to discuss their counselling regularly with one or more people who have an understanding of counselling and counselling supervision/consultative support. Its purpose is to ensure the efficacy of the counsellor–client relationship.

Kaberry (1992) has given a good description of supervision as it applies to practising counsellors, and suggests that the counselling supervision model is one which can usefully be applied in nursing, where a formal approach to supervision is less common. It is encouraging to see that the importance of clinical supervision in nursing is now beginning to be recognised, with the Department of Health's (1993) *A Vision for the Future* acknowledging that nurses need support, and identifying targets which include consideration of different models of clinical supervision.

For the mental health nurse whose role may only be partly counselling, it is important to ensure that the very specific nature of the supervision relationship is not overlooked. More general supervision may (or should) be provided, but this should not be seen as a substitute for appropriate counselling supervision, and indeed the politics of the employing body may necessitate separate supervision arrangements, other than those provided by line management.

Training Requirements

Appropriate training is also essential if counsellors are to perform at a competent level. Nurses in their initial training will begin to learn and develop many of the communication and interpersonal skills necessary for a counselling approach, but they will need to monitor their own levels of competence before embarking on a more formal counselling relationship. This is where the input of an appropriate supervisor is particularly helpful. Together with her supervisor the nurse will be able to look at her skills, identify strengths and weaknesses, determine areas of development and decide how best to proceed. For nurses who are interested in developing their general counselling skills, in-service training courses or an introductory course in counselling may be appropriate, but for those who are developing a specialist interest in this field, or who are likely to do a great deal of counselling in their particular area of work, a more extensive training will be necessary. Currently a number of organisations provide diploma courses in counselling. Although a more systematic approach to training is now developing in Britain, with accreditation by the British Association for Counselling being the main yardstick, courses vary widely in terms of philosophy, content, organisation and cost. Counselling courses aimed specifically at nurses tend to be rare, although Clift and Magee (1992) have described the development of the English National Board's Certificate in Counselling Skills. This course is Rogerian in approach, but looks at counselling skills particularly from the perspective of the health care worker. Tschudin (1983) and Buckroyd and Smith (1990) have also described approaches to teaching counselling to nurses. Determining an appropriate course may at first seem to be a daunting task, and to a large extent will be a matter for personal choice, but the help and advice of supervisors, colleagues and training departments within the employing agency may be invaluable here.

Most training courses will require the trainee counsellor to see clients as part of the course commitments, and close supervision will be particularly important during these early stages. As long as appropriate safeguards are in place, there is no reason why the counsellor in training cannot provide the highest standard of work which is compatible with her level of skill.

Personal Growth in the Counsellor

A third aspect of development which is necessary for the competent counsellor to consider is in the area of personal growth. This is perhaps a more contentious area, particularly when it comes to whether the counsellor should be in counselling or therapy herself. 'Self Awareness' has been a popular catchphrase in the nursing world in recent years, but it has not always been so clear how this is developed and maintained. Certainly both supervision and training will contribute substantially in this area, but this is not the primary function of either. In supervision the primary focus is the counsellor's work with the client, and although looking at what is going on for the counsellor will be an essential part of this process, it is not the main purpose. As Kaberry (1992) has put it:

. . . Supervision is not counselling for the counsellor – it is different – it is about the client/patient. Nevertheless, it may highlight issues of the supervisees which could be addressed in counselling therapy. For many trainee counsellors, therapy or counselling for themselves is essential (Kaberry, 1992).

Similarly during training, personal awareness and self development will occur and be encouraged, but will not be the primary focus.

Involvement in personal counselling or therapy is a necessary requirement of many counselling training courses. Perhaps one of the reasons why this tends to be more controversial in the mental health field relates to a feeling that mental health workers need to keep themselves 'separate' from their clients or patients. Unfortunately the 'us versus them' philosophy has not entirely disappeared in all areas of mental health, and it is often the fears of health professionals themselves which intrude here. Understandably we all have some anxieties about what we might find out about ourselves in therapy, but we owe it to our clients to do so. The personal growth and development which occurs when the counsellor is the primary focus leads to a level of richness in her work which cannot easily be achieved by other means. Not only does the counsellor gain insight into what it feels like to be in the client's place, but she also discovers aspects of herself that may enhance or interfere with her work with clients. This in turn allows a more careful and respectful approach to the counselling relationship.

ETHICAL ISSUES IN COUNSELLING

Ethical issues have been referred to several times in this chapter, and the British Association for Counselling Code of Ethics and Practice for Counsellors has been quoted more than once. The emphasis that has been placed on this is no accident; all counsellors must pay particular attention to ethics, and the nurse who is counselling will need to look closely at a number of issues. Two in particular are briefly mentioned here, because of their particular relevance to nurses working in a mental health setting.

Confidentiality

'Counsellors treat with confidence personal information about clients, whether obtained directly or indirectly by inference. Such information includes name, address, biographical details, and other descriptions of the client's life and circumstances which might result in identification of the client'. This means not revealing any of the above information to anyone, except for the purposes of supervision or appropriate consultation with colleagues: 'If counsellors include consultations with colleagues and others within the confidential relationship, this should be stated to the client at the beginning of counselling' (British Association for Counselling Code of Ethics and Practice for Counsellors, 1990).

These exceptions may cause ethical concerns for the mental health nurse, as reporting arrangements within an organisational structure may raise concern about what information is shared with whom. How confidentiality is properly protected will largely be a matter for the organisation to consider, but this needs to be thought through carefully before counselling is offered. Most importantly, nurses who are counselling should be careful to be as clear and as explicit as possible with their clients as to what confidentiality means and who it includes. In this way the client is able to make an informed choice about what he divulges to the counsellor.

A further ethical dilemma which may arise relates to the situations where it may become necessary to break confidentiality, in circumstances where the counsellor believes that there is a risk of serious harm occurring to the client or to others, and the client does not agree to extending confidentiality. Situations such as these will always be a challenge to the most competent counsellor. Respect for the client's wishes needs to be carefully balanced against the safety of the individuals concerned, and the counsellor will need to act decisively but sensitively, and with support.

Role Conflicts

Working within any organisation raises issues of various kinds for the counsellor, and this will be particularly so in the case of nurses who are working in the capacity of counsellors as well as nurses. It is important that where this is the case the issues and possible areas of conflict are carefully considered. For example, some aspects of the nurse's role (such as giving injections) may be seen by the client as conflicting with the role of counsellor, and where the nurse comes into contact with the client in other situations or through other interventions it is also possible that role conflict will occur.

The implications of such conflicts need to be carefully thought through, and it may be necessary to find other ways around them (for example, arranging for the injection to be administered by another nurse rather than the one whose relationship with the client is one of counsellor).

COUNSELLING IN A MENTAL HEALTH SETTING: SOME EXAMPLES FROM PRACTICE

The following examples of clients who have been helped using a counselling approach are taken from real-life situations in a community-based mental health unit in East London. They are included here in order to give a flavour of the kind of situations in which a counselling approach may be helpful. For reasons of confidentiality, names have been excluded and some relevant details have been changed to ensure anonymity.

Mrs A

Mrs A was a married woman in her early fifties who had been experiencing severe anxiety characterised by acute panic attacks, particularly in crowded areas such as supermarkets or on public transport. She came looking for help to control her symptoms and began by attending an anxiety management workshop in which an educational approach was used, consisting of physiological, cognitive and behavioural methods for coping with anxiety.

During her initial assessment, however, it had been noticed that Mrs A was struggling with a variety of feelings which appeared to relate to the deaths of her mother and brother some years previously. The option of counselling was given, but Mrs A decided that the main priority was her anxiety, and opted for the workshop. Once this work was done, however, she was again offered counselling and this time felt ready to accept this kind of help. She was seen by a nurse working as a counsellor over a period of 3 months, during which time Mrs A gradually became able to express her feelings, and also gave herself 'permission' to have them. Once she felt accepted as she was, she was able to identify how she had shut herself off from the feelings of sadness and anger that she felt about these two deaths. She became more in touch with herself, and came to realise that there was a relationship between her anxiety and her inability to work through her grief. Once this had happened her anxiety symptoms, already reduced following the workshop, virtually disappeared, and she was able to go out and cope with those situations that had previously been a nightmare to her.

The flexibility which allowed Mrs A to face her problems in a practical way gave her the opportunity to accept counselling when she felt ready for it. She was given control over what she chose to do, and this allowed her to take the further steps which enabled her to complete the mourning process, delayed for so many years.

Mr B

Mr B was in his early thirties when he began counselling after he and his wife separated. At the time that his wife left him, Mr B felt so devastated that he took a serious overdose and almost died. Subsequently he became involved in another relationship which was very up and down, and Mr B's mood was very up and down in line with this.

His pattern during the early sessions was one of irregular attendance (particularly at the beginning), and arriving late to sessions. He would invariably start with the problems in his current relationship, but would usually return to his relationship with his wife by the end of the session. Once Mr B had 'engaged' with his counsellor, he began being able to look at what was going for him, how he was feeling, and how he dealt with his fears, particularly about being alone. He started to look at his ambivalence as expressed by his lateness and non-attendance, and to look at his own patterns of behaviour for the first time. Gradually he was able to develop a greater understanding of what his relationship with his wife meant to him.

As Mr B came to understand himself better, he became more able to accept the loss of the relationship with his wife and began to work through his feelings about this loss. He also recognised that he had found it hard to understand his feelings for his new girlfriend while he was still so tied up in mourning the loss of his wife. After almost a year of weekly counselling sessions, Mr B felt that he was able to cope with these feelings on his own, and was ready to move on. His mood was no longer so up and down, and although he thought that there were still a number of issues that he needed to resolve about his present relationship, he considered that he was now on top of things and in control of his life again.

Ms C

Ms C was a young woman in her late twenties, who lived with her parents. From her teenage years, Ms C had experienced a number of psychotic episodes. At these times her mood became either excessively 'high' or she was extremely aggressive towards others. This resulted in her causing disturbances both at home and in public, and she ended up being taken to hospital by the police and detained under various sections of the 1983 Mental Health Act. The doctors who saw her thought that she was suffering from a manic-depressive psychosis.

At the time that she began counselling, Ms C was 'well' and had been discharged from hospital with a combination of interventions in the community. These included input from a social worker, attendance at a psychiatric out-patient clinic (she was on regular medication) and attendance at the day centre for individual counselling, as well as for a relaxation class. At this time Ms C was very receptive to the counselling approach and her mental state was such that she was able to cope with working on her problems in this way. She was very keen to explore her reactions to her illness, and to look for ways of coping more effectively with the stresses that she faced in her life in order to avoid future break-downs. The counselling relationship appeared to give Ms C a sense of control which she felt was starkly absent in other parts of her life. This seemed to be a vital ingredient in helping Ms C, because there were times when, in order to protect herself and others, control had had to be taken from her.

While she was accessible to this way of working, Ms C worked very hard to regain control over her own life, to adjust to the new role of being in employment again, and to cope with the pressures she felt her family imposed on her (although they were very supportive, they tended to treat every sign of emotion in her as a sign of psychosis). She was also able to identify this fear of the return of her illness as a fear that she had within herself. In the short period of this initial counselling relationship, she was able to begin making sense of her situation, and attributing meaning to what were a series of highly distressing events.

Subsequently Ms C did have a further psychotic breakdown which necessitated admission to hospital. However, she recovered quickly, and was able to resume counselling again before she was discharged. At this time family therapy was also commenced, and since that time (approximately 18 months ago at the time of writing), Ms C has remained well and appears to be coping effectively with the problems that she has experienced during this time.

CONCLUSION

In this chapter, I have provided a brief outline of the nature of counselling. Person-centred counselling has been presented as an example of an effective counselling approach, which also has many applications in the mental health nursing field as well as in multidisciplinary settings. Some basic counselling skills have been described and the development of the counselling relationship has been outlined. Issues of accessibility have been discussed, and the importance of listening carefully to the client and trusting in his 'innate capacity to grow' have been stressed. Various professional aspects of being a competent counsellor have also been identified, including the need for good supervision and personal development and growth. Some examples of counselling work carried out by mental health nurses have been described in order to give a flavour of this approach in action.

In such a short space as this it is not possible to give a fully comprehensive account of what is in itself a huge topic. Such an account is and has been the task of others. That being said, however, I hope that in these short pages I have been able to capture something of what counselling is all about. For those whose task is to work with and try to help others, and in particular the mental health nurse who has an interest in working with clients in this way, this chapter will perhaps provide a perspective on counselling from which that interest can develop.

ACKNOWLEDGEMENTS

The completion of this chapter would not have been possible without the advice and support of many people. Thanks are due in particular to Charlotte Sills from the Metanoia Psychotherapy Training Institute and Elizabeth Bennett from the Newham District Psychology Department. The author would also like to express his appreciation to other friends and colleagues who have given their support, and to the clients and staff at the East Ham Centre.

REFERENCES

British Association for Counselling (1990) *Code of Ethics and Practice for Counsellors*. Rugby: BAC.

Buchan R (1991) An integrated model of counselling. *Senior Nurse*, **11**(4): 32–33.

Buckroyd J and Smith E (1990) Learning to help. *Nursing Times*, **86**(35): 54–57.

Burnard P (1989) *Counselling Skills for Health Professionals*. London: Chapman and Hall.

Clift I and Magee T (1992) Developing a new counselling course. *Nursing Standard*, **6**(18): 34–36.

Department of Health, NHS Management Executive (1993) *A Vision for the Future. The Nursing, Midwifery and Health Visiting Contribution to Health and Health Care*. London: Department of Health.

Egan G (1986) *The Skilled Helper*. Belmont, California: Brooks/Cole.

Heron J (1986) Six Category Intervention Analysis, 2nd edn, *Human Potential Research Project*. Guildford, Surrey: University of Surrey.

Hershenson D B and Power P W (1987) *Mental Health Counseling, Theory and Practice*. New York: Pergamon Press.

Hopper L and Jesson A (1991) A definite role. *Nursing Times*, **87**(9): 41–43.

Jeavons B (1991) Developing counselling skills. *Nursing: The Journal of Clinical Practice, Education and Management*, **4**(37): 28–29.

Kaberry S (1992) Supervision – support for nurses? *Senior Nurse*, **12**(5): 38–40.

Mearns D and Thorne B (1988) *Person-Centred Counselling in Action*. London: SAGE Publications Ltd.

Munroe E A, Manthei R J and Small J J (1983) *Counselling, A Skills Approach.* Auckland: Methuen Publications (NZ) Ltd.

Rogers C R (1967) *On Becoming a Person. A Therapist's View of Psychotherapy.* London: Constable and Company Ltd.

Rogers C R, Gendlin E T, Kiesler D J and Truax C B (eds) (1967) *The Therapeutic Relationship and its Impact. A Study of Psychotherapy with Schizophrenics.* Madison, Wisconsin: University of Wisconsin Press.

Rolfe G (1990) The assessment of therapeutic attitudes in the psychiatric setting. *Journal of Advanced Nursing*, **15**: 564–570.

Swaffield L (1990) Patient power. *Nursing Times*, **86**(48): 26–28.

Truax C and Mitchell K (1971) Research on certain therapist interpersonal skills in relation to process and outcome. In: *Handbook of Psychotherapy and Behaviour Change*, eds Bergin A and Garfield S. New York: Wiley.

Tschudin V (1981) A question of mind over matter? 2: The response of the nurse using counselling skills. *Nursing Times*, **77**(11): 455–459.

Tschudin V (1983) A feasibility study for a counselling training package. *Nurse Education Today*, **3**(4): 95–96.

Tschudin V (1991) Just four questions. *Nursing Times*, **87**(39): 46–47.

Ware P (1983) Personality adaptations (Doors to therapy). *Transactional Analysis Journal*, **13**(1): 11–19.

Wright J (1991) Counselling at the cultural interface: is getting back to roots enough? *Journal of Advanced Nursing*, **16**: 92–100.

11

Community Care

Marilyn Paynter

INTRODUCTION

In this chapter three main themes – deinstitutionalisation, role of the Community Psychiatric Nurse (CPN) and relationships with other members of the Mental Health Team – are explored within the context of Community Care. Cameos from clinical practice in the community are illustrated.

WHAT IS A COMMUNITY?

The meaning of the term 'community' has been difficult to define. It portrays meanings such as locality, the interaction of people, their common bonds and their combined actions. In sociological terms, it simply implies a social group (Bennett and Freeman, 1991). It also implies that 'community' could be referred to both treatment in the hospital and outside its walls. According to Acheson (1985), it also refers to the public health approach to care. These differing views may cause confusion. However, since the early 1960s, after much debate about the meaning of the term, it has been used mainly to differentiate between aspects of mental health care, as opposed to the physical care provided by district nurses.

CONCEPTS OF COMMUNITY CARE

This is another term which comes under heavy criticism, since it seems to imply different meanings to different people. Sladden (1974) criticises the use of this term and says that it is 'indiscriminately used' to denote either a 'principle of administration' or the actual 'range of services provided'. She breaks down the concept of community care into three principles:

1. The *care of social problems* by social agencies, thus highlighting the need/responsibility of local authorities for the provision of services (Titmus, 1963; Harrison, 1973).
2. The *care or treatment* given to an individual without recourse to a psychiatric hospital. This form of treatment was encouraged since the much-publicised works of Barton (1959) and Goffman (1961) highlighted the 'harmful aspects' of institutional care which caused psychological damage to the individuals.
3. The *comprehensive system of preventive psychiatry.* The philosophy behind preventive psychiatry was based on Caplan's views, in that he advocated a community mental health approach (or public health model), so that the level of mental health among the people in the community could be raised by using several techniques of prevention and thus minimise the incidence of mental disorders in the community (Caplan, 1961).

Caplan's proposals resulted in the prolific development of Community Mental Health Centres in the USA. The focus of these centres was two-fold: (i) to provide treatment and rehabilitation of mentally ill individuals in community-based settings as opposed to the State Mental Hospitals and (ii) to promote mental health throughout the nation (Larsen and Jerrell, 1983).

A more practical and social care perspective to community care was outlined by Payne (1986). He viewed community care as a way of reducing the dependence on others and cautioned against simply abandoning the clients to their fate, but suggested that opportunities should be made available for clients and their carers to learn to act independently. He positively advocates that community care should involve people in providing care which is 'relevant to their wishes and culture' instead of fitting the individuals into a 'service' which is unsuitable. His views are now being equally reinforced by the government's legislation of the Citizen's Charter and by the principles of the Community Care Act (1990), whereby users of the mental health services are asked for their views and encouraged to participate in the planning of the provision of these services. Goldman *et al* (1983) suggest that 'community care' may imply a change in the locus of the care, and that the care may be by the community, and in the community.

DEINSTITUTIONALISATION

The trend towards deinstitutionalisation has accelerated within the last 15 years in Britain due to the various health and social policy reforms. This concept – deinstitutionalisation – has been defined by Gruenberg (1977) as the diminution of mental hospital populations, while the sociologist Bachrach (1983) viewed it as 'the eschewal, shunning or avoidance of traditional institutional settings . . . for the care of the chronically mentally ill, and the concurrent expansion of non-institutional facilities for the care of this population' (Bachrach, 1983, p.10). She goes on to explain that deinstitutionalisation should not only be viewed as if it refers exclusively to patients leaving hospitals, since the process itself has more far-reaching consequences, even on people who have never been hospitalised.

Bennett and Freeman (1991) have added more weight to her views and argue that the philosophy behind deinstitutionalisation is 'still being formulated incorrectly' in that it is viewed as the physical reconstructuring of units in new ways and in new places, instead of trying to change staff attitudes and promote better relationships between staff and patients. It may be deduced that the philosophy behind deinstitutionalisation is good, but the way in which it is being done poses the question as to whether, in effect, there will be any positive benefits for the clients if the staff take a traditional approach to view their roles. One of the possible reasons for the above comment is that there is an ambiguity in the definition of the term deinstitutionalisation. Although from a sociological perspective it merely indicates the breakdown of traditional ways of dealing with the problems of the mentally ill, its main principle implies a social change in a 'least restrictive' environment, or 'humanising' mental health care, that is, providing community-based facilities.

NORMALISATION

In Britain, one of the most successful schemes to date on mental hospital closures and the provision of alternative localised services for people with mental health problems is in Torbay. Here, its first hospital – Exminster – was closed in July 1987, in response to both the government's policy on mental health and the comprehensive approach as was embodied in the World Health Organisation's strategy for attaining Health for All. Its success story is well documented in the book *Community Care Works* (Beardshaw and Morgan, 1990).

One of the guiding lights behind Torbay's dehospitalisation process, was to incorporate the principles of 'normalisation' – which have been very influential in the development of services for People with Learning Difficulties (formerly known as mentally handicapped people) – in the planning of residential services in the community (Wolfensberger, 1972). Briefly, his approach emphasises the importance of minimising social disadvantage for already disadvantaged groups, and prevent them from encountering the increasingly personal and social marginalisation that is felt by people who experience mental distress.

Principles of Normalisation Theory

The main principles of normalisation theory which emerged from Sweden and North America have been summarised by Tyne (1982) to include:

1. assisting the handicapped individual to gain skills;
2. supporting and enabling the handicapped person to participate genuinely in the mainstream of life;
3. providing services in settings which are valued by society;
4. providing age-appropriate and culturally valued social activities.

The central concern of the theory was to highlight the 'rights' of the mentally disabled to live a full life in the community, especially those who had been discharged from large institutions and to provide culturally sensitive provision for care by enhancing the individual's social image and personal competence (Pilling, 1991). Although the above principles related initially to people with learning difficulties, they are also applicable to individuals with psychiatric disabilities. However, the process of deinstitutionalisation will be fraught with problems for all concerned: the patient/client, the carer and the community at large, if it is not properly implemented.

Phases of Deinstitutionalisation

Kingsley and Towell (1988) assert that the process of deinstitutionalisation needs active involvement by the direct care workers who are involved in the planning, implementation and monitoring of the care. They further stated that they (direct care workers) are the 'stakeholders', and should have a legitimate interest in the transition from the hospital to the community setting, by ensuring that their opinions are sought in the planning process. The literature suggests that there are four main phases in the deinstitutionalisation process, and they are identified in Table 11.1.

Table 11.1   Showing phases in the process of deinstitutionalisation

Phase	I	Rehabilitation of patients
	II	Assessment for the move and subsequent treatment planning
	III	Preparation of the staff
	IV	Preparation of the community

(Adapted from Hume and Pullen, 1986; Pilling, 1991.)

Phase I – Rehabilitation and Resettlement of the Patient

A working definition of rehabilitation is given by Hume and Pullen (1986) as the 'process through which a person is helped to adjust to the limitations of his disability' (p.43). This definition also takes into consideration that the aim of rehabilitation is on restoring the individual to his 'maximum level of independence' psychologically, socially, economically and physically. In this context, the 'maximum level' refers to the optimum level for the individual. Therefore success is measured against the goals set for that person (Hume and Pullen, 1986). The focus of rehabilitation should encompass the quality of a person's life and must also consider the realities of the world outside. This therefore involves a systematic approach to rehabilitation over a period of time, and must involve both the staff and patients.

Once the acute symptoms of the illness have subsided, there will be a need to discuss with the patient his future in the community. Here it is important that the patient shows some motivation to leave the hospital, since he may sabotage all attempts at rehabilitation and resettlement (Hume and Pullen, 1986). In the first instance, the patient will be assessed provisionally by the ward clinical team to determine whether he is ready for referral to the Community Resettlement Team. The Consultant Psychiatrist, on behalf of the Team, will then send in the official referral for an assessment by the Community Resettlement Team. When the patient has been accepted by the Resettlement Team, he may be transferred to a designated Resettlement Training area which may be within the hospital or purpose-built facilities in the community (Community Health Services Unit, 1991).

Phase II – Assessment for the Move and Subsequent Treatment Planning

This assessment will be conducted over a period of time by all the professionals working in the multidisciplinary team with on-going self-assessment by the patient. Since assessment is the foundation of any treatment regime, it requires a baseline from which to monitor the patient's progress. Hence there will be measurement of the patient's skills, achievements, deficits and problems, using several methods (Hume and Pullen, 1986). Some examples of methods include personal care and mental state assessments by the nurses; IQ testing by the clinical psychologists; and domestic and work skills measurement by the occupational therapist. The treatment planning stage will involve the patient, naturally, and it must have clear goals with identifiable steps to be taken towards the patient's rehabilitation. This involves team work and accurate documentation of the patient's progress through formative and summative evaluations. At a later stage, a discharge planning meeting will be arranged by the Multidisciplinary Resettlement Team, to include the client, his relatives/carers and other relevant staff. Prior to the final move into a community-based facility, e.g. group home or flat, the patient would have undergone a 'trial' period of coping in a pre-discharge flat, for example, or a hostel ward. The latter is a ward based in the community and is used for long-term patients who do not need hospital care, but are unable to cope with the unstructured environment of the group home and have the support and supervision from nursing staff (Hume and Pullen, 1986; Pilling, 1991).

Phase III – Preparation of the Staff

For community care to be successful the staff need to be involved in the deinstitutionalisation process, since it can be viewed as a sort of bereavement by the staff. Bender (1986) makes the point in reminding us that there is a need for the social recognition of the pain and trauma of institutional termination. One has to consider that it may be a painful experience, since it may involve loss of familiar and predictable status and roles. The problems created by the impending closure or 'death' of an institution are similar to the stages of grief (Allan and Hall, 1988) (see Tables 11.2 and 11.3, for the 'effects' of deinstitutionalisation on the hospital and implications for staff).

Part of the staff's preparation will include reorientating them to the community facilities available, as they may not originally be from the areas in which the new community units will be set up. They will also need to visit other community units that are fully functioning, in order to understand the philosophy of community care and their roles in this new environment (Pilling, 1991). They may also need additional psychological preparation, and the necessary skills to increase their autonomy in the new setting, and cope with the possible isolation that the move to the community facilities will bring, as it may reduce the personal and social support that the hospital provided.

Phase IV – Preparation of the Community

Because of the stigma attached to mental illness, there may be a great deal of resentment and fear from the members of the public. Part of the CPN's role will be to educate members of the public about the factors causing mental illness and the philosophy behind community care. Due to ignorance, some of the members of the community may attempt to veto planning permission for some of the community facilities, that is, the group homes, community mental health centres, drop-in centres and sheltered work facilities. Other facilities used in the community care programme include luncheon clubs, counselling and crisis intervention services and Day Hospital provisions. Part of the preparation could include having open meetings with the professionals, prospective residents and members of the public. Clerkenwell, Islington, is a good example of a locally based residential project for the mentally ill, in which there was full consultation and involvement from the local community

Table 11.2 Effects of deinstitutionalisation on the manifest functions of psychiatric hospitals

Function	Effects of transferring function to community services
Active treatment for short- to intermediate stay patients	Function maintained or improved: but data from model programmes may not be generally applicable
Custody for long-stay patients	Function maintained in residential homes: quality of care variable
Physical assessment and treatment	Function may be better transferred to GP
Protection of patients from exploitation	Function markedly impaired: increased physical, sexual and financial vulnerability
Respite for family	Function equivocal: locus of treatment at home, offset by potential for increased professional support to family
Haven/asylum for patient	Function maintained in crisis/foster homes, or impaired in home treatment
Research and training centre	Function partially decentralised: greater coordination and flexibility required
Provision of day- and out-patient	Function decentralised and may be impaired if successor services not established: renegotiation if responsibilities of health and social services for day care. Opportunities to work from health centres
Secure provision for involuntary and assaultive patients	Function vulnerable: clear commitment needed to provide well-staffed units
Occupation and vocational rehabilitation	Function at risk if industrial and occupational therapy not transferred
Shelter, nutrition, basic income and clothing	Function decentralised and at risk without continuity of care

(From Thornicroft and Bebbington, 1989.)

in overseeing the development of the project (Pilling, 1991).

When the new community facilities are in operation, the various members of the Mental Health Team will need to continue giving support as appropriate, to the former hospital patients and to the various staff working in these new facilities. The process of deinstitutionalisation will only be successful if the staff, patients and the community are adequately prepared.

THE ROLE OF THE COMMUNITY PSYCHIATRIC NURSE

Historical Development of the CPN's Role

The most frequently quoted published papers giving an account of the Community Psychiatric Nurse's (CPN's) role are those of May and

Table 11.3   Effects of deinstitutionalisation on the latent functions of psychiatric hospitals

Function	Effects of transferring function to community services
Job security to professional	Function less secure: staff roles, numbers, location and pay may change
Segregation from society of deviant or dangerous members	Function impaired: behavioural deviance more visible in urban areas.
Economies of scale from block treatment	Function vulnerable: dependent upon size of residential settings and staff: patient ratios
Local tax base and consumer of local goods and services	Function loss: redevelopment of hospital site may offset loss
Segregation within psychiatry of less attractive patients	Function impaired: but two-tier community services may develop
Structured roles and identities for staff and patients	Function eroded: risks of role blurring and patient anonymity
Providing the illusion of comprehensive care	Function reduced: consequences of inadequate care more publicly visible

(From Thornicroft and Bebbington, 1989.)

Moore (1963) and Hunter (1974). Briefly, these papers identified that the first 'outpatient nurse' or Community Psychiatric Nursing Service was established in 1954 at Warlingham Park Hospital, Surrey and at Moorhaven Hospital in Devon. The identified roles of the CPN at that time were to provide 'after care' for discharged patients with long-term psychiatric problems and to administer long-acting (depot) injections.

However, a more recent study by Gasson (1991) identified that psychiatric nurses were working in the community in Birmingham as early as 1913, from Winson Green Hospital. This therefore supersedes reports that Miss Peat (Warlingham Park Hospital) was the first 'outpatient nurse'. Gasson's study also highlighted that a report in 1913, by Dr Cecil Roscrow (Medical Superintendent of Birmingham City Asylum), to the Committee of Visitors, asserted that: '. . . a new office was created by the appointment of Miss A F Wightwick as a special nurse and after care visitor . . .'.

This recent development highlights that the nursing and medical professions had, very early in the century, recognised the dangers of institutionalisation, and were advocating community care for patients with mental health problems. The role and functions of the CPN have since developed enormously to cover the broad categories as outlined in Figure 11.1. A detailed description of these roles follow later in the chapter.

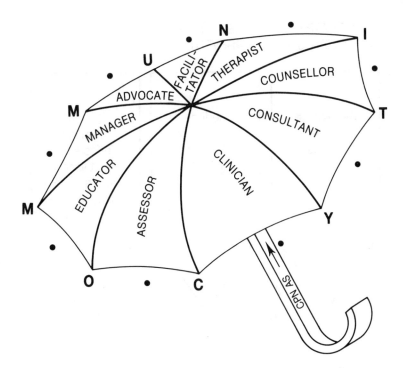

Figure 11.1 Roles of the CPN (adapted from Barker, 1977; Sladden, 1974; Carr *et al*, 1980; Flaye, 1990).

Principles of Preventive Psychiatry and Psychiatric Nursing

As mentioned earlier, Caplan's approach to preventive psychiatry greatly influenced the way in which all health professionals attempted to prevent illness within their sphere of community work. The main focus was not on the 'cure' of the mentally ill, but on identifying the factors which contributed to mental illness, and minimising the impact on the sufferers and their families (Caplan, 1964).

Caplan's three-pronged approach at preventing mental illness covered primary, secondary and tertiary prevention, as shown in Figure 11.2. Therefore, the CPN working in the domain of *primary prevention* will be trying to reduce the risk of mental illness among 'mentally well' individuals and groups, by counteracting stressful circumstances before they can produce an illness. Many CPNs are attached to Primary Health Care Teams, and are therefore in a position to take direct referrals from General Practitioners (GPs), or other primary health care colleagues. Examples of preventive work include teaching relaxation techniques to stressed individuals, offering bereavement counselling, dealing with factors leading to psychosocial problems and giving supportive advice to

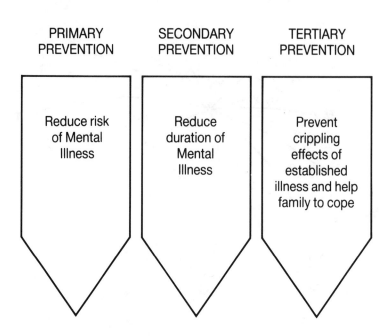

PRIMARY PREVENTION	SECONDARY PREVENTION	TERTIARY PREVENTION
Reduce risk of Mental Illness	Reduce duration of Mental Illness	Prevent crippling effects of established illness and help family to cope

Figure 11.2 Caplan's theory: principles of preventive psychiatry (adapted from Caplan, 1961).

community self-help groups, e.g. the Asian Women's Therapy Group. The latter example also helped the CPN to learn more about Asian cultures and gave the clients an opportunity to act as a 'teacher' to the CPN, thus enhancing the principle of 'side by side' psychiatry (Khandwalla, 1984; Jervis, 1986).

In _secondary prevention_, the focus is on the early identification of clients suffering from mental illness, and providing them with the care and support needed, in order to minimise the severity and duration of the illness. Exemplars from practice include assessing the client's mental state, monitoring the side-effects of medication and offering advice as necessary. These activities can be done either during Domiciliary Visits (DVs), at outpatient clinics or drop-in Mental Health Clinics, where clients may also be afforded the opportunity to 'socialise with a cup of tea', while the CPN undertakes the assessment and tries to identify any other current stresses the client may be experiencing and, where appropriate, mobilise the resources to deal with it.

Tertiary prevention is an area of increased growth within the Community Mental Health services, since it focuses on the 'after care' rehabilitative aspects of preventive Psychiatric Nursing. Changes in the 1983

Mental Health Act state that clients who had been detained in hospital under sections 3, 37, 47 and 48 of the Act, and are being discharged into the community, should be allocated a 'key worker' to coordinate and monitor the 'after care' given to these clients. Section 117 of the Act also outlines the statutory obligations of the Health Authority and the Social Services Department. Therefore, as good practice the CPN (as a member of the multidisciplinary team) may be involved in the 'after care planning meeting' and, where appropriate, may be nominated to monitor the discharged client's mental state, and report back to the multidisciplinary team on the success or failure of the client's ability to cope in the community.

The following section gives a more detailed account of the CPN's roles. It is known from research (Barker, 1977; Sladden, 1979; Carr *et al*, 1980) and a small-scale study by Flaye (1990), that the CPNs have many roles. These roles are outlined in Figure 11.1.

ROLES OF THE COMMUNITY PSYCHIATRIC NURSE (CPN)

Clinician

In this role, the CPN utilises her various psychiatric nursing skills. Here she can operate at several levels – (i) during her Domiciliary Visits (DVs), and (ii) during the periods when she operates from any of her bases, which could be in a Mental Health Centre, the outpatients' clinic or as a member of the Primary Health Care Team in the GP's surgery. However, before any intensive work is undertaken, the CPN needs first to establish a therapeutic relationship with her client, regardless of the treatment setting. This development of interpersonal relations is crucial to the formation of a nurse–client relationship. Through working with clients in their homes the CPN is better able to understand the lifestyle and interests of the family, observe the family dynamics and perhaps reduce the social stigma of hospitalisation by giving care and treatment in the home (Pollock, 1989).

The care could involve monitoring progress or relapse of the client's illness, by observing his or her mental state or behaviour, and identifying when the client needs to be re-referred to the GP or psychiatrist for assessment. As a clinician, the CPN is able to offer a range of therapeutic interventions. Pollock (1983) cited that as part of her role as a clinician (working with individuals suffering from emotional stress ('in dis-stress') would be to listen, counsel and facilitate emotional problem-solving, which may be in the form of 'talking therapy' in the home situation. The CPN also needs to encourage the client to identify his/her needs, participate in formulating care plans, and to provide opportunities for clients to discuss their feelings with respect to 'engaging' in any therapeutic work.

Another aspect of her role is to monitor the desirable and undesirable effects of the medication taken by the clients. In addition, the CPN may need to persuade clients to accept and continue taking medication, and educate them about the benefits and side-effects of the drugs (Samarasinghe, 1986). Therefore, it is important that the CPNs are conversant with current psychopharmacology in order to give their clients and families advice and guidance to recognise the undesirable effects of the medication.

A few Health Authorities – for example Barnet – provide weekend visiting and twilight services for the Elderly Mentally Infirm clients, in keeping with its general philosophy of providing 24-hour crisis intervention facilities for the district (Scott, 1980; Barnet Health Authority, 1988; Riley, 1988). Hence some CPNs may be involved in clinical 'crisis' work at the weekends.

During a routine DV by a CPN to a middle-aged client, the author noted that after administering the depot injection, the CPN made a point of asking the client's carer about how he was coping with his wife's illness. When asked by the author if she usually sees both client and carer together, she (CPN) indicated that most of the time she aimed to see them together and offer her husband support, because '. . . I can pick up very quickly when she (client) is becoming very disturbed, since that is very much part of how she presents when she is ill, as her behaviour towards her husband seems different . . .'.

Simmons and Brooker (1986) highlighted that CPNs should pay attention to what family members tell them about their situation, since many are not used to being asked about their own experiences, only about the person who has been identified as having the problem. In this instance, the CPN was giving the carer valuable psychological support. The fact that the carer was listened to, and complimented on his methods of coping, helped to reduce the resentment and burdensome duty felt by some relatives. Gottlieb (1983) asserted that when carers receive nothing back, they may withdraw from the situation to protect their own psychological well-being. This may, in turn, lead to a 'crisis' for the client, and the return to hospital for additional care. In a situation such as the above the nurse has to use her past experience with the family, and clinical judgment to determine when it is appropriate to offer additional support to the carer and the family as a whole.

Assessor

The CPN as an assessor has the ongoing responsibility of client's needs in the clinical setting, and acting as an assessor of student nurses during their clinical placements. As part of her assessment of client's needs, she uses the framework of the Nursing Process and a model of nursing, and subsequently plans with the client the appropriate care. Here some form of 'contract' may be negotiated within the care plan and opportunities are made available to have ongoing discussions with the client about the way in which the treatment is progressing.

With respect to assessing clients, it is very important that the CPN is versed in the 'special' instruments to assess cultural diversity in attitudes and perceptions of health care. An American tool by Tripp-Reimer *et al* (1984) provides an example of a *cultural assessment tool*. However, they point out that when using this tool, one does not require information on every element of the culture, but information on the *major values, beliefs* and *behaviours* which may have some influence on a *particular health problem, in a specific clinical setting*. Therefore, when the nurse is conducting an assessment of the client's mental state, she needs to bear in mind aspects of *transcultural psychiatry* which highlight that each culture has its own *language of distress*, since *normality* and *abnormality* are expressed differently in different cultures (Helman, 1984).

Despite Britain's multicultural make-up, there are no specific cultural assessment tools available to psychiatric nurses to use when assessing clients' needs from different cultural backgrounds. The assessment tools developed by Brink (1976) and Tripp-Reimer *et al* (1984) help to promote intercultural understanding; however, there is a paucity of literature in British textbooks to assist the nurse. In a recent British text on *Transcultural Nursing* Susan Dobson, a Health Visitor, urges nurses to '. . . become skilled at bridging cultural barriers, and adept at discovering cultural information that is relevant to their clients' health . . .' (Dobson, 1991, p.10). Unless the CPN is aware of the cultural factors that impinge on the health and well-being of her client, it is questionable whether an accurate assessment could be conducted, thus reducing the CPN's capacity to fulfil her role in the early detection and primary prevention of mental illness. This cultural knowledge will help the CPN to view the client as a 'holistic' entity (Simmons and Brooker, 1986), be able to decide between the various courses of action and refer the client to appropriate agencies, if she is unable to deal adequately with the problem.

The CPN also plays an important part in the facilitating and assessing of student nurses, to determine whether they have achieved the learning outcomes of their clinical placements, especially as the students now have a small 'caseload'. This facilitative and assessing process is enhanced by regular 'clinical supervision' with the learner. Simmons and Brooker describe this as an educational tool which promotes learning and increases confidence. It also helps the learner to develop a different perspective on her work with clients, by encouraging greater self-awareness, by building on her strengths and therapeutic and coping skills.

Therapist

Due to the current growth of community-based, as opposed to hospital-based, facilities CPNs are in an ideal position to be innovative to develop mental health care programmes for groups and individuals. The fact that the CPN is able to have an extended period of time with clients, as opposed to the hospital-based nurse, means that she may be able to develop a therapeutic relationship much quicker with her clients. Part of her role as a therapist will include using alternative therapies, where appropriate to the client's needs. Examples include behaviour therapy, family therapy and counselling.

To enhance their clinical abilities and deal with the demands of their caseloads, most CPNs have become specialists in areas of psychiatric nursing which could be of benefit to clients. These specialist areas are developed during postregistration, and may include child psychiatry and complementary medicine therapies such as aromatherapy and reflexology.

Counsellor

Inherent in the role of the psychiatric nurse is the ability to develop and use counselling skills. This role is a specialist one with the CPN using the principles of counselling and applying them to specific situations; for example, the CPN may use these skills to help individuals during periods of emotional trauma. It is well documented that some CPNs are attached to Primary Health Care teams and provide counselling services on a sessional basis at health centres. In other instances, the CPN may provide counselling as a specialist service to other professionals, for example the police force, at MIND drop-in centres or be part of the recently created specialist teams dealing with post-traumatic events.

Consultant/Resource Person

As a nurse consultant the CPN can work with statutory and voluntary groups and provide them with specialist skills, either as a resource, or directly into client care; for example, working with other disciplines to set up group work for individuals dealing with the problem of tranquilliser withdrawal (Flaye, 1990). In her role as consultant, the CPN may undertake health education activities in primary and secondary schools; these activities could include talks on drug or sexual abuse.

The dual roles of nurse consultant and resource person enable the CPN to promote mental health awareness and help to 'demystify' psychiatric nursing to other professionals in the primary health care team, to individuals and other agencies. Pollock (1983) cited that she was able to help health visitors set up a support group for new mothers following the birth of their babies. Here she was able to share some of her specialised psychiatric nursing skills with these professionals, and in return was able to tap into new community resources that could become available to individuals with mental health problems, such as babysitting groups.

This liaison also helped to increase the CPNs knowledge of the wealth of statutory and voluntary agencies, which she could use later for clients who may have a paucity of social support. This is in keeping with Caplan's principle, in which he strongly suggested to professionals working in the community to identify the 'indigenous patterns of lay support in the community', and to strengthen them, in order to foster more 'person-to-person' support and reduce stress (Caplan, 1964). Other writers support Caplan's views by stating that social support acted as a 'buffer' between the stressor and an 'illness reaction in the individual', hence this support may insulate the individual from the harmful effects of stress (Simmons and Brooker, 1986; Gottlieb, 1983).

Manager

The CPN must be able to manage her own time effectively and that of junior colleagues, use the resources available to her, and carry a caseload in the community. Therefore, as a manager she should be able to liaise and link resources effectively. Inherent in this role is a high degree of professional autonomy, but the CPN is still accountable to a line manager. Hence there is a need for her to be an effective communicator within the team and with other professionals, by maintaining accurate records and statistical information about visits and therapeutic work undertaken (Flaye, 1990). Another management function of the CPN concerns participation in the development of the Community Psychiatric Nursing Service (CPNS). Due to the solitary nature of the job, most Community Nursing Services provide clinical supervision for its qualified members of staff. Pollock (1989) asserts that supervision increases the awareness of potential difficulties and problems, thus enabling the CPN to make more effective decisions.

Educator

The modern CPN's role as an educator is becoming increasingly important, since the World Health Organisation (WHO) has advised that all health professionals should try to achieve 'Health for All' by the year 2000. The CPN also has to respond to the needs of the nursing profession, and help to prepare the future Project 2000 practitioners to work competently in a range of care settings (Project 2000, English National Board, 1989).

CPNs are now actively involved in curriculum planning for all pre- and postregistration nursing courses, especially Project 2000 (P2K), since they are expected to contribute updated philsophical changes in the principles of community/public health nursing, and enable the trainees to achieve the required competencies. Husband (1991) astutely reminds the profession that by including community nurses on curriculum planning teams the profession will be able to ensure ongoing 'course corrections', and maintain up to date clinical placements for the learners. The CPNs are also actively involved in the block/study day preparation for the student nurses prior to and during their 'community' placements, since it is expected that the future P2K practitioner will be qualified to work within the community setting.

From the author's experience (as a non-participant observer of a group of CPNs), a local initiative was set up by the CPN attached to the Forensic Psychiatric Services, to have health education workshops with a group of local magistrates, in order to heighten their awareness about mental illness. The workshop was co-facilitated by the local psychiatrist and probation officer. This workshop was in response to a 'felt need', since the needs of the mentally disordered offender patients are not always fully understood by the presiding magistrate (Paynter, 1991). As a community worker, the CPN is exposed to having a variety of 'trainees' from other allied professions observing her role. Here, she has the ideal opportunity to update their knowledge and skills in respect to aspects of mental health care.

CPN as an Advocate

With the increased attention paid to the powerful and valuable concept of normalisation (which in mental health has been closely associated with the rights and representation of the individuals' need for services), nurses have been encouraged to act as the client's advocate. From the CPN's perspective, advocacy is 'a means of transferring power back to the patient to enable him to control his own affairs' (Walsh, 1985, p.24). This, in principle, is what the CPN is aiming to do in her role, since she is trying to minimise the effects of the client's disability, and empowering him to regain control by offering support and advice. As the CPN is viewed as a resource person, she is able to point the patient in the right direction for access to the care needed to resolve his problems. As an advocate, the CPN can help to 'destigmatise the role of the psychiatric patient', by enabling him to live his life in the community (Flaye, 1990).

CPN as a Facilitator

This role is viewed as providing a bridge in the integration of community and hospital services. In some instances CPNs are nominated as 'key workers' to specific clients who may be undergoing a rehabilitation programme. In order to avoid duplication of effort as a key worker the CPN, according to Pilling, '. . . is charged with responsibility for the coordination of the care and involvement of the range of other professionals and agencies . . .' (Pilling, 1991, p.63). This could involve liaising with voluntary agencies such as MIND (National Association for Mental Health), the Salvation Army and various mental health self-help groups. Due to her facilitative skills, the CPN will be able to provide specialised therapy and education for clients, and help to reduce vulnerability to mental illness. Some CPNs have undergone additional post-basic training, and are therefore able to use those additional skills to set up 'support' or 'self-help' groups, which help to develop self responsibility and independence in the clients (Flaye, 1990).

The above are just some examples of the role and functions of the Community Psychiatric Nurse. The last two roles – facilitator and advocate – were identified by Flaye during a small-scale study of CPNs in selected areas of England and Wales. These roles will naturally change in response to developments in Community Psychiatric Nursing, and Community Care generally. The next section of the chapter focuses on the CPN's relationship with the other members of the Mental Health Team.

Relationships With Other Members of the Mental Health Team

As health care workers, CPNs make up the membership of different teams with several professionals. The recent Cumberlege Report (DHSS, 1986) stipulates that 'the care of people in the community with chronic or severe mental disorders, should be the primary concern of specialist multidisciplinary teams, in collaboration with General Practitioners' (DHSS, 1986, p.39). The report goes on to say that all health care workers should familiarise themselves with the roles of the specialist multidisciplinary teams, and 'know how and when' to make referrals or seek advice. This concept of multidisciplinary team is not new, and has been in existence in various forms since the inception of the National Health Service (NHS).

Within the domains of Community Psychiatry, the Mental Health Team consists of several professional groups working together for the benefit of the clients, with each professional group recognising that each member is a professional in his or her own right, and must share the responsibility of client care. These teams are sometimes referred to as Community Mental Health Teams (CMHTs) (Adams, 1990), Multidisciplinary Clinical Teams (MDCTs) (Royal Commission, 1979); or simply Multidisciplinary Teams (MDTs). The CPNs, besides relating to their own line management structures, have to interact with several members of the Mental Health Team as identified in Figure 11.3. More recently, these teams have expanded to include Home Care Organisers and Ethnic

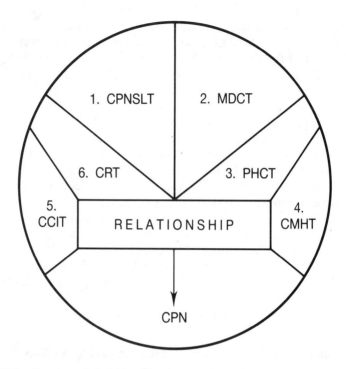

Figure 11.3   Showing relationship with other members of the Mental Health Team.

Development Workers. With the changes in mental health care provision from hospital to community-based facilities, there is a devolution of traditional medical autocracy to multidisciplinary democracy, as represented by the CMHTs (Adams, 1990). This therefore enables the CPN to increase her professional autonomy within the team, with its appropriate clinical responsibilities.

The CPN can operate in, and liaise with, several teams. These include the following.

1. *The Community Psychiatric Nursing Services locality team* (the nursing line-management structure).
2. *The Ward/Unit MDCT* (nurses, doctors, approved social workers, clinical psychologists and occupational and industrial therapists).
3. *Primary Health Care Teams* (GPs, district nurses, health visitors).
4. *Community Mental Health Teams* (CPNs, occupational therapists, approved social workers, psychologists and psychiatrist).
5. *Community Crisis Intervention Team* (CPN, approved social worker and psychiatrist).
6. *Community Resettlement Team* (CPN, members of the MDCT, home care organiser, ethnic development workers, physiotherapist,

probation officer, disablement resettlement officer and job search officer).

The Community Psychiatric Nursing Services Locality Team

Within this team structure it is very important that the CPN is able to be an effective communicator, and pass on the relevant information to other members of the care team. This communication is essential in all aspects of the care process, i.e. the assessment, planning, implementation and evaluation. It also means that CPNs must maintain good intraprofessional relationships in order to enhance the development of the Community Psychiatric Nursing Services (Barnet Health Authority, 1988).

The Ward/Unit MDCT

Part of the CPN's role is to liaise with the hospital clinical team on a regular basis, and during the weekly ward rounds. Here the CPN may assess prospective clients for follow-up care and treatment in the community. This may be the first contact of the CPN and client, and it is a crucial part of the future nurse–patient relationship. At these meetings, also, the CPN may give feedback to the ward team on the progress of recently discharged patients. By attending these meetings, the CPN is able to get a global picture of the client's previous treatment in the hospital.

Primary Health Care Teams

As an affiliated member of the Primary Health Care Team (PHCT), the CPN can contribute by providing a specialist support service. In some instances, the GPs make direct referrals to the CPNs who may have a sessional input at the surgery, and may provide counselling to individuals or families. Part of the CPN's role in the team could be to provide expert advice to other members of the PHCT if needed.

Community Mental Health Team

Within this multidisciplinary framework, the CPN's role may vary from providing some form of mental health education to clients with mental health problems, to conducting specific sessional therapy at the community mental health centre, which could be the operational base for the team.

Community Crisis Intervention Team

In Britain a few health authorities provide additional community support by setting up specialist crisis intervention teams to deal with urgent calls from GPs, Accident and Emergency departments, members of the public and the police force. The membership of the team varies, but in most instances it consists of a CPN, an approved social worker and a consultant psychiatrist. The team provide a 24-hour service, 7 days per week. Their main role is to respond to any crises within the district. Members of the team provide emergency mental health assessments on clients showing acute mental health problems. This assessment could take place in the clients' homes, Accident and Emergency centres or at a police station.

Prior to the actual assessment, the team meet to decide on who will be the key person to conduct the assessment, with the other members taking a secondary role. Depending on the situation, the team may suggest immediate hospitalisation or containment of the crisis in the individual's home (Scott, 1980). Following the assessment, a nominated person will be designated to follow up the client and make arrangements for subsequent care. Because of the nature of the work it is important that mutual respect is shown by all members of the team, since this could cause friction, and patient care may suffer due to fragmentation (Riley, 1988).

Community Resettlement Team

As part of the CPN's specialist role she may be attached to the Resettlement Team. Part of her role will be to monitor the progress of the clients on the rehabilitation/resettlement programmes. She will need to liaise with the home care organiser and social worker, to assist the client in applying for rehousing or the associated Social Security benefits. The ethnic development worker, in some instances, assists the CPN and other members of the team in providing 'link workers' or interpreter facilities for clients with poor command of English. The development worker will liaise with Ethnic Minority mental health groups, in order to provide 'culturally sensitive' care and resources, where appropriate. This is an area of neglect by the Mental Health Services, but recent government legislation has emphasised the importance of paying attention to the mental health needs of Ethnic Minority groups (National Association of Health Authorities, 1988). It may be deduced that the CPN is a key person in the Community Mental Health Services, and therefore she needs to maintain a satisfactory professional relationship with all of the other members of the team.

CURRENT PERSPECTIVES IN COMMUNITY CARE: AN UPDATE

Finally, an update for the reader on the effects of changes which have resulted in community care policies from the 1989 White Paper on community care, up to the implementation of the NHS and Community Care Act in 1993.

The areas which will be briefly addressed are:

Case management/care management approach
Care assessments
Compulsory Treatment Orders
Development of services – deinstitutionalisation

1 April 1993 heralded the full implementation of the NHS and Community Care Act of 1990. The Act had transitional stages for different policies before full implementation (see Table 11.4).

The Act, in 1993, made Social Services Inspectorates the 'lead' agencies to undertake social care assessments, with inbuilt mechanisms for clients to appeal against the results of these assessments. Hence, in June 1993 Lineham reported that a local authority – London Borough of Tower Hamlets – was fined £550 and was criticised for failing to assess the needs of a client with mental health problems, who was discharged from hospital without support.

It would appear that this ruling by the local government ombudsman was the 'first fine' against a local authority under the NHS and Community Care Act 1990. The Council was apparently found 'guilty of maladministration causing injustice in the form of worry and stress' (Lineham, 1993, p.4).

A worrying aspect of the case cited by Lineham is that it might have future implications for some community mental health workers (for example CPNs), especially if they have been nominated as 'lead assessors' by the Social Services Inspectorates and are involved in the assessment of both the health and social care needs of an individual prior to the formulation of the individual care plans, thereby demonstrating the Department of Health view that care agencies and practitioners must have a common understanding of the term 'need' as it relates to this new needs-led concept (Department of Health, 1991, p.14).

The above instance highlighted that clients have a recourse to appeal against their mental health care packages and also reinforces that under the 1992 Patient's Charter, patients have the right to have any complaint about NHS services investigated (Department of Health, 1991).

Within the provisions of the NHS and Community Care Act was the compulsory directive of the care programme approach that arrangements must be made for clients to be supported outside hospital and that these

Table 11.4   Community care policies, aspects of mental health and consultative documents

Community care	Mental health
1. 1983: Care in the Community, DHSS	1. 1983: New Mental Health Act (MHA) introduced
2. 1985: Community Care: with specific reference to mentally ill and mentally handicapped people, Social Services Select Centre	2. 1985: Hallstrom Judgment (re: Sec. 17 MHA 1983, Extended Leave)
3. 1986: Making a Reality of Community Care, Audit Commission Report	3. 1986: Compulsory Treatment in the Community: A Discussion Paper, MHA Commission 1987: Community Treatment Orders: A Discussion Document, Royal College of Physicians
4. 1988: Community Care: Agenda for Action, Sir Roy Griffiths report	
5. 1989: White Paper: Caring for People: Community Care in the Next Decade and Beyond	
6. 1990: National Health Service and Community Care Act	
7. 1991: Practice Guidance on Inspection Units and Complaints Procedures – Guidance on Mental Illness Specific Grants (MISG)	7. 1991: Working Group on Community Supervision Order, Royal College of Psychiatrists
1992: Community Care Plans Produced by Social Services Department, Health Authorities and FHSAs Community Care Support Force set up by DOH	7. Publication of two Controlled Studies of Compulsory Community Treatment Order, Sensky, Hughes and Hirsch (1991)
8. 1993 (April) NHS and Community Care Act (full implementation) 1993: Health and Social Care Assessments implemented by Social Services Department (Lead Agency) • Care Management implemented • Purchaser/Provider split • Residential and Nursing Home Care Act • Income Support transferred to Social Services Authorities • 1993 (Spring) First Local Authority 'fined' for inadequate assessment of psychiatric patient prior to discharge (NHS and Community Care (1993)	8a. 1993: Royal College of Physicians Publish Report on Community Supervision Orders b. Commons Health Select Committee rejects possible use of Community Treatment Orders. Use of voluntary crisis cards (July 1993) c. Calls for review of supervision of discharged psychiatric patients (Guardianship Orders), Department of Health (June 1993) d. Research and Development for Psychiatry (Mental Health Charity): evaluates treatment options of four projects e. Department of Health conducts survey on public opinion of Community Care of the Mentally Ill *Public opinion:* 'best therapy for mental illness is to be part of the community' (published results, July 1993)

arrangements are made prior to discharge from hospital (Onyett, 1992).

With all these recent community care legislations, the CPN's role and relationships with other members of the mental health teams could be fraught with difficulties. In 1990, White and Brooker suggested that the care programme approach might reintroduce a closer working relationship between the CPNs and psychiatrists, and might threaten the autonomous practice of CPNs in primary care. More research is needed to confirm whether their predictions are correct.

In the interim, however, research from the LSE by Wilson produced some evidence which implied interprofessional conflicts between the different professionals involved in community care, using the case management model, especially when there was an overlapping of professional boundaries (Wilson, 1993).

Wilson goes on to say that 'the lack of clarity over tasks and the absence of clearly defined boundaries between professionals will affect the organisation and delivery of community care in the future' (Wilson, 1993, p.119). She also commented on the fact that unless day to day working practice contracts can be negotiated to include staff from different agencies and professions, clients will suffer, which will reinforce that case (care) management is time-consuming.

There has been a resurgence of concern relating to the care of individuals with chronic mental health problems, living in the community unsupervised. Since the unfortunate incident with Ben Silcock being mauled in the lions' den in December, 1992 and subsequent reported cases in the media about clients with mental health problems being discharged into the community and fatally wounding innocent people, there have been increased clamours by mental health pressure groups and psychiatrists to enforce changes in the 1983 Mental Health Act, and introduced compulsory treatment orders (Brooker, 1993; Royal College of Psychiatrists, 1991).

A recent article by Charles Brooker entitled 'A Hindrance to Care?' does not support more changes in mental health legislation in the form of compulsory treatment orders, since it will not, in his view, develop appropriate services for people with serious mental health problems (Brooker, 1993). A similar view is partly shared by the Royal College of Psychiatrists which also feels that the Department of Health should not be considering these treatment orders as an alternative to other methods of care (Bluglass, 1993).

The Royal College of Psychiatrists (RCP) has debated compulsory treatment orders (CTOs) since the 1980s, which resulted in a Court of Appeal decision in 1985 widely referred to as the 'Hallstrom Judgment'. (Brooker, 1993). However, more recently the RCP was advocating a compulsory *supervision* order and not a compulsory *treatment* order (Bluglass, 1993). The final changes in this mental health legislation, if any,

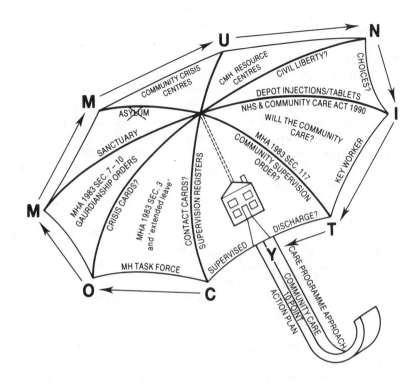

Figure 11.4 Mental health community care – the future: 2001?

will be sanctioned by the Department of Health, and one waits with interest the results of their deliberations. However, the Government in August 1993 in a press release, announced a ten point plan for comunity care, which included proposals for the supervised discharge of mentally ill clients from hospital to the community, and the establishment of a Mental Health Task Force to publicise good practices in community care. The most recent legislation in October 1994 was the introduction of supervision registers for patients who are seriously mentally ill. It is hoped that the supervision registers will be an 'integral part' of the care programme approach, thus protecting the public and vulnerable patients. (Figure 11.4 suggests future trends.)

Brooker again focuses attention on the serious professional and ethical implications that any changes in legislation will have on CPNs who might have to administer treatment to patients against their will (Brooker, 1993).

As an alternative to legislative changes he recommends changes from a nursing perspective and says that 'strenuous efforts must be made to continue encouraging CPNs (and all other mental health professionals) to target those suffering from severe mental illness', to use 'a variety of approaches' to increase clients' compliance to medication (Brooker 1993, p.35; Brooker *et al*, 1992).

Brooker also welcomed the recent research-funding monies contributed by the Sir Jules Thorne Charitable Trust, which may enable the research-based training of CPNs to deliver psychosocial interventions to clients with severe mental health problems (Brooker, 1993).

As the process of deinstitutionalisation continues, several large asylums are being closed – lately Friern Hospital in Friern Barnet, North London. Onyett provides an update of some of the alternative community arrangements, most of which are based on case management models in the UK and other parts of the world.

The British examples include the Early Intervention Service (EIS) provided by an ethnically and socially diverse inner London community mental health team. The approach to a 'comprehensive mental health service' was outlined by a service planning team in Kent, the DISC approach (Developing Individual Services in the Community); The Daily Living Programme in Camberwell, London which focused on people living at home and an overview of the various government-funded care in the community demonstration projects (Onyett, 1992).

REFERENCES

Acheson E D (1985) That over used word 'community'! Health Trends. In: *Community Psychiatry: The principles*, p.4, eds Bennett D H and Freeman H L. Edinburgh: Churchill Livingstone.

Adams T (1990) A model of multidisciplinary team working. *Senior Nurse*, **10**: 13–16.

Aguilera D and Messick J (1982) *Crisis Intervention*. St Louis: Mosby.

Allan J and Hall B (1988) Between diagnosis and death. The case for studying grief before death. *Archives of Psychiatric Nursing*, **1**: 30–34. Cited in: Kavenagh K and Johnson L (1990) When an institution dies – Nursing's role in closing a facility. *Journal of Psychosocial Nursing*, **28**(9): 11–15.

Bachrach L (1983) Concepts and issues in deinstitutionalisation. Patients in the community. In: *The Chronic Psychiatric. Principles of Treatment*, eds Barofsky I and Budson R. New York: Spectrum Publications Inc.

Barker C (1977) A Community Psychiatric Service. *Nursing Times*, 14 July: 1075–1079.

Barnet Health Authority (1988) *Profile of Community Psychiatric Nursing Services*.

Barton R (1959) *Institutional Neurosis*. Bristol: Wright.

Beardshaw V and Morgan E (1990) *Community Care Works – Learning from the Torbay Experience*. London: Mind Publications.

Bender M (1986) Crisis of closure. *Health Service Journal*, **17**: 524–525.

Bennett D and Freeman H (eds) (1991) *Community Psychiatry – The Principles* Edinburgh: Churchill Livingstone.

Brink P (ed.) (1976) *Transcultural Nursing: A book of readings*. Englewood Cliffs New Jersey: Prentice-Hall.

Brooker C (1993) A hindrance to care? *Nursing Times,* **89**(6): 34–35.

Brooker C, Tarrier N, Barrowclough C *et al* (1992) The outcome of training community psychiatric nurses to deliver psycho-social intervention; results of a pilot study. *British Journal of Psychiatry,* **160**: 836–844.

Bluglass R (1993) The case for supervision. *Nursing Times,* **89**(6): 32–33.

Caplan G (1961) *An Approach to Community Mental Health*. New York: Grieve and Stratton Inc.

Caplan G (1964) *Principles of Preventive Psychiatry.* New York: Bani Books Inc

Carr P, Butterworth C and Hodges B (1980) *Community Psychiatric Nursing Caring for the Mentally and Mentally Handicapped in the Community.* Edinburgh: Churchill Livingstone.

Community Psychiatric Nurses Association (CPNA) (1989) *Moving Out: A Discussion on Resettlement Issues.* Kingswinford, West Midlands: CPNA Publications.

Community Health Services Unit (1991) Standard Guidelines for Nursing Staff (clinical): *Referral for Community Resettlement*, London, Colney: Napsbury Hospital, Barnet Health Authority.

Damde A (1989) Transcultural issues in community psychiatry. *Community Psychiatry,* **2**: 22–25.

Department of Health (1990) National Health Service and Community Care Act. London: HMSO.

DHSS (1986) Neighbourhood Nursing. A Focus for Care. *Report of the Community Nursing Review for England.* The Cumberledge Report. London: HMSO

Dobson S (1991) *Transcultural Nursing*. London: Scutari Press.

Flaye A (1990) *A Study to Examine the Role and Function of the Community Psychiatric Nurse.* London: Royal College of Nursing. In: Brooker C and White E (eds) (1993) *Community Psychiatric Nursing – A Research Perspective, Vol. 2.* London: Chapman and Hall.

Francis E (1991) Out of sight, out of mind. *Open Mind,* **53**: 9.

English National Board (ENB) (1989) *Project 2000. New Preparation for Practice, Part A. (1.21).* London: ENB

Gasson B (1991) Community psychiatry nursing: looking into the past. *Community Psychiatric Nursing Journal,* **11**: 17–21.

Goldman H, Adams N and Tause C (1983) Deinstitutionalisation: the data demythologised. *Hospital and Community Psychiatry,* **34**(2): 129–134.

Goffman E (1961) *Asylums – Essays on the Social Situation of Mental Patients and other Inmates*. Harmondsworth: Penguin.

Gottlieb B H (1983) *Support Social Strategies.* London: Sage Publications. In: Simmons S and Brooker C (eds) (1986) *Community Psychiatric Nursing,* p.98. London: Heinemann Nursing.

Gruenberg E (1977) Community care is not 'deinstitutionalisation'. In: *New Trends of Psychiatry in the Community*, Serban G ed. Cambridge Mass: Ballinger.

Hall P and Brockington I (1991) *The Closure of Mental Hospitals.* The Royal College of Psychiatrists: Gaskell.

Harrison P (1973) The careless community. *New Society*, **24**: 742–745.

Helman C (1984) *Culture, Health and Illness*. Bristol: Wright.

HMSO (1989) *Caring for People. Community Care in the Next Decade and Beyond*, CM849. London: HMSO.

Hume C and Pullen I (1986) *Rehabilitation in Psychiatry – An Introductory Handbook*. Edinburgh: Churchill Livingstone.

Hunter P (1974) Community psychiatric nursing in Britain – an historical review. *International Journal of Nursing Studies*, **2**(4): 223–233.

Husband L (1991) The Level One nurse and community practice. *Senior Nurse*, **11**(4): 25–27.

Huxley P (1990) Community Mental Health. A challenge to care. *Community Psychiatric Nursing Journal*, **210**(3): 12–15.

Jervis M (1986) Female, Asian and isolated. *Open Mind*, **20**: 10–12.

Jones K and Poletti A (1985) Understanding the Italian experience. *British Journal of Psychiatry*, **146**: 341–347.

Kavanagh L and Johnson L (1990) When an institution dies – nursing role in closing a facility. *Journal of Psychosocial Nursing*, **28**: 11–15.

Kenny B, Couchman W and Gray B (1986) Normalisation theory and practice. *Health and Social Services Journal*, 16 Jan: 80–81.

Khandwalla M (1984) Asian women's therapy. *Nursing Times*, 28 November, 44.

King D (1991) *Moving on From Mental Hospital to Community Care. A case study of change in Exeter*. London: The Nuffield Provincial Hospitals Trust.

Kingsley S and Towell D (1988) Planning for high quality local services. In: *Community Care in Practice*, Lavender A. London: John Wiley & Sons.

Korman N and Glennerster H (1990) *Hospital Closure – A Political and Economic Study*. Milton Keynes: Open University Press.

Larsen J and Jerrell J M (1983). Mental Health Services in Transition, Technical Report 83–84. In: *Community Psychiatry*, eds Bennett D and Freeman H, p.568. Edinburgh: Churchill Livingston.

Lineham T (1993) News: first fine. *Community Care: The Independent Voice of Social Work*, **972**: 4.

Longo D and Chase G (1984) Structural determinants of hospital closure. *Medical Care* **22**: 388–402.

Mares P, Larbie J and Baxter C (1987) *Trainer's Handbook for Multiracial Health Care. Training in Health and Race*. Cambridge: National Extension College.

May A and Moore S (1963) The mental nurse in the community. *Lancet*, **1**(7274): 213–214.

Mohammed S (1991) N.H.S. reforms? How will black people fare? *Ethnic Minorities Health Current Awareness Bulletin*, i–iii.

National Association of Health Authorities (NAHA) (1988) Action not words. A strategy to improve Health Services for Black and Minority Ethnic Groups. Birmingham: NAHA.

Onyett S (1992) *Case Management in Mental Health*. London: Chapman & Hall.

O'Riordan P (1987) A review of professional attitudes on the context of deinstitutionalisation. The Eire perspective. *Community Psychiatric Nursing Journal*, March/Apr: 11–19.

Ovretveit J (1986) *Organisation of Multi-disciplinary Community Teams. A Health Service Centre Working Paper*. Uxbridge: Brunel University.

Parry G (1990) *Coping with Crises. Problems in Practice*. Leicester: BPS Books, Routledge.

Payne M (1986) *Social Care in the Community*. London: British Association of Social Workers.

Paynter M (1991) A Study: How do CPNs Decide Practice Priorities and Make Clinical Judgements? University of Sussex, Unpublished paper.

Pilling S (1991) *Rehabilitation and Community Care*. London: Routledge.

Pollock L (1983) Community psychiatric nursing – a review and au revoir! *Community Psychiatric Nursing Association Journal*, 3(3): 30–36.

Pollock L (1989) *Community Psychiatric Nursing: Myth and Reality*. London: Scutari Press.

Ramon S and Giannichedda M (eds) (1988) *Psychiatry in Transition. The British and Italian Experience*. London: Pluto Press.

Rathwell T (1991) The N.H.S. Reforms and Britain's ethnic communities. *Ethnic Minorities Health and Current Awareness Bulletin*, 3(1): i–iv.

Riley T (1988) The Napsbury Community Crisis Intervention Service. *Community Psychiatry*, 1(2): 19–20.

Ritter S (1989) *Manual of Clinical Psychiatric Nursing Principles and Procedures. Bethlem Royal and Maudsley Hospital*. London: Harper and Row.

Royal College of Psychiatrists (1993) *Community Supervision Orders*. London: Royal College of Psychiatrists.

Royal Commission (1979) *Royal Commission on the N.H.S.* London: HMSO.

Samarasinghe N (1986) The Role of the C.P.N. and the Skills Required to Perform the Role Effectively. Barnet Health Authority, Unpublished paper.

Scott R (1980) A family oriented psychiatric service to the London Borough of Barnet. *Health Trends*, 12: 65–68.

Sensky T, Hughes T and Hirsch S (1991a) Compulsory treatment in the community 1. A controlled study of compulsory community treatment with extended leave under the Mental Health Act: Special characteristics of patients treated and impact of treatment. *British Journal of Psychiatry*, 158: 792–799.

Sensky T, Hughes T and Hirsch S (1991b) Compulsory treatment in the community 2. A controlled study of patients whom psychiatrists would recommend for compulsory treatment in the community. *British Journal of Psychiatry*, 158: 799–804.

Shepherd G (1984) *Institutional Care and Rehabilitation*. London: Longman.

Simmons S (1988) Community psychiatric nurses and multidisciplinary working. *Community Psychiatric Nursing Journal*, September: 14–18.

Simmons S and Brooker C (1986) *Community Psychiatric Nursing. A Social Perspective*. London: Heinemann Nursing.

Sladden S (1979) *Nursing in the Community. A Study of a Working Situation*. Edinburgh: Churchill Livingstone.

Titmus R (1963) Community Care – fact or fiction? In: *Trends in the Mental Health Service*, eds Freeman H and Farndale J. Oxford: Pergamon.

Thornicroft G and Bebbington P (1989) Deinstitutionalisation – from hospital closure to service development. *British Journal of Psychiatry* (Review Article), **155**: 739–753.

Tripp-Reimer T, Brink P and Saunders J (1984) Cultural assessment: Content and process. *Nursing Outlook*, **32**(2): 78–82.

Tyne A (1982) Community Care and mentally handicapped people. In: Walker A (ed.) *Community Care: The Family, the State and Social Policy*. Oxford: Blackwell. Cited in: Korman N and Glennersten H (1990) *Hospital Closure*. Milton Keynes: Open University Press.

United Kingdom Central Council (UKCC) for Nursing, Midwifery and Health Visiting (1991) *Report on Proposals for the Future of Community Education and Practice (PREPP)*. London: UKCC.

Vousden M (1968) Closing time (News Focus). *Nursing Times*, 19 March: 16–18.

Walsh P (1985) Speaking up for the patient. *Nursing Times*, 1 May: 24–26.

Weleminsky J (1990) Community mental health. A way of meeting the challenge. *Community Psychiatric Nursing Journal*, **10**(3): 35–36.

White T (1990) Emerging issues in community psychiatric nursing. *Community Psychiatric Nursing Journal*, **10**(3): 34.

White E (1990) *Community Psychiatric Nursing. The 1990 National Survey*. Nuneaton: Community Psychiatric Nursing Association.

White E and Brooker C (1990) The future of community psychiatric nursing: what might 'The Care Programme Approach' mean for practice and education? *Community Psychiatric Nursing Journal*, **10**(6): 27–30.

Wilson G (1993) Conflicts in case management: the use of staff time in community care. *Social Policy and Administration*, **27**(2): 109–123.

Wing D (1989) Community participant observation. Issues in addressing diverse cultures. *Journal of Community Health Nursing*, **6**(3): 125–133.

Wolfensberger W (1972) The principle of normalisation in human services. In: *Moving out: A discussion on resettlement issues*.

FURTHER READING

Audit Commission (1992) *Homeward Bound: A New Course for Community Health*. London: HMSO.

Brooker C and White E (eds) (1993) *Community Psychiatric Nursing: A Research Perspective*. London: Chapman and Hall.

Davis B (1986) Culture and psychiatric nursing: implications for training. In: Cox J (ed). *Transcultural Psychiatry*, pp.218–233. Beckenham: Croom Helm.

Crepaz-Keay D (1994) 'I wish to register a complaint. . .'. *Open Mind*, 71: 5.

Cresswell J (1994) Register needs a vote of confidence: Supervision Registers. *Community Care*, (1038): 8–9.

Department of Health (1990) *National Health Service and Community Care Act*. London: HMSO.

Department of Health (1993) *The Health of the Nation. Key Area Handbook: Mental Illness*. London: HMSO.

Department of Health (1994) *Legislation to Provide Supervised Discharge of Psychiatric Patients*. London: HMSO.

DHSSI (1991) *Care Management and Assessment Managers' Guide*. London: HMSO.

DoH/RCN (1993) *Community Care*. London: Royal College of Nursing.

Dobson S (1991) *Transcultural Nursing*. London: Scutari Press.

Faugier J (1993) Falling through the holes. *Nursing Times*, **89**(3): 20.

Faulkner A (1994) Mental Health: Policy. Mission Impossible. *Community Care*, (1033): 22–23.

Francis E, David J, Johnson N *et al* (1989) Black people and psychiatry in the U.K. *Psychiatic Bulletin*, **13**, 482–485.

Ford R (1993) *Case Management: Does it Work?* London: The Brewery.

House of Commons Select Committee (1994) *Better Off in the Community: The Care of People who are Seriously Mentally Ill*. London: HMSO.

Knapp M, Cambridge P, Thomason C *et al* (1992) *Care in the Community: Challenge and Demonstration*. Aldershot: Gower.

Leader A (1993) Step by step: Brixton community sanctuary. *Open Mind*, **62**: 24.

Long C, Mackle E and Monaghan J (1989) What happens when the hospital closes? Repatriation of chronic patients. *Journal of Psychosocial Nursing*, **27**(4): 11–14.

Massey P (1991) Institutional loss: an examination of a bereavement reaction in 22 nurses losing their institution and moving into the community. *Journal of Advanced Nursing*, **16**: 573–585.

National Health Service Management Executive (1994) *The Introduction of Supervision Registers for Mentally Ill People*. Leeds: NHS Management Executive.

North East Thames Regional Health Authority (1994) *The Report of the Inquiry into the Care and Treatment of Christopher Clunis*. (The Ritchie Report). London: HMSO.

Parliament (1993) *Community Supervision Orders: Government Response to the Fifth Report from the Health Committee, Session 1992–93*. CM 2333. London: HMSO.

Parliament (1994) *Working in Partnership: A Collaborative Approach to Care*.

Report of the Mental Health Nursing Review Team (Professor Butterworth). London: HMSO.

Petch A (1990) *Heaven Compared to a Hospital Ward: An evaluation of eleven supported accommodation projects for those with mental health problems.* Stirling University, Scotland: Social Work Research Centre.

Ramon S (ed.) (1991) *Beyond Community Care: Normalisation and Integration Work.* Basingstoke: Macmillan Education Ltd/MIND Publications.

Reynolds W and Cormack D (1990) *Psychiatric and Mental Health Nursing. Theory and Practice.* London: Chapman and Hall.

Roach F (1992) Research report: community mental health services for black and ethnic minorities. *Counselling Psychology Quarterly,* 5(13): 277–290.

Ryan T (1994) The risk business. *Nursing Management,* 1(6): 9–11.

Rye D (1993) Editorial: Reforming community care. *Senior Nurse,* 13(3): 3.

Sassoon M (1993) A voice for black users. *Open Mind,* 62: 25.

Smith H (1990) *Developing Individual Services in the Community (DISC). Discussion Paper.* Canterbury: University of Kent.

Utting W, Sir (1994) *Creating Community Care.* London: Mental Health Foundation.

Wallcraft J and Read J (1992) *Guidelines for Empowering Users of Mental Health Services.* London: COHSE/MIND Publications.

Wilson M (1993) *Mental Health and Britain's Black Communities.* London: King's Fund Centre.

12

Research in
Mental Health
Nursing
Graham Stew

INTRODUCTION

This chapter aims to introduce the reader to aspects of research in mental health nursing in a straightforward fashion, minimising unnecessary jargon and obscure terminology. It does not assume any previous knowledge of research design and methodology, but simply addresses a number of relevant questions, and will indicate where further reading may be helpful. Following a short discussion on the nature and importance of research and its relationship to theory and practice, research design and the stages of the research process will be described. The chapter will end with a review of specific areas where research has contributed to mental health nursing, and suggestions for further study and reading.

WHAT IS RESEARCH?

Research can be defined in many ways, but for the purposes of this chapter it is seen as a systematic method of collecting information, in order to increase understanding and knowledge. Clark and Hockey (1989, p.4) also define research as:

> an attempt to increase available knowledge by the discovery of new facts or relationships through systematic enquiry.

In short, it is an organised way of asking questions and seeking answers. The actual word *re-search* implies that one is looking again at something, in an attempt to know it better.

Research can describe, explain, predict and prescribe events and phenomena, and the result of these processes is *theory*. Theory can be seen as making statements about the relationships between concepts and constructs within a field of knowledge. Theory can be tested, confirmed or refuted, and developed further, contributing not only to our awareness and understanding, but also to a body of knowledge.

WHY DO WE NEED RESEARCH IN NURSING?

Many people have expressed the view that the only qualities that nurses need are caring and common sense, and that there is nothing 'scientific' about caring. It may well be that research findings confirm what many people intuitively believe, but before the systematic study of a topic, there is no way of really 'knowing' what the facts are. For example, you may have 'felt' that mental disorder affects mainly the lower social classes, but until research studies present the statistics to prove this, your 'knowledge' stays at the level of 'common sense'. You may then wish to ask further questions: why are the lower social classes affected more? Is social class an effective way to distinguish between populations? What does social class mean? . . . and so on. To a 'research-minded' individual, one answer only provokes another question.

To a great many practising nurses, research has a poor image. It is regarded as an elitist activity for a small number of academic nurses, difficult to understand and implement, and irrelevant to everyday reality. Some of these criticisms are valid, and it is unfortunately true that many researchers have produced work which is obscure and jargonistic in terms of language and presentation, and which is incapable of application to practice. The primary purpose of the nurse is to provide the highest possible quality of care, and unless research enables nurses to improve the service they offer, it will continue to be regarded as remote and impractical.

If nurses are to become 'reflective practitioners', as the UKCC (1986) hopes, they will need to ask questions about the value and efficacy of their care. In developing the skills of critical thinking, nurses will need to challenge and question previously accepted customs and practice, which have remained at the level of ritualised routine for many years. They may need to examine how various activities and therapies influence the course of patients' disorders; for example, how do art therapy or sociodrama sessions affect patients? What are their perceptions of group activities? How can the principles of the therapeutic community be applied in an acute admission unit? Is the ward's daily routine designed to meet the staff's or patients' needs? Which patients are best referred to the Community Psychiatric Nurse?

In order to provide effective care, nurses need to possess and develop a body of nursing knowledge which is research-based and capable of critical scrutiny. Their knowledge should provide rationales when challenged, and allow them to engage in informed debate with other members of the multidisciplinary team. In these times of financial and political pressures, nurses must be able to define and defend their role alongside other health care professions; for this, a sound knowledge base is essential.

Research has also been promoted as the means to elevate nurses' status as an occupational group to that of a profession. Increased status, important as it is, can be achieved through improved care, which is research-based and justified in a rational and informed manner. Professional status, with its consequent changes in role and image for the nurse, will inevitably affect the nurse–patient relationship, may detract from essential interpersonal and caring skills and may not be in the interests of nursing as a whole.

WHAT NEEDS TO BE RESEARCHED?

What areas of mental health nursing are appropriate for research studies? It may well be argued that as nursing is a skills-based occupation, the principal interest of researchers should be in the field of nursing practice. In order to better understand and develop the skills used by the psychiatric nurse, research needs to examine a multitude of questions raised by practitioners in the course of their work. The findings need to illuminate and explain the processes within practice, and suggest ways in which nurses can improve the care they provide.

Nursing research can provide information and theory in three areas where nurses take on roles and responsibilities: practice, management and education.

Research into Nursing Practice

Research questions can be asked about particular forms of treatment: which patients are best helped by referral to behavioural psychotherapists? When is electro-convulsive therapy prescribed, and what are staff and patient perceptions of this treatment? How common are unwanted side-effects from psychotropic drugs and how may they best be detected? And so on . . . the list is as long as the 'research-mindedness' of the nurse makes it. Topics of interest for research may be stumbled upon in the course of practice, or may arise out of critical incidents where important questions were asked, but answers were not forthcoming. Nurses may choose to research areas where a good deal is already known (e.g. chemotherapy), or question an issue which has rarely, if ever, been examined before (e.g. how institutionalised patients cope with relocation in the community). In each case, the research design will differ according to the question asked.

Research into Nursing Management

In addition to research into clinical areas of practice, nurses also need to ask questions about the management of care. Nurse managers are becoming increasingly aware of the need to be efficient and cost-effective in terms of manpower and resources. They will need answers to questions about staffing needs, quality assurance, performance reviews, recruitment and service requirements. Research findings can shed light on these and other areas, and help nurses to assert and justify their needs in these times of financial stringency.

Research into Nursing Education

Much research has been undertaken within nurse education, but a good deal remains to be explored, particularly in psychiatric nursing. The introduction of Project 2000 courses and Branch Programmes in mental health nursing has generated a great need for research into the effects of these reforms. The socialisation of student nurses into their chosen field of nursing is an area of interest, as is their status and experience during the new courses. The well-established problem of integrating theory and practice requires further investigation, and the effects of new schemes of continuous assessment will need ongoing research and evaluation.

WHAT IS THEORY?

If nursing research is concerned with the generation of nursing theory, what then is the nature of *theory*? A broad definition is offered by Chinn and Jacobs (1987), who define theory as:

> a set of concepts, definitions, and propositions that projects a view of phenomena by designating specific interrelationships among concepts for the purposes of describing, explaining and predicting phenomena.

Taking this definition, we can further divide theory into two main types: inductive and deductive.

Inductive Theory

Inductive theory is concerned with 'bringing knowledge into view' (Field and Morse, 1985). It is mainly descriptive, identifying features of the phenomenon being studied and then suggesting relationships between them. Starting with particular instances and situations, the researcher tries to identify patterns or themes, which then have the potential for generalisation to other instances and situations. The aim is to increase understanding of the setting or event, and to suggest relationships between the named concepts and constructs. These tentative explanations may take the form of hypotheses, which are simply statements of the expected relationship between one or more factors (known as variables), which can then be tested deductively. Inductive theory thus moves from the particular case to the general, and is usually descriptive and interpretive.

Deductive Theory

The laws of logical reasoning are based upon the principles of deduction, insofar as deduction produces new knowledge by inferring from what has preceded. The starting point is known fact or theory, from which an hypothesis is developed, and then tested under experimental conditions for confirmation or refutation. The resulting findings are incorporated as new theory into the body of knowledge. The traditional scientific approach to research has been built upon this foundation of deductive reasoning, which moves from the general to the particular, and is concerned with prediction and prescription.

Types of Theory

Dickoff and James (1968) described four types of theory which can be produced by research studies: factor-isolating (descriptive); factor-relating (explanatory), situation-relating (predictive); and situation-producing (prescriptive). It may be worth looking at examples of each in more detail before we go on to discuss other aspects of research.

Factor-isolating theory derives from description of the most basic kind. Here the researcher attempts to identify and name observable features of a social phenomenon. Names or labels are the first step in conceptualising key components of the situation under study. They may be abstract concepts that can be used by nurses to construct a meaningful picture of their workplace, and help them understand the people for whom they are providing care. Altschul (1972) used a factor-isolating approach to identify the types of contact nurses have with their patients. She found that the nurses viewed their interactions with patients as based upon common sense, and that there was little evidence or acknowledgement of any therapeutic ideology or philosophy of care.

Factor-relating theory goes one step further in making connections between the identified concepts, rather than simply describing them. Causal relationships are suggested, but not tested, as this level of theory remains basically descriptive. Cormack (1983), in an exploratory study of the psychiatric nurse's role, identified a large number of factors concerned with interactions between nurses and patients. From this collection of factors, he went on to suggest that the psychiatric nurse's role was multifaceted, and consisted of therapeutic, administrative, technical, educational and other components.

Whereas factor-isolating and factor-relating theories are principally concerned with the discovery of previously unknown concepts and features, situation-relating and situation-producing theories can be seen as seeking to confirm or verify the existence of something already discovered, and then to predict and prescribe actions. An example of *situation-relating* theory could be the research of Berrios and Sage (1986), who studied the problem of patients who did not comply with fasting before ECT treatments. They found that patients who were unmarried, detained, non-consenting and disagreed with the use of ECT were more likely to break their fast.

Situation-producing theory often results from experimental research which is rigorously controlled and seeks to confirm, for example, the advantages of a particular form of treatment. Marks (1985) set out to study the efficacy of nurse behavioural therapists compared to General Practitioner treatment. The findings demonstrated the advantages of nurse therapists as shown in clinical follow-up studies. Thus, the case for increased referral to behavioural therapists was strongly made, in what could be regarded as an example of 'prescriptive' research.

It should be emphasised that there is a close relationship between all four types of theory; in fact, they could be regarded as being positioned along a continuum that moves from inductive to deductive approaches to theory generation. The most important factor in determining the choice of approach is the extent of current knowledge of the phenomenon being studied. If little is known, then an inductive approach may be more appropriate; if established facts are known, then deductive methods may be more suitable.

What is important in all nursing theory is its relationship to practice. Many 'grand' unifying theories and models of nursing have been produced which do not have their origin in actual practice, but in the minds of academics. This has exacerbated the problematic 'theory–practice' gap, whereby '*know that*' theory has been regarded as irrelevant and 'out of touch' by practising nurses, who continue to use '*know-how*' theory in their work. The problem arises from the fact that this practical '*know-how*' theory is rarely made explicit or written down, and although it reflects real skills and expertise fails to influence the work of colleagues other than by role-modelling. Theory derived inductively from practice offers the best chance of acceptance and implementation by nurses, as it will enjoy both credibility and relevance.

Thus it should be seen that practice, research and theory are interconnected and interdependent. Each one supports and nourishes the others. As Stevens (1984) states:

theory arises out of practice and, once validated, returns to direct or explain that practice [and that] further practice under the guidance of a given theory leads to theory refinement.

The relationship can be depicted as a cyclical process which one can take up at any stage of the cycle, and move in either direction (see Figure 12.1).

WHICH RESEARCH APPROACH?

Having looked at the types of theory which can be developed through research activities, it is now worth examining the approaches which can be taken by researchers. Here a distinction can be made between qualitative and quantitative approaches and designs (see Field and Morse, 1985, for a fuller discussion).

Qualitative Research

Qualitative methods are best suited to the discovery and description of features within settings about which little is known. Here the researcher attempts to enter the field of study and depict what is found in a 'naturalistic' manner; that is, without imposing any controls or experimental conditions upon the subject. The focus is upon individual cases/situations (or on a small number only), and the researcher acts as the research 'instrument' and tries to reflect the perspective and perceptions of the participants within the setting.

For example, the experiences/perceptions of young people admitted to an adolescent unit may be studied using qualitative method of inquiry. Significant patterns or themes may emerge using unstructured interviews and periods of observation, and enable the researcher to 'tell it as it is' from the point of view of the participants (the 'emic' perspective). The information, or data, will be 'grounded' in that reality and will be unique and not necessarily generalisable, but may be used inductively to develop tentative hypotheses concerning causal relationships, which can be tested out in further research.

Quantitative Research

Quantitative methods are suited to areas of study that already possess an established body of theory, from which hypotheses can be developed. This approach seeks to confirm causal relationships and produce 'facts' by generalising from specific cases, using deductive reasoning. The research design is predetermined and adopts the external or 'etic' viewpoint, as

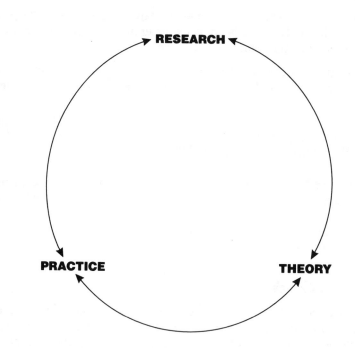

Figure 12.1   The research cycle.

experimental conditions with strict control of variables may be imposed
upon the setting/subjects. The purpose of this type of research is verification of hypotheses, and the production of data which is objective, measurable, replicable and capable of being presented statistically. As an
example, physiological changes indicating stress, following admission to
a psychiatric unit, may be measured and used to confirm an hypothesis
relating stress to admission.

WHAT IS THE RESEARCH PROCESS?

Whether a qualitative or a quantitative approach is adopted, the process
of the research itself must follow a prescribed sequence of steps to ensure
a systematic and thorough investigation. The research process enables
questions to be asked within a framework which handles data in a meth-
odical and logical fashion and discourages assumptions and guessing.

   Cormack (1984) and Burnard and Morrison (1990) both present very
readable accounts of the research process, but it should be stressed that
simply reading about research is no substitute for actual research work
under adequate supervision. Only in this way can students obtain the

valuable 'hands-on' experience that facilitates the development of research skills. Although it is not possible to give an exhaustive account of the steps that researchers need to consider, there is room here to address seven stages of the research process, expressed in terms of the questions that should be asked.

1. *Asking the Research Question*: Why is the question necessary? What will be the possible benefits of the research? Has it been researched before? If so, is a replication study needed? Can an hypothesis be developed from existing theory? If a new field of study, what needs to be investigated?

2. *Searching the Literature*: What has been written and published before in this field? How much is relevant? Where to start? When to stop?

3. *Gaining Access*: Where will I find answers to my questions? If a social setting, how do I negotiate access? What kind of sample from the population is needed? Are there ethical considerations, or matters of confidentiality?

4. *Designing the Research*: Is a quantitative or qualitative approach best suited to my research question (or a combination of both)? Which methods of data collection are appropriate (interview, questionnaire, observation, etc.)? Can several methods be used to 'triangulate' my findings?

5. *Collecting the Data*: Is a pilot study necessary? How much time is available? Can the research question(s) be refocused in the course of fieldwork? When to stop?

6. *Handling the Data*: How do I make sense of the data? What has been found? Can quantitative data be analysed statistically? Do categories/themes emerge from qualitative data? What about validity and reliability?

7. *Presenting the Research*: How do I show what has been found? What type of theory has been produced? Can quantitative findings be presented as graphs and tables? Can qualitative findings be presented accurately and sensitively? How to discuss conclusions and recommendations for further research? How to disseminate findings (publication, seminar papers, conferences, etc.)?

RESEARCH IN MENTAL HEALTH NURSING

Research in the field of mental health nursing is still relatively new, but is developing rapidly. Much has been written about the importance of 'research-based' theory in nursing, and the need for a body of knowledge which is specifically related to nursing. It is certainly true that mental health nurses should possess a body of knowledge which is not only derived from, but also informs, their professional practice. The way to achieve this is through practice-based research which is viewed as relevant and realistic by psychiatric nurses, and which assists them in their work.

The following section looks at a selection of research studies which have been completed in the field of mental health nursing, and is divided again into the three areas of practice, management and education.

Nursing Practice

In a now classic study, David Towell (1975) used participant observation to examine nursing practice in three different settings: an admission ward, a psychogeriatric ward and a therapeutic community. He found that the nurses' role differed in each area, and that the attitudes and values of the nurses were largely influenced by the doctors' treatment ideologies. The findings still have implications today, as nurses need to examine their own therapeutic orientations and professional philosophies when working within multidisciplinary teams.

On the topic of nursing ideologies, Savage (1991) has examined the function of patient assessment in psychiatric nursing within the context of appropriate nursing models, and found that most assessment is a task-based information-gathering procedure. He suggests that assessment could be used as a more holistic and diagnostic process, taking into consideration broader social and psychological factors.

Focusing upon specific clinical situations, MacIlwaine (1983) looked at how nurses communicated with female neurotic patients within psychiatric units. Most interactions were brief and seemed to be practical and administrative in nature, and simple conversation was regarded as relatively unimportant. Coupar and Conway (1986) studied the problem of clinical depression, and the factors which influenced its severity, both at home and in hospital. Morrison (1990) has described the use of seclusion for the management of disturbed and difficult behaviour in acute settings. Retrospective examination of seclusion records revealed unexpected patterns in the practice of seclusion, with factors including the sex and status of the patient, and staffing levels. In a recent study, Gilloran *et al* (1993) discuss how the quality of care in psychogeriatric wards may be assessed through the use of standardised observation schedules. This is linked to a larger study which aims to identify factors affecting levels of job satisfaction, as well as factors influencing the quality of care.

Community Psychiatric Nursing

With the transition from a hospital to a community-based mental health service, there is a need for research to identify issues and effects which relate to both patients and staff. Platt (1990) describes an experiment in community care where a relatives' group was developed, and examines the changing relationship between the consumers and providers of mental health services. The views of carers in the community have also been studied, and Adams (1987) used diaries and interviews with the carers of sufferers from Alzheimer's disease to find that as the patient's problems became the family problems, a family-centred approach to care was desirable. In another study, Norman and Parker (1990) used qualitative methods to describe the experiences of a group of long-stay patients as they moved from a large institution to a staffed community hostel.

Community psychiatric nursing, the most important growth area in mental health nursing, has been the subject of numerous research studies. Two valuable anthologies of research studies in community psychiatric nursing have been edited by Brooker (1990c) and by Brooker and White (1993). These collections demonstrate a wide range of research methods, and focus on issues of practice, education and management.

Relationships between community psychiatric nurses (CPNs) and General Practitioners were examined by White (1986), who found great diversity in the nature and quality of interactions. Referral policies were influenced by a number of factors, but primarily the personal relationships formed between the individuals concerned. Two studies by Brooker (1990a, b) describe the role of the CPN, from the viewpoint of students attending the CPN course (ENB 811), and more specifically the potential role of the CPN in meeting the health education needs of families caring for a schizophrenic relative.

Treatment approaches used by CPNs have also been the subject of recent research studies. Hughes (1991) argues that the use of cognitive therapy would make a positive contribution to the care of the depressed elderly in the community, and Gournay (1991) examines the optimum use of exposure treatment for agoraphobic clients by nurse behaviour therapists and CPNs. One recent study by Sheppard (1993) looks at the interpersonal skills used by psychiatric nurses working in a community mental health centre. The concept of client satisfaction is explored in relation to certain skills such as empathy, listening, openness and genuineness. Strategies for effective CPN interventions in the community care of anorectic and bulimic clients are discussed in a study by Meades (1993), who identifies two major issues in these disorders, namely distorted body image and stressful interpersonal relationships. He goes on to suggest that CPNs are well-placed to observe and supervise people with eating disorders who are potentially vulnerable to relapse following discharge from hospital.

Nursing Management

There is a small but growing number of studies in the area of management issues. Action research by Lemmer (1986) demonstrated how change can be brought about by feedback on performance to ward staff working with the elderly mentally ill. Strengths and weaknesses were identified, and staff were then able to move from a task-based custodial nursing role towards individualised, problem-solving care. This project is a good example of how research can be derived from, and then used to inform, practice.

The subject of job stress was examined by Jones *et al* (1987), who used structured interviews together with a questionnaire, and showed that stressors for psychiatric nurses were primarily organisational and administrative, and that negative patient characteristics were not regarded as particularly stressful. In a further study, Jones (1988) demonstrated that nurses working in an environment which was highly stimulating showed higher levels of morale than those working in a more traditional area. Occupational stress for psychiatric nurses was also the subject of a recent study by Sullivan (1993) who described stressors in two acute admission wards, the effects of stress and the types of coping strategy used by nurses.

McKenna (1990) reported the perceptions of psychiatric ward sisters/charge nurses towards nursing models, as part of a larger study aimed at enabling ward managers to select an appropriate model for their practice. The majority of respondents were positive in their views of models, although 23.2 per cent voiced negative perceptions. The implications for nursing practice, education and administration are discussed. In another interesting study, Massey (1991) examined the 'grief' reactions of nursing staff to the closure of a large mental hospital, and the important implications for the rehabilitation of long-term patients discharged into the community. More recently, Long *et al* (1992) compared two systems of in-patient care in a general hospital, focusing upon staff and patient perceptions and attitudes. The preferred continuous care system offered an improved 'ward atmosphere', where involvement, support and spontaneity were regarded as positive features.

Nursing Education

A significant number of research studies fall into this category, but six will be singled out as examples. Reynolds and Cormack (1985) and Reynolds and Presly (1988) looked at the teaching of interpersonal skills to student nurses, and the concept of empathy in particular. Nurse teachers were interviewed, and although major differences were found in the teaching methods across three schools of nursing, the value of the teachers as role models was recognised.

Davis (1986) studied the socialisation process that student nurses experience, examined the students' perceptions of themselves and of psychiatric nursing, and shed light upon the important issue of student stress. Chambers (1988) showed how a qualitative research approach can be used to evaluate a course, involved both students and teachers in gathering information and identified strengths and weaknesses in the programme, which assisted in future planning.

Drummond (1990) has analysed the work methods of students of mental health nursing undertaking Project 2000 courses. He argues the case for supervised primary nursing because it 'engenders a professional cognitive style and a heightened sensitivity to the empirical, research-based culture'. It is suggested that team nursing produces a bureaucratic style of learning which may constrain students in gaining mastery of the cognitive skills required by Project 2000 programmes.

More recently, a number of post-basic training courses have been evaluated by researchers, and two examples are given here. Lam *et al* (1993) examined a course in the skills of family work with schizophrenics, and found that attitudes and beliefs changed in the desired direction, and that an effective model of family work for patients with schizophrenia can be developed. Brooker and Butterworth (1993) analysed the effects on CPNs of a short part-time course. CPNs were trained to deliver psychosocial intervention to families caring for a relative with schizophrenia at home. A number of variables, including attitudes, skills, relationships and aspects of their role, were examined and the outcomes are described in some detail.

REFERENCES

Adams T (1987) How does it feel to be a caregiver? *Community Psychiatric Nursing Journal*, **7**: 11–17.

Altschul A (1972) *Patient–Nurse Interaction: A Study of Interaction Patterns in Acute Psychiatric Wards*. Edinburgh: Churchill Livingstone.

Berrios G E and Sage G (1986) Patients who break their fast before ECT. *British Journal of Psychiatry*, **149**: 294–295.

Brooker C (1990a) A description of clients nursed by community psychiatric nurses whilst attending English National Board Clinical Course No. 811: clarification of current role? *Journal of Advanced Nursing*, **15**: 155–166.

Brooker C (1990b) The health education needs of families caring for a schizophrenic relative and the potential role for community psychiatric nurses. *Journal of Advanced Nursing*, **15**: 1092–1098.

Brooker C (ed.) (1990c) *Community Psychiatric Nursing – A Research Perspective*, Volume 1. London: Chapman & Hall.

Brooker C and Butterworth T (1993) Training in psychosocial intervention: the impact on the role of community psychiatric nurses. *Journal of Advanced Nursing*, **18**: 583–590.

Brooker C and White E (eds) (1993) *Community Psychiatric Nursing – A Research Perspective*, Volume 2. London: Chapman & Hall.

Burnard P and Morrison P (1994) *Nursing Research in Action*, 2nd edn. Basingstoke: Macmillan.

Chambers M (1988) Curriculum evaluation; an approach towards appraising a post-basic psychiatric course. *Journal of Advanced Nursing*, **13**: 330–340.

Chinn P L and Jacobs M K (1987) *Theory and Nursing: A Systematic Approach*, 2nd edn. St Louis: C V Mosby.

Clark J M and Hockey L (1989) *Further Research for Nursing*. London: Scutari Press.

Cormack D F (1984) *Psychiatric Nursing Described*. Edinburgh: Churchill Livingstone.

Coupar A and Conway A (1986) Hospital admission for depression. *Journal of Advanced Nursing*, **11**: 697–704.

Davis B D (1986) The strain of training being a student psychiatric nurse. In: *Psychiatric Nursing Research*, ed. Brooking J I. Chichester: Wiley.

Dickoff J and James P (1968) Researching research's role in theory development. *Nursing Research*, **17**: 197–203.

Drummond J S (1990) The work style of students of mental health nursing undertaking the Project 2000 schemes of training: a logical analysis. *Journal of Advanced Nursing*, **15**: 977–984.

Field P A and Morse J M (1985) *Nursing Research: the application of qualitative approaches*. London: Croom Helm.

Gilloran A J, McGlew T, McKee K, Robertson A and Wight D (1993) Measuring the quality of care in psychogeriatric wards. *Journal of Advanced Nursing*, **18**: 269–275.

Gournay K J M (1991) The base for exposure treatment in agoraphobia: some indicators for nurse therapists and community psychiatric nurses. *Journal of Advanced Nursing*, **16**: 82–91.

Hughes C P (1991) Community psychiatric nursing and the depressed elderly: a case for using cognitive therapy. *Journal of Advanced Nursing*, **16**: 565–572.

Jones J G, Janman K, Payne R L and Rick J T (1987) Some determinants of stress in psychiatric nurses. *International Journal of Nursing Studies*, **7**: 129–144.

Jones R G (1988) Experimental study to evaluate nursing staff morale in a high stimulation psychiatry setting. *Journal of Advanced Nursing*, **13**: 352–357.

Lam D H, Kuipers L and Leff J P (1993) Family work with patients suffering from schizophrenia: the impact of training on psychiatric nurses' attitude and knowledge. *Journal of Advanced Nursing*, **18**: 233–237.

Lemmer W (1986) *The Management of Change: an Evaluation of Work Upon Five Psychogeriatric Wards of a London Psychiatric Hospital*. London: West Lambeth Health Authority.

Long C G, Blackwell C C and Midgley M (1992) An evaluation of two systems of in-patient care in a general hospital psychiatric unit I: staff and patient perceptions and attitudes. *Journal of Advanced Nursing*, **17**: 64–71.

MacIlwaine H (1983) The communication patterns of female neurotic patients with nursing staff in psychiatric units of general hospitals. In: *Nursing Research: Ten Studies in Patient Care*, ed. Wilson Barnett J. Chichester: Wiley.

McKenna H P (1990) The perception of psychiatric-hospital ward sisters/ charge nurses towards nursing models. *Journal of Advanced Nursing*, **15**: 1319–1325.

Marks I M (1985) *Psychiatric Nurse Therapists in Primary Care*. London: Royal College of Nursing.

Massey P (1991) Institutional loss: an examination of a bereavement reaction in 22 mental nurses losing their institution and moving into the community. *Journal of Advanced Nursing*, **16**: 573–583.

Meades S (1993) Suggested community psychiatric nursing interventions with clients suffering from anorexia nervosa and bulimia nervosa. *Journal of Advanced Nursing*, **18**: 364–370.

Morrison P (1990) A multidimensional scalogram analysis of the use of seclusion in acute psychiatric settings. *Journal of Advanced Nursing*, **15**: 59–66.

Norman I and Parker F (1990) Psychiatric patients' views of their lives before and after moving to a hostel: a qualitative study. *Journal of Advanced Nursing*, **15**: 1036–1044.

Platt C (1990) An experiment in psychiatric community care in north Staffordshire: the experience of working with relatives of mentally-ill people. *Journal of Advanced Nursing*, **15**: 1315–1318.

Reynolds W and Cormack D F S (1985) Clinical teaching of group dynamics: an evaluation of a clinical teaching programme. *Nurse Education Today*, **5**: 101–108.

Reynolds W and Presly A S (1988) A study of empathy in student nurses. *Nurse Education Today*, **8**: 123–130.

Savage P (1991) Patient assessment in psychiatric nursing. *Journal of Advanced Nursing*, **16**: 311–316.

Sheppard M (1993) Client satisfaction, extended intervention and interpersonal skills in community mental health. *Journal of Advanced Nursing*, **18**: 246–259.

Stevens B J (1984) *Nursing Theory: Analysis, Application, Evaluation*, 2nd edn. Boston: Little & Brown.

Sullivan P J (1993) Occupational stress in psychiatric nursing. *Journal of Advanced Nursing*, **18**: 591–601.

Towell D (1975) *Understanding Psychiatric Nursing: a sociological study of modern psychiatric nursing practice*. London: Royal College of Nursing.

United Kingdom Central Council (1986) *Project 2000: a New Preparation for Practice*. London: UKCC.

White E (1986) Factors influencing general practitioners to refer patients to community psychiatric nurses. In: *Psychiatric Nursing Research*, ed. Brooking J I. Chichester: Wiley.

FURTHER READING

This chapter has outlined the purpose and process of nursing research, and hopefully has motivated the reader to find out more. It was not the intention to provide a comprehensive guide to research in mental health nursing, nor to furnish the reader with a skills manual for carrying out research fieldwork. Students should learn about research by doing it, naturally under appropriate supervision. Research, like nursing, is a practice-based occupation, and the necessary skills can only be developed through involvement in research activities.

A number of texts are suggested below which students may find helpful in pursuing their interest in research. Reading is obviously a personal matter of taste and choice, and students' decisions about reading should also be supported by advice from tutors/supervisors, where necessary.

Nursing Research

Cormack D F S (1984) *The Research Process in Nursing*. Oxford: Blackwell Scientific Publications.
Burnard P and Morrison P (1990) *Nursing Research in Action*. Basingstoke: Macmillan.

Quantitative Research Methods

Abdellah F G and Levine E (1986) *Better Patient Care Through Nursing Research*, 3rd edn. New York: Macmillan Publishing Company.
Polit D F and Hungler B P (1987) *Nursing Research – principles and methods*, 3rd edn. Philadelphia: J B Lippincott.
Seaman C H C (1987) *Research Methods: principles, practice and theory for nursing*, 3rd edn. Norwalk, Connecticut: Appleton & Lange.

Qualitative Research Methods

Field P A and Morse J M (1985) *Nursing Research: the application of qualitative approaches*. London, Sydney: Croom Helm.
Leininger M (ed.) (1985) *Qualitative Research Methods in Nursing*. New York: Grune & Stratton.
Strauss A and Corbin J (1990) *Basics of Qualitative Research: grounded theory procedures and techniques*. Newbury Park: Sage Publications.

Mental Health Nursing Research

Brooker C (ed.) (1990) *Community Psychiatric Nursing – A research perspective,* Vol. 1. London: Chapman & Hall.

Brooker C and White E (eds) (1993) *Community Psychiatric Nursing – A research perspective,*Vol. 2. London: Chapman & Hall.

Brooking J I (ed.) (1986) *Psychiatric Nursing Research.* Chichester: Wiley.

Brooking J I (1989) The care of psychiatric patients. In: *Further Research for Nursing,* Chapter 4, eds. Mcleod Clark J and Hockey L. London: Scutari Press.

Davis B D (1990) Research and psychiatric nursing. In: *Psychiatric and Mental Health Nursing: Theory and Practice,* Chapter 21, eds. Reynolds W and Cormack D. London: Chapman and Hall.

13

Nurse–Patient Relationship

Peggy Martin

INTRODUCTION

Nursing has been defined by Brodish (1982) as the therapeutic use of self for the benefit of others, having first acquired both the knowledge and the skills to identify needs. The problem, however, of identifying a unique body of knowledge for nursing still exists; Kenny (1991) has observed that professions outside nursing appear to have structure and purpose while nursing still remains uncertain and divided.

The pursuit of professionalism in nursing is an attempt to remove the uncertainty and re-establish the uniqueness in nursing. Kitson (1985) suggests that the disease model has largely been replaced by equally impersonal concepts such as Johnson's behavioural model or Roy's adaptation model. Although these theories sought to describe in a systematic and logical way what nurses do, Kitson argues that none have considered the affective relationship between the nurse and patient.

Draper (1992) recommends that nurses move away from models which at some stage have been based on models from other disciplines. She proposes that we should be looking at the discipline of nursing itself. Only by doing this can we generate unique nursing theory. Dick (1983) reminds us that nursing is directly related to the real world and dependent on the real world for its subject matter.

Biley (1992) argues that it is necessary to start discovering the true essence of nursing without entirely forgetting our empirical inheritance. He proposes that we follow our intuition, pay less attention to our earlier follies, place greater value on practical experiences and move on to explore the human sciences and nursing concepts that include 'presencing', 'being with', 'caring' and 'loving'. Perhaps only then, he suggests, can we discover the real essence of nursing and have a positive impact on improving the quality of patient care. The therapeutic use of self permeates all the activities that the nurse engages in with the patient. The nurse who is aware of her own thoughts, feeling and attitudes is in a better position to help another person.

Psychiatric nurses have always been less easily observed in their work, and therefore their practice less understood. There has been much debate over the years about what psychiatric nurses do in relation to other health professionals within a multidisciplinary team. In describing the influence of psychology and sociology on the knowledge base of nursing in the latter part of the twentieth century Barker (1990) suggests that despite developments in recent years the concepts of psychiatric nursing in Britain still remains an insecure and somewhat hazy concept. Many important concepts in mental health nursing remain somewhat elusive and warrant further study. The earlier work of Brown and Fowler (1971, (Table 13.1)) in describing 'High and Low Visibility Functions in Nursing', emphasised those tasks which were easily observed when carried out; these tasks were highly valued and rewarded. Low Visibility Functions, which related to the psychosocial aspects of nursing, were not readily observed and therefore not highly rewarded despite the high degree of cognitive and affective skill required for their delivery. Consequently, nurses have often been trained to believe that they are most effective when 'doing' for a patient (Benner and Tanner, 1987).

Low Visibility nursing actions are now being recognised as the focus of authentic nursing practice; research shows that these actions are significant and valued by patients. Wright (1991) suggests that the therapeutic nurse has a very clear idea of what constitutes nursing and recognises

Table 13.1   Degree of Visibility in Nursing (after Brown and Fowler, 1971)

High Visibility Easily observed by others	Low Visibility Not readily seen by others
Lifting and advising patients Feeding patients Wound dressings Taking temperatures Bed-making Recording blood pressure Attending to patient's hygiene needs	Listening Presence Availability Body language Genuineness Honesty Empathetic understanding

that these acts, often dismissed as basic, are actually complex, intricate and value elements in their own right. Without them the essence of nursing is lost. He calls it nursing of a sort but emphasises that it is not therapeutic nursing. The challenge is to combine both facets, the instrumental and the expressive, into a healing whole which serves the patient.

According to Powell (1991) therapeutic practice is that in which the nurse has made a positive difference to a client's health state. He emphasises the importance of the nurse being aware of how and why these positive differences have occurred.

THE NURSE–PATIENT RELATIONSHIP

The nurse–patient relationship is central to nursing. It is the basis of all nursing activity and can act as a tool to facilitate self-learning and promote the patient's recovery. Peplau (1952) emphasises the importance of the patient being the focus of such a relationship. A professional relationship only concerns certain aspects of a patient's life, while personal relationships may involve greater sharing between the parties concerned. The nurse–patient relationship can enable the nurse to institute professional closeness, education, advocacy or other identified needs (Cooper, 1981).

Kitson (1985) describes the nurse–patient relationship as a caring relationship. She identifies three integral parts of such a relationship: a need for commitment – the carer undertakes to provide the support necessary to sustain the other person on emotional, practical and time dimensions. Possession of appropriate knowledge and practical skills which will contribute to the performance of caring activities. The total interaction is given shape and direction through the respect the carer has for the recipient of care.

PRESENCE

The nurse's presence has been defined as a powerful phenomena, described by Gardener (1985) as an elusive concept which is challenging to measure in quantitative terms yet is recognised by both nurses and patients. Paterson and Zderad (1976) define presence as being available or open in a situation with a wholeness of a person's unique individual being. Presence is a gift of self; it means being there in a psychological as well as a physical sense for the purpose of meeting the client's health care needs.

Gardener (1985) suggests that the nurse's presence, as a nursing intervention, can meet outcomes for support, comfort, encouragement and motivation. Presence is closely related to other low visibility concepts such as empathy, listening and touch. According to Gardener these concepts are intricately interwoven into the reality of nursing knowledge and skill, and are essential antecedents to the nurse's use of presence as a nursing intervention. Shannon (1991) suggests that the nurse is the person who is there, who knows what the disturbance in function has interrupted for the client; who understands and feels with him the frustrations of disability and who can cope with the pain of another. Shannon believes that presencing requires knowledge of the path to be taken, and the ability to help the individual or family to find meaning in an experience. Furthermore, she believes that presencing requires knowledge of the biophysical and behavioural sciences, and of ethical dilemmas which are present in health care situations.

LISTENING

Listening requires a total kind of perceptiveness and is an important observational skill. When a nurse listens to a patient she is immersing herself in his frame of reference, and she is hearing much more than words. There is a need to focus on what is seen so that it can be put together with what is heard. Consideration needs to be given to the tone of voice, fluency of speech, language, facial expression, posture and movement. A patient will not be encouraged to talk about himself if he senses that the nurse is not really listening. A voluntary effort is needed to understand what the patient is really saying and the meaning of the words. Unencumbered listening involves understanding and patience. Listening is particularly important in assessment and can help to reduce tension and improve a person's self-perception and confidence.

In order to listen it is necessary to be silent; some people feel highly uncomfortable when they are not actually speaking. A few moments of silence can seem like a long time and a person may feel a need to fill the void with words. Learning to be comfortable with silence is one of the most difficult skills to accomplish in interactions with others (Hein, 1980). The nurse who uses the self therapeutically will use silence intentionally and purposefully in maximising interactions with patients.

INTUITION

When examining nursing process literature, intuition is rarely mentioned. Benner and Tanner (1987) suggest that intuition has seldom been granted legitimacy as a sound approach for clinical judgment and has been viewed as the basis for irrational acts, guesswork or unfounded knowledge. They argue that intuition appears to have a legitimate role to play in clinical judgment; the most insightful and significant judgments may be overlooked, undervalued or disbelieved because of an apparent lack of concrete evidence.

Both Cooper (1981) and Jennings (1986) emphasise the importance of intuition. Cooper suggests that the data obtained from seeing and listening are often inadequate; she feels that the true practice of nursing lies in the nurse's ability to see, to listen and to feel beyond the ordinary person.

Jennings also stresses the importance of subjective, creative, humanistic and holistic dimensions within the art of nursing.

TRUST

Trust is the foundation upon which effective nursing is based. A trusting relationship may be defined as the connection that exists between two persons who are in close association with one another and have a firm belief in each other's honesty, integrity, reliability and accountability (Wiedenbach and Falls, 1978).

Byrne and Thompson (1978) define trust as a feeling of safety in sharing one's own thoughts and feelings with another. An individual will limit the information he shares in order to protect the integrity of his self concept; and will only share information about his thoughts and feelings when he feels it is relevant and safe to do so.

The nurse should have the appropriate communication skills to establish a trusting relationship with the patient. Thomas (1978) suggests that the person who trusts accepts others who deviate from his or her own ways of feelings and behaving without having an intense need to change them. Nurses can often put on a professional front wishing to appear efficient, competent and devoid of any emotion. The front is often acquired as a means of coping with anxiety and permits the nurse to go about her duties unaffected by any disturbing feelings. Such stereotyped interpersonal behavioural patterns can lead to consequences which are in opposition to the aims of a caring profession. Engledow (1987) suggests that one of the greatest barriers to developing a relationship with a patient is inauthenticity, not experiencing ourselves but denying our very humanness.

TIME

The concept of time is a significant phenomenon in nursing. All behaviour takes place within the dimension of time; the commitment of time is in itself a component of communication. The giving of time has been shown to be highly valued by patients (Brown, 1986).

Nurses provide a 24-hour service every day of the year. The sustained and continuous contacts in nursing are characterised by a quantity of presence on the part of the nurse (Botteroff and D'Cruz, 1984).

TOUCH

Touch is one aspect of the nurse's therapeutic use of self. While there are cultural differences in the use of touch, it is socially permitted for a nurse to touch a patient although he may be a total stranger to her. Through touch the nurse can indicate care and concern and provide reassurance in a crisis situation. Touch can indicate to a patient that he is perceived and valued as a person. Some nurses are not aware of the value of touch as a therapeutic intervention. Indeed, some nurses may have to overcome previous learning that touch is taboo. Touch can be a valuable tool in the assessment, planning and implementation of care. Touch can enhance the meaning of verbal messages and in some instances replace verbal messages completely.

Kreiger (1979) carried out research into the therapeutic value of touch. She describes therapeutic touch as a healing process involving the laying-on of hands, on or close to the body of a sick person by someone who intends to help or heal that person. The excess energy from the helping person is directed towards the patient who, because of his illness, is not in possession of his full optimal energy state. The transfer of energy from the helper to the sick person is purposeful; the helper's thoughts, actions and energies are focused on the other person and his needs. If this intentional focus is operative a transfer of energy takes place. During the transfer the helper's energy re-patterns the patient's lowered energy level so that it is raised towards the level of the helper's energy level. When the energy transfer is complete Kreiger noted that the patient experienced the helper's touch as a feeling of heat in the areas being touched; he felt relaxed and experienced a sense of well-being. Haemoglobin values increased following treatment.

The re-patterning of energy levels appear to have a physiological basis and involves some kind of electron transfer resonance.

Feelings can be shared through touch and a close bond can exist between people when they share feelings with one another. Touch is a highly valued intervention in a wide range of nursing situations.

EMPATHY

Empathy has been defined by Disiker and Michiellute (1981) as the ability to understand what another person is experiencing and to communicate that understanding to the person. Empathy is a crucial element in the establishment of facilitator relationships and a desirable characteristic for health professionals. Layton (1979) suggests that without the skill of empathy, other skills and abilities that nurses possess are less effective.

Truax and Carkhuff (1967) reported on a series of studies concerning the relationships between empathy and outcome and found the level of empathy to be significantly higher in successful therapy.

An interesting study by Forsyth (1979) demonstrated that empathic ability was not related to areas of practice. Similar scores were found among medical, surgical, orthopaedic and psychiatric nurses. It was anticipated that psychiatric nurses would display the highest levels of empathy since their area of practice involves conscious efforts to make empathic responses. However, it was found that nurses can make empathic remarks without actually experiencing empathy. Forsyth suggests that the meaning of the findings may indicate that clients' perceptions of psychiatric nurses' empathic abilities is high, whereas the nurses' empathic abilities were lower than expected. Forsyth supports her reasoning by analysis of data on nurse empathy as perceived by patients. Barrett-Lennard (1962) Relationship Inventory scores were used while nurses' scores were measured on the Hogan (1969) Empathy Scale.

CARING

Morse *et al* (1991) suggest that caring is emerging as a significant concept for the nursing profession and is rapidly influencing nursing theory and practice as well as education and research. They maintain that if caring really is the essence of nursing then it must be demonstrated and not merely proclaimed. It must be relevant to the patient and to practice, and not merely an internalised feeling on the part of the nurse.

Although nursing is concerned primarily with caring, it has relied substantially on scientific knowledge to define its knowledge base. Farmer (1992) argues that caring is not a series of predetermined isolated actions, but manifests as patterns of interactions that are not regulated by rules. Kelly (1988) expressed concern about the disturbing signs that the public image of nursing reflects a profession that has lost its ethic of caring.

Kenny (1991) believes that nurses have not only played down their caring role but allocated it away. Now the realisation dawns that it is the caring and interpersonal processes that are unique to nursing. Similarly Kitson (1985) shares the belief that nurses have denied their caring function. Being unable to identify what professional caring is, they have looked to grand theories and esoteric notions concerning health and individualised care.

Watson (1981) suggests that it is crucial for nursing in its quest for finding itself to know the important functions that science cannot perform for practice behaviour, and the important functions that the humanities and arts cannot perform for the knowledge base. She suggests that an understanding of the differences may help the profession reclaim and combine both perspectives.

Watson (1981) also advocates that the art of nursing demands that those who practice it form and hold to a strict set of human values. Furthermore, she suggests that the artistic activities of nursing allow unlimited expansion of humanistic creativity. She describes as a truly artistic endeavour the active search and discovery of reaching out and making contact with another human being. Watson argues that discoveries in art are just as important as discoveries in science. There is however an important difference: certain values generated by an art are not generated by the practice of a science; these are the values of tenderness, of kindliness, of caring and of concern for another human being. For nurses to be effective carers, caring needs to be viewed from the patient's perspective, and the caring behaviours that patients particularly value should become an integral part of their practice.

Mayeroff (1971) suggests that caring is sometimes spoken of simply as a matter of good intention or warm regard, as if caring is an act that does not require knowledge. He suggests that knowing is a major ingredient of caring. To care for someone, the carer needs to know many things; who the other person is, his strengths and limitations, what his needs are and what is conducive to his growth. The carer must know how to respond to the other person's needs as well as having a knowledge of his own powers and limitations.

Barber (1991) feels strongly that unaware carers give unaware care. He argues that a nurse's ability to develop an effective therapeutic relationship with patients is related directly to his or her own degree of self-insight and understanding.

A number of studies have looked at caring behaviours; Wolf (1986) devised a Caring Behaviour Inventory by selecting from the literature words and phrases that represented caring. Nurses ranked 75 caring words on a four-point Likert scale selecting words or phrases evident in caring situations with patients. The 10 highly ranked caring behaviours were: attention, listening, comforting, honesty, patience, responsibility, providing information for the patient to make informed decisions, touch, sensitivity, respect and calling the patient by name.

Brown (1986) used tape recordings to provide patients' perspectives of feeling cared for, while hospitalised for treatment of acute medical or surgical conditions. Patients were asked to describe an experience in which they felt cared for by a nurse. Analysis of the transcripts enabled eight caring themes to be identified, which may well be applicable to other care settings.

1. *Recognition of Individual Qualities and Needs.* This theme was characterised by perceptions of the nurse adapting the usual way of doing things to meet the unique needs of the individual. There was a common perception of the service being personalised and not routine.

2. *Reassuring Presence* was indicated by perceptions of the nurse as being comforting, supporting and reassuring others.
3. *Provision of Information* was characterised by nursing actions taken to inform and teach the patient.
4. *Demonstration of Professional Knowledge and Skill* was characterised by the nurse taking immediate action in a situation that was perceived by the patient as urgent or an emergency. The action was seen as effective and appropriate.
5. *Assistance With Pain* was characterised by two kinds of nursing actions: the first were direct actions by the nurse to relieve pain and included giving medication. The second group of actions focused on helping the patient to manage pain, for example teaching relaxation techniques.
6. *Amount of Time Spent* was indicated by the nurse taking more time than was actually necessary to do something for the patient.
7. *Promotion of Autonomy* was defined by interactions that enabled the patient to participate in decision-making.
8. *Surveillance* was characterised by interactions in which nursing activities were experienced by the patient as keeping him under observation with the emphasis being on his physical condition and safety.

Brown (1986) concludes that these hospitalised patients' views of care support theoretical descriptions of care and the findings of empirical studies. Patients emphasised the importance of nurses meeting their treatment needs (instrumental activities) and carrying out these activities in such a way as to protect and enhance the unique identity of the individual (expressive activities).

In a research project conducted by Yoder and Rode (1990) the focus was directed towards nursing actions thought to be helpful to patients experiencing psychosocial difficulties. The purpose of the study was to identify nursing actions which were seen as being helpful to the patients and those which were less helpful, and to what extent patients perceived nursing staff as actually performing these actions. Identification of nursing actions was based on a review of current psychiatric nursing textbooks which emphasised specific therapeutic interventions. The most helpful nursing actions perceived by patients included comments on the patient's progress, friendliness, being knowledgeable, being able to explain medication and giving physical care when necessary. The nurse helped the patient to see the good things in himself. Unhelpful nursing actions were identified as doing things for the patient instead of making him do them for himself, or telling the patient to do things he felt he was not able to do. Yoder and Rode (1990) concluded that the quality of patient care could be enhanced if nursing actions perceived as helpful by patients were implemented into care.

REFERENCES

Barber P (1991) Caring: the nature of a therapeutic relationship. In: *Nursing. A Knowledge Base for Practice*, eds Perry A and Jolley M. London: Edward Arnold.

Barker P J (1990) The conceptual basis of mental health nursing. *Nurse Education Today*, **10**: 339–348.

Barret-Lennard G (1962) Dimensions of therapist response as causal factors in therapeutic change. *Psychological Monographs*, **76**(43): 562.

Benner P and Tanner C (1987) How expert nurses use intuition. *American Journal of Nursing*, 24–31 Jan.

Biley Francis (1992) Editorial, Nursing models redundant in practice. *British Journal of Nursing*, **1**(5): 219.

Bottorff J L and D'Cruz J V (1984) Towards inclusive notions of 'patient' and 'nurse'. *Journal of Advanced Nursing*, **9**: 549–553.

Brodish M S (1982) Nursing practice conceptualised: an interaction model. *Image*, **14**: 5–7.

Brown L (1986) The experience of care: patient perspectives. *Topics in Clinical Nursing*, **8**(2): 56–62.

Brown M and Fowler G R (1971) *Psychodynamic Nursing*. Philadelphia: W B Saunders.

Byrne M L and Thompson L F (1978) *Key Concepts for the Study and Practice of Nursing*. St Louis: C V Mosby.

Cooper S (1981) What is nursing. *Nursing Times. Occasional Papers*, **77**(34): 136.

Dick J (1983) What makes an excellent practising nurse? *Canadian Nurse*, **79**(11): 44–47.

Disiker R and Michiellute P (1981) An analysis of empathy in medical students before and following clinical experience. *Journal of Medical Education*, **56**: 1004–1010.

Draper J (1992) The impact of nursing models. *Senior Nurse*, **12**(3): 38–39.

Engledow P (1987) Psychotherapeutic skills in nursing. *Senior Nurse*, **7**(3): 40–41.

Farmer E (1992) Promoting caring in nursing. *British Journal of Nursing*, **1**(11): 537.

Forsyth G L (1979) Exploration of empathy in nurse client interaction. *Advances in Nursing Science*, **1**: 2.

Gardner D L (1985) Presence. In: *Nursing Interventions*, eds Bulechek G M and McCloskey J. New York: W B Saunders.

Hein E C (1980) *Communication in Nursing Practice*, 2nd edn. Boston: Little Brown and Co.

Hogan R (1969) Development of an empathy scale. *Journal of Counselling and Clinical Psychology*, **33**: 307–316.

Jennings B M (1986) Nursing science; more promise than threat. *Journal of Advanced Nursing*, **11**: 505–511.

Kelly L (1988) The ethic of caring: has it been discarded? *Nursing Outlook*, **36**(1): 17.

Kenny T (1991) A search for identity. *Senior Nurse*, **11**(2): 3–4.

Kitson A (1985) Education for quality. *Senior Nurse*, **3**(4): 11–16.

Kreiger D *et al* (1979) Therapeutic touch. Searching for evidence of physiological change. *American Journal of Nursing*, **79**: 660.

Layton J (1979) The use of modelling to teach empathy to nursing students. *Research in Nursing and Health*, **2**: 164–176.

Mayeroff M (1971) *On Caring*. New York: Harper and Row.

Morse J, Bottorff J, Neander W and Solberg S (1991) Comparative analysis of conceptualizations and theories of caring. *Image, Journal of Nursing Scholarship*, **23**(2): 119–126.

Paterson J G and Zderad L T (1976) *Humanistic Nursing*. New York: Wiley.

Peplau H E (1952) *Interpersonal Relations in Nursing*. New York: G P Putnam's Sons.

Powell J (1991) Reflection and the evaluation of experience: prerequisites for therapeutic practice. In: *Nursing as Therapy*, eds McMahon R and Pearson A. London: Chapman and Hall.

Shannon (1991) The future of nursing. *Nursing*, **4**(41): 26–28.

Thomas M D (1978) Trust. In: *Behavioural Concepts and Nursing Interventions*, eds Carlson C E and Blackwell B. Philadelphia: J B Lippincott Co.

Truax C B and Carkhuff R R (1967) *Towards Effective Counselling and Psychotherapy*. Chicago: Aldine.

Watson Jean (1981) The lost art of nursing. *Nursing Forum*, **XX**(3): 244–249.

Wiendenbach E and Falls C E (1978) *Communication: Key to Effective Nursing*. New York: Tiresias Press.

Wolf Z R (1986) The caring concept and nurse identified caring behaviours. *Topics in Clinical Nursing*, **8**(2): 84–93.

Wright S (1991) Facilitating therapeutic nursing and independent practice. In: *Nursing as Therapy*, eds McMahon R and Pearson A. London: Chapman and Hall.

Yoder D S and Rode W M (1990) How are you doing? Patient evaluation of nursing actions. *Journal of Psychosocial Nursing*, **28**(10): 26–30.

14 | Specific Mental Health Problems
Peggy Martin

NOTES ON INTERVENTION

There are some mental health problems where general principles of management and intervention may be useful. Such approaches may be beneficial when incorporated into a patient's individual care plan.

ANXIETY

Anxiety is an emotion aroused by actual or symbolic threat of danger. Anxiety gives a person feelings of uneasiness and apprehension; it is an uncomfortable feeling. Mild anxiety can produce a heightened awareness and sharpness of the senses. It can provide an impetus for learning and change. This type of anxiety is viewed as constructive, promoting growth for an individual. At the other extreme, severe anxiety may be so destructive for a person that it leads to dysfunctional patterns of behaviour in which the perceptual field is greatly reduced, and personal and environmental safety threatened. Although anxiety is not directly observable, it is conveyed through a person's behaviour, and is accompanied by psychological changes in the body which give rise to unpleasant symptoms. These symptoms include dry mouth, nausea, raised blood pressure, palpitations, frequency of micturition, diarrhoea, muscle tension, increased pulse and respiratory rates. The psychological symptoms vary from person to person but are usually more intense in severe levels of anxiety.

The first priority for the nurse when caring for a severely anxious patient is to ensure he has a quiet, safe environment where stimuli is minimised. Anxiety levels can be increased by external stimuli. The patient is more likely to feel secure if the nurse adopts a calm approach towards him. If she is self-aware and can recognise any anxiety in herself, this may help to ensure that her own behaviour will not be disadvantageous to the patient (Collins, 1983). The person who is anxious has limited abilities to deal with abstraction or problem-solving; the nurse who recognises this will keep communication to a simple level. Her use of presence as a therapeutic intervention can help the patient to feel safe and secure, whereas the patient's anxiety will escalate if he is left alone.

Medical examination is important and can eliminate any possible physical condition which could produce symptoms similar to those of anxiety, e.g. thyrotoxicosis. The patient needs to understand the relationship between stress and anxiety and the physiological responses that occur. Whenever possible it will be helpful if the nurse can use the patient's own experiences as part of the learning process. He will need to learn about his own negative responses in stressful situations, how to become more confident and exercise self-control.

The patient can be helped by learning to control his anxiety through the use of relaxation techniques. Occasionally, in the short term, prescribed drugs can be beneficial, particularly in severe anxiety. However, the patient's condition will need to be regularly assessed, otherwise he may come to rely on 'chemical courage'. Some patients develop focused anxiety in relation to some specific object or situation, resulting in severe feelings of anxiety or panic when exposed to an object or situation that they fear. The list of exaggerated or irrational fears that people may have is a long one.

People may fear open or closed spaces, insects, animals, darkness, supermarkets, social occasions, and so on. A person who fears the enclosed space of a lift may walk up numerous flights of stairs to avoid the situation. A person suffering from a severe phobia will actively take measures to avoid the circumstances which arouse that fear; usually he is unable to confront the situation without professional help. Behavioural techniques under the direction of a trained therapist can help by gradually exposing the person to the problem situation through both imaginary and reality confrontation.

Community Psychiatric Nurses may also help patients to increase their confidence and coping abilities through referral to support groups.

DEPRESSION

Depression is a term commonly used to describe feelings of sadness which are experienced from time to time by many people, usually in response to some event that has some significant bearing on their lives. Feeling states and emotion help a person towards the process of adaptation; for example, coming to terms with the loss of a loved one. The signs and symptoms of depression may be extremely variable and can be viewed as a continuum, ranging from feeling 'down', feeling 'blue', unhappy, to a more severe expression when an individual is consumed by self-denigration and hopelessness.

Depression can also be hidden behind a smiling façade. Depression may occur in relation to other disorders, such as drug and alcohol withdrawal, schizophrenia, anorexia nervosa and in the child victims and adult survivors of incest. Jasmin and Trygstad (1979) describe depression as a biological, psychological and social phenomenon, as it affects the sufferer in all these dimensions.

The depressed person frequently experiences disturbances in sleep patterns, such as early waking, difficulty in sleeping or excessive tiredness; physical problems are common, such as lack of concentration, constipation, poor personal hygiene and listlessness. The depressed person may harbour thoughts about suicide or openly express his ideas and intentions. The nurse's immediate goal must be to ensure the patient's safety. He must be cared for in a safe enviroment where he is unable to inflict self harm.

A plan of care should pay attention to the physical as well as the psychological needs of the patient. It is important to ensure that he has adequate nutrition and fluids; to monitor eliminatory functions and to make certain that he has adequate activity, rest and sleep. The nurse plays an essential and valuable role in helping the depressed person towards recovery. While the severely depressed patient may communicate very little, the presence of the nurse can communicate interest and concern, and help the patient to feel that he is an acceptable and worthwhile person. Non-verbal responding is an important and valued nursing intervention.

The nurse has to learn to be comfortable with a patient who may be silent. Some nurses experience feelings of guilt because they view the time as unproductive. On the contrary, the use of silence as a therapeutic intervention can be very beneficial; it allows for the development of trust, it shows respect for the patient's feelings and creates space for him to express his innermost thoughts in his own time and when he feels ready to do so.

Relating to a person who is experiencing feelings of sadness and hopelessness can be difficult and painful for the nurse concerned. The dynamics and related behaviours associated with depression may generate feelings in the nurse that are hard to face. The nurse's understanding of her own feelings and experience may enable her to work more objectively with the patient. Interventions should be directed towards increasing the patient's self-esteem.

The depressed person should never be pressurised by being asked a lot of questions. Communications should involve simple words and sentences. Complex questioning may discourage the patient from communicating; he may feel confused and unable to cope and consequently retreat further into himself. Time spent with the depressed patient is amply rewarded when the individual is restored to health.

The role of the nurse is critical when a patient is potentially or actively suicidal. Suicidal risk must be assessed, see 'Assessment of Suicidal Risk'. When the risk is high, the priority of care is to ensure that the patient is managed within a safe environment. This means removing and controlling any objects or means by which the patient may attempt to end his own life. Sharp objects such as glass, china and crockery which could be broken, razor blades and polythene bags should be removed. Belts, neckties, tights and other articles of clothing which could be used for suffocation should also be excluded from the environment. Close observation is essential; a nurse must remain with the patient at all times. The ward manager needs to plan a staff rota which provides for continuous observation while at the same time allowing relief for participants. A number of key nurses will have a better opportunity to develop a helping relationship with the suicidal person, and may contribute effectively towards the resolution of depressive and suicidal thoughts.

The suicidal person needs to be able to talk about his feelings without being judged. He needs to know that the nurse is spending time with him because she perceives him as a worthwhile human being. However, she must be honest about the need to be with him to maintain his safety and prevent him from harming himself.

There are times when a determined patient succeeds in the act of suicide. It arouses all kinds of emotions for professional carers as well as for the patient's family and friends. As Alison Wertheimer (1991), who lost her own sister through suicide, suggests, death can disrupt family life and relationships, but when one member commits suicide the effects can be particularly devastating.

Alexander (1991) suggests that suicide is unlike other deaths; it is an untimely chosen death carried out alone and often secretly. She describes the isolation, secrecy and disconnection of suicide as the survivors' legacy, survivors being those people who experience the loss in their own lives.

Suicide is usually difficult to discuss outside the family; discussion within the family may be equally difficult. All kinds of emotions may be aroused with regard to the deceased person and the meaning and impact on each individual will be different. In contrast to the aftermath of 'normal' deaths Lukas and Seiden (1987) state that friends and relatives are often reluctant to talk about events surrounding suicide. Family members may find it difficult to expose the blame and guilt that they feel, either towards themselves or other members. Some individuals may react by being silent. Lukas and Seiden (1987) suggest that when silence surrounds suicide it can impede healing. Professional counselling can help the survivors of suicide to express and work through feelings associated with the

---

ASSESSMENT OF SUICIDAL RISK

Some factors are known to contribute towards the incidence of suicide and may be considered under the following headings.

History
Has the person a history of depression or other mental illness? Has he or she made previous suicidal attempts and what were the methods used?

Life Span
Into which age group does the person belong?
There is a higher incidence of suicide among adolescents and the elderly.

Health
In addition to the person's present mental and physical state is there any serious progressive illness that has or will result in a loss of mobility/independence? Has there been drug or alcohol abuse?

Behaviour
Has the person been tying up loose ends – giving away possessions? Has the person given verbal warnings concerning his or her intentions to commit suicide? Has the person actually thought out a plan in order to carry out these intentions?

Support Systems
How does the person receive support as part of his or her daily living – family, friends or significant others?

Loss
Has there been a loss of a loved one or significant person in the individual's life, or some other loss such as loss of employment, children leaving home or a change in financial circumstances?

---

death. When a suicide occurs in hospital or under the auspices of community carers, then staff who are affected by the death will also need help to come to terms with the loss.

THE ELATED PATIENT

Caring for the person who is elated is a very challenging task indeed, particularly as he will usually deny being ill and claim that he has never felt better in his life. The elated patient is amusing and fun-loving. Thoughts flow through his head rapidly. He may use words which rhyme or miss words out altogether. His thoughts and ideas change rapidly and his span of attention is brief. He is indiscreet and may make embarrassing personal remarks about the staff or other patients. He is overactive and sexually disinhibited; he is out of control, lacking judgment and rational thinking; he interferes in other people's affairs and is extremely distractable. He misidentifies and misinterprets stimuli and may have grandiose ideas or delusions; he is unable to perceive actual or potential danger.

His mode of dress is usually in keeping with his elevated mood – colourful and expressive and frequently inappropriate. His needs for personal hygiene, nutrition, elimination and rest will be poorly met if he is left to his own devices. However, the nurse can use his distractability to facilitate the meeting of basic needs, bearing in mind that the patient cannot and will not be fitted into ward routines. Food and fluids can be offered frequently. Because of the patient's short span of attention, he will lose interest quickly and want to move on to some other pressing task. The patient can become very noisy and excitable, and his mood can change rapidly from joviality to irritability. He may be argumentative or aggressive.

Nursing interventions are challenging and require a great deal of tolerance, patience and good humour on the part of the nurse. Lacking social constraints, the patient may make hurtful or embarrassing remarks. The most beneficial approach for the nurse is to remain non-retaliatory and non-defensive, to behave in a calm manner and to be aware of and to control body language. All stimuli within the patient's environment should be reduced as far as possible. The nurse can listen to what the patient says but should not promote conversation. What the patient needs is rest; his boundless physical and mental energy can lead to exhaustion. Rest is achieved by giving prescribed medication. The patient who is elated needs to feel accepted as a person and to be cared for in a safe environment.

CONFUSION

Confusion is a condition characterised by bewilderment, disorientation, loss of memory, poor conceptual boundaries and inappropriate verbal statements.

Confusion may be acute or chronic and may occur, for example, as a consequence of physical illness, chemical imbalance or head injury. In some individuals confusion is caused by dementia, a cerebral disease which results in an altered mental state and progressive mental deterioration. Dementia is characterised by alterations in the cognitive areas of memory, orientation, judgment, affect and intellectual functioning.

There is often a history of absent-mindedness and a deterioration in levels of self-care. A progressive loss of contact with reality is highlighted by intellectual, emotional and memory disturbances. The patient's world is one of strangeness and bewilderment, unfamiliar places, faces and sounds. The nurse can do much to alleviate the patient's anxiety and distress. Non-verbal communication is particularly significant in lessening the patient's distress. The nurse's use of touch and presence can provide reassurance for the patient. Practical measures, such as caring for the patient in a small group with key nurses can reduce the amount of stimuli to which the person is exposed and aid orientation. Independence and individuality should be preserved, as far as possible, within a safe environment. Reminiscence therapy can be valuable, enabling a person to recall from memory things of significance which happened a long time ago. This can enhance a person's self-esteem by compensating for a lack of short-term memory. Reality orientation can help the patient to maintain contact with the environment, enabling him to benefit from his surroundings and reduce confusion. Disorientation in time, place and person is particularly distressing for relatives. The confused person may fail to acknowledge their presence or make statements such as 'Where am I?', 'Who are you?', 'I certainly don't know you'. These announcements can be especially upsetting for the patient's family, who may feel socially isolated. When relatives experience feelings of helplessness, guilt or anger the nurse can provide support through her presence and her ability to listen and understand their situation.

SUSPICIOUSNESS

The suspicious person has an attitude of doubt towards the trustworthiness of objects or people. He may think others are out to trick or harm him in some way; he may be secretive, jealous, question the loyalty of others or be overconcerned about what he believes to be hidden agendas or special meanings. The person is often highly sensitive and easily offended; he may show no wish for social involvement, with a tendency towards being reserved and reclusive. Patients who have a diagnosis of Paranoid Disorder may show evidence of actual delusional thinking and may, for example, believe that they are being poisoned or persecuted by others.

The nursing care of the suspicious patient is very challenging. During initial contact with the patient the nurse needs to be aware that there may be an attempt by the patient to maintain distance and control, because of underlying fears of harm or rejection; therefore all interactions should be characterised by a sense of objectivity. Communications should be clear, simple and concise. If the nurse faces the patient directly when speaking there will be less chance for misinterpretations to occur.

The patient's need for concrete space must also be considered. Physical closeness will usually arouse his anxiety and heighten his suspiciousness.

Developing a relationship with a suspicious patient requires time and effort. It requires that the nurse behaves in a consistent manner, is non-judgmental and non-threatening. Without the development of a relationship, the achievement of goodwill will be limited. Focusing on positive aspects of the patient's personality can help to increase his self-esteem. Time spent on suspicious cognition can be limited for the patient when the nurse provides non-competitive activities. The nurse who acts as the key person in the development of a worthwhile relationship may enable the patient to test out relationships with others.

THE PATIENT WITH PROBLEMS OF ADDICTION

Drug-taking among the younger population is an increasing problem. Young people may take drugs to experiment; these may be isolated incidents or the beginning of behaviour which may lead to addiction. Drug-taking may be seen as daring and exciting or used to blot out personal and family problems. The consequences can sometimes be fatal. There is a wide range of substances that can be misused, with varying effects. Some are illegal and some are not. Alcohol is commonly used and in the long term can lead to serious health problems. Solvent sniffing may involve various widely available solvent-based glues, dry cleaning fluid, paint thinners, butane gas, correction fluids and petrol. However, cannabis is the most widely used illegal drug and is usually smoked mixed with tobacco.

The nurse needs to accept that the patient who abuses drugs is a person who is worthy of her help. This is of fundamental importance, because the person with problems of addiction is very often stigmatised within society and his problems are not understood.

When engaged in a therapeutic relationship with a person who abuses alcohol or drugs it is essential for the nurse to direct the patient towards specific goals; this enables him to feel a sense of achievement. This is important because the person with problems of addiction is often surrounded by a feeling of chaos. Life-cycle events infringe on a person's health–illness continuum and there may be different stresses to overcome. The patient has to develop new patterns of living, as much of his time will have been spent on drink- or drug-related activities. The nurse can help the patient to fill this void by enabling him to discover new interests and abilities. One of the nurse's major functions is to educate the patient about the detrimental effects of his addiction. She needs to do this honestly and factually and to be guided by how he perceives his problems and situation, and the difficulties he and his family have to face.

Robinson (1983) suggest that people with addictive personalities do not think their way through problems. They use alcohol and drugs as substitutes for thinking about and resolving problems. Developing a relationship with the patient is of paramount importance; interpersonal relationships of a therapeutic nature are one of the patient's greatest needs. Establishing such a relationship is not easy; the patient may have difficulty in facing up to his problems and will tend to minimise and rationalise concerning his drinking or drug-taking.

As the nurse helps the patient to identify problematic areas in his current situation and to discover and understand what is happening to him during his illness, not only does she help the person to grow; she also expands her own insights (Peplau, 1952).

When the nurse can use herself therapeutically in her relationship with the patient she can help the patient to make corrections in his own faulty communications processes. She can use the relationship as a vehicle for learning and exploration of experiences in his everyday life.

AGGRESSION

Aggression is a drive that exists in all individuals and serves as a mechanism for self-protection. Aggressive behaviour, either verbal or physical, may be directed towards others. Such behaviour may be rational or irrational and may result from real or imagined fear, anxiety or anger.

Boettcher's (1983) assaultive incident assessment need tool provides a valuable framework for the planning of nursing care for the aggressive or potentially aggressive person and enables the nurse to identify the patient's needs in the following areas: need for territoriality, communication, self-esteem, safety and security, own time, autonomy, personal identity, comfort and cognitive understanding. The nurse should be aware of the patient's needs for space or personal territory. Pluckham (1978) describes space as the most significant 'nothing' that affects interpersonal communication. In relationships space has the power to convey meaning. She suggests that each person has an interior space plan which determines his spatial tolerance. Personal space is invisible and the nurse must infer from the patient's body language whether he desires closeness or whether he is distressed by it. Usually, a person with a potential for violence has a greater body-space requirement. Effective communication is important; breakdowns in communication can lead to frustration and anger. The patient's self-esteem should always be protected and he must be treated with respect.

The behaviour of aggressive patients may be sudden and unpredictable as consequence of a sudden build-up of tension. Nursing intervention should focus on prevention; the nurse needs to recognise indications of the patient's anxiety and frustration. Body language, facial expression, verbal and non-verbal language reveal rising levels of frustration. Physical signs such as flushing or pallor of the skin, tremor or muscle tension may give similar forewarning. Acceptable outlets for the patient's aggressive energy, such as physical activity in the gymnasium or on the sports field, occupational therapy and leisure activities, can be provided. External stimuli should be reduced, particularly factors which may trigger an assaultive incident.

The nurse should have some knowledge concerning what might enhance irritability and frustration in certain situations. If she can help the patient to identify sources which have caused frustration previously, she can then help him to explore socially acceptable alternative ways of dealing with frustration and anger. Alternative strategies can be tried out through role-play, psychodrama group work, cognitive therapy and through learning relaxation techniques. It is essential for staff who manage aggressive or potentially aggressive patients to work as a team. Close co-operation, effective communication and consistent approaches are essential in implementing care plans. Staff must adhere to policies and procedures for handling and removing an aggressive person, as these are designed to maximise safety for both patients and staff and to maintain the safety of other patients.

The patient may agree to enter into a contract which explicitly sets out in writing the limits of his behaviour. This should be realistic, attainable and reinforceable. All staff concerned with the patient and his family should be aware of this. In this way the patient knows quite clearly what is expected of him and how he can be helped.

THE HALLUCINATED OR DELUDED PATIENT

Hallucinations are false sensory perceptions which occur in the absence of any external stimuli and involve the five sensory processes of the body: hearing, sight, taste, touch and smell. The person may hear voices giving him commands or a running commentary on his behaviour; he may see things which do not exist; complain of tactile experiences such as people touching him or of sexual interference; he may taste or smell substances: none of which exist in actuality. However, it is important to emphasise that although hallucinations constitute a break with reality, the patient's experience is a very real one; it cannot be emphasised too strongly just how real a hallucinating experience is to the patient.

The nurse needs to be sensitive to what the patient is feeling and experiencing and should never argue about validity. At the same time it is necessary to state quite firmly that she does not share his hallucinatory processes. Developing a trust relationship with the patient is vital. It is through this relationship that the nurse can use opportunities to reinforce reality, by enabling the patient to touch real things and be in contact with people. Touch as a nursing intervention should be used if appropriate. The patient can be taught to interrupt auditory hallucinations and to learn to devalue his voices (Field, 1985).

Although hallucinations occur in the more severe forms of psychotic mental illness, they can also occur in individuals who have been deprived of sleep, starved or suffered from prolonged isolation, in states of electrolyte imbalance, delirium, physical exhaustion or as a result of taking hallucinogenic drugs.

REFERENCES

Alexander V (1991) *Words I Never Thought To Speak. Stories of Life in the Wake of Suicide.* New York: Lexington Books.

Boettcher E G (1983) Preventing violent behaviour. An integrated theoretical model for nursing. *Perspectives in Psychiatric Care*, **21**(2) 54–58.

Collins M (1983) *Communication in Health Care.* Missouri: C V Mosby Co.

Field W E (1985) Hearing voices. *Journal of Psychosocial Nursing*, **23**(1): 9–14.

Jasmin S and Trygstad L N (1979) *Behavioural Concepts and the Nursing Process.* Missouri: C V Mosby Co

Lukas C and Seiden H M (1987) *Silent Grief. Living in the Wake of Suicide.* London: Papermac Macmillan Publishers Ltd.

Peplau H E (1952) *Interpersonal Relations in Nursing.* New York: G P Putnam's Sons.

Pluckhan M L (1978) *Human Communication: The Matrix of Nursing.* USA: McGraw Hill, Inc.

Robinson L (1983) *Psychiatric Nursing as a Human Experience.* Philadelphia: W B Saunders Co.

Wertheimer A (1991) *A Special Scar. The Experience of People Bereaved by Suicide.* London, New York: Tavistock/Routledge.

Index